**Rickey H Bullard, D.P.M. LLC**
**Podiatrist**
**1902 West Main Street**
**Tupelo, MS 38801**

# Podiatric Medicine and Surgery
## A Monograph series


*Managing Editor:* **Morton D. Fielding, D.P.M.**

# Soft Somatic Tumors of the Foot

## Diagnosis and Surgical Management

*by*

**Steven J. Berlin,** D.P.M., Chairman
and Members of the Maryland Podiatric
Residency Research Committee

**Futura Publishing Company, Inc.**
**Mount Kisco, New York**
**1976**

## Dedication

This book is dedicated to my wife, Eileen,
and to all of the wives of those involved
in the Maryland Podiatry Residency Program.

# Special Acknowledgment

The subject of oncology in relation to the foot offers a broad spectrum for all interested persons, yet there is a lack of literature on this specific subject in podiatry. We hope this book helps fill the existing void and stimulates greater accomplishments for both our patients and the podiatric profession.

Successful research in this area depends on an understanding and harmonious relationship with our medical colleagues. Special acknowledgment for their assistance in the preparation of this book goes to: William Amoss, M.D., Donald Barrick, M.D., Guy Choi, M.D., Bradley King, M.D., Edward Krufky, M.D., Joseph Orlando, M.D., Selvin Passen, M.D., and William V.R. Shellow, M.D.

We also wish to thank other members of the Maryland Podiatry Residency Committee for their guidance and support of the program: Robert Bewley, D.P.M., Douglas Butler, D.P.M., Leonard Janis, D.P.M., Robert Perez, D.P.M., and John Stroh, D.P.M.

Once again, our sincerest thanks to the special individuals who labored so efficiently in its preparation: Mrs. Eileen Berlin, Mrs. Elizabeth Heisler, Mrs. Carolyn Lynch, and Mrs. Eva Plude, our secretaries.

# Preface

"Soft Somatic Tumors of the Foot: Diagnosis and Surgical Management" is the first book on the pathology and management of soft tissue tumors of the foot. It was conceived by and dedicated to podiatrists.

In the efforts to define soft tissue tumors of the foot, an extensive literature survey was undertaken; but in the wealth of literature available on soft tissue tumors, relatively little was found which dealt with the foot. However, this need not be disheartening, because soft tissue tumors, especially malignant ones, may be very difficult to handle. Tumors in the foot that are of soft tissue origin may also be found anywhere in the body where that same soft tissue exists; and this includes skeletal and smooth muscles, the connective tissues, including bone, cartilage, fibrous tissue, adipose tissue, vascular and neural tissues, synovial tissue, and skin. The only soft tissue tumor that may be considered unique to the foot is Morton's neuroma of the plantar fibromatoses, although, of course, other fibromatoses are found elsewhere.

An effort has been made to be as thorough in the consideration of these tumors as possible by including discussion of presenting signs and symptoms, laboratory work and x-ray studies useful in diagnosis or follow-up, pertinent gross and microscopic pathology, and treatment and prognosis. Because of the relatively limited number of references to tumors specifically arising in the foot, prognostic considerations were necessarily limited.

In general, the diagnosis and treatment of soft tissue tumors of the foot is much like the treatment of similar soft tissue tumors elsewhere in the body, except for the problems intrinsic to the unique anatomical structure of the foot. Two real differences in diagnosis and treatment of tumors of the foot include the clinical appearance of plantar lesions which may be different than those on the dorsum of the foot, because of weight-bearing, possibly masking an otherwise relatively easy diagnosis; and the importance of any operative procedure on weight-bearing—and, therefore, ambulation of the patient—both of which factors have to be seriously considered in the decision as to how extensive a procedure to undertake. Obviously, for malignant tumors, the problem requires less consideration, for most malignant tumors have to be treated promptly with radical surgery if any hope for cure is to exist.

It should be noted that the anatomic diagnosis of soft tissue tumors may be especially difficult, and specific diagnosis of tiny biopsy specimens may be almost impossible in some situations. Therefore, it is important that when consideration is being given to the possibility of a malignant soft tissue tumors of the foot, the patient should have the best possible setting for definitive therapy at the time of surgery—namely, a hospital operating room, where the services of a pathologist for Frozen Section diagnosis are readily available and where facilities for radical surgery are also at hand. Since the favorite route of dissemination of cells from a malignant tumor of the soft tissues is the blood stream, office biopsy and definitive surgery days or weeks later, following a specific diagnosis, may not offer the patient the best chance. Further, the rapid growth potential of many soft tissue malignancies in itself should encourage promptness in surgical extirpation of the neoplasm, with the hope being that the earlier the surgery, the more likely the possibility of complete removal and the more likely the possibility that larger portions of the foot will be preserved for future weight-bearing. Prompt diagnosis and therapy are very important with these tumors.

A "first" in any endeavor is, perforce, subject to omissions of data or presentation of data which is less than complete, not by intent, but, rather, by the problems involved in reviewing all the literature. The volume of literature on this subject, the relatively small number of rerferences relating specifically to neoplasms of the foot, and the relatively infrequent occurrence of such tumors in and on the foot made the writing of this book especially difficult.

It is the hope of the authors that this book, while admittedly less than ideal and perhaps incomplete in its approach to and solutions for some of the problems of soft tissue tumors which present to podiatrists, will serve as a nucleus or, at least, as a guide to stimulate greater interest in foot pathology, both among podiatrists and others interested in feet and foot problems; that it will provide a source book of information as of this date; that it will encourage reporting of successes and failures in therapy of foot problems which revolve around the presence or treatment of soft tissue tumors; that it will encourage more reporting of definite information on the specific management of tumors of the foot; and that, above all, it will encourage interest in defining more specifically the gross and microscopic anatomy of neoplasm of the foot for podiatrists and their associates. It is hoped that thereby the specialty of Podiatric Pathology will be helped to assume an importance commensurate with the importance of the feet and that patients everywhere will benefit.

**W. Bradley King, Jr., M.D.**

*Assistant Professor of Pathology, University of Maryland School of Medicine, Pathologist-in-Chief and Director of Laboratory, Maryland General Hospital*

# Contributors

**Steven J. Berlin, D.P.M., F.A.C.F.S.**
Diplomate National Board of Podiatric Surgery; Fellow American College of Foot Surgeons; Director Podiatry Research, and Assistant Director of Podiatric Surgery, Maryland Podiatry Residency Program; Chairman, Tissue Committee, American College of Foot Surgeons; Special Consultant in Oncology, Journal American Podiatry Association; Chief of Podiatry Service, Spring Grove Hospital Center; Podiatry Staff: Fallston General Hospital, Provident Hospital, Rosewood and Mt. Wilson Hospital Centers, and Fort Howard V.A. Hospital.

**Lawrence D. Block, D.P.M., A.A.C.F.S.**
Associate American College of Foot Surgeons; Assistant Director of Podiatric Surgery, Maryland Podiatry Residency Program; Chief Podiatry Services, Henryton and Rosewood Hospital Centers; Podiatry Staff: Fallston General Hospital, Provident Hospital and Springfield Hospital Center.

**Harvey Brown, D.P.M.**
Surgical Instructor, Maryland Podiatry Residency Program; Podiatry Staff: Provident Hospital, Rosewood and Springfield Hospital Centers, and Crownsville Hospital Center.

**Anthony J. Costa, D.P.M., A.A.C.F.S.**
Surgical Instructor Maryland Podiatry Residency Program; Director, Department of Podiatric Surgery, Maryland House of Correction at Jessup; Podiatry Staff: Maryland General Hospital, Spring Grove Hospital Center; Good Samaritan Hospital, Fort Howard V.A. Hospital, Mt. Wilson and Springfield Hospitals.

**Irvin I. Donick, D.P.M., F.A.C.F.S.**
Diplomate National Board of Podiatric Surgery; Fellow American College of Foot Surgeons; Director, Maryland

Podiatry Residency Program; Chief of Podiatry Staff, Maryland General Hospital and Fallston General Hospital; Podiatry Staff: Rosewood Hospital Center, Spring Grove Hospital Center, Provident and Ft. Howard V.A. Hospitals.

### Michael Feinstein, D.P.M., A.A.C.F.S.
Associate American College of Foot Surgeons; Surgical Instructor, Maryland Podiatry Residency Program; Podiatry Staff, Provident Hospital, Howard County General Hospital, Springfield and Crownsville Hospital Center.

### Bruce Lebowitz, D.P.M.
Surgical Instructor, Maryland Podiatric Residency Program; Podiatry Staff Provident Hospital and Springfield Hospital Center.

### Lanny Rubin, D.P.M., F.A.C.F.S.
Diplomate National Board of Podiatric Surgery; Fellow American College of Foot Surgeons, Co-Director, Maryland Podiatric Residency Program; Podiatry Staff: Fallston General Hospital, Howard County General Hospital, Provident Hospital, Podiatry Consultant: Rosewood and Springfield Hospital Centers, and Crownsville State Hospital Center.

### Neil M. Scheffler, D.P.M., A.A.C.F.S.
Associate American College of Foot Surgeons; Surgical Instructor, Maryland Podiatry Residency Program; Chief of Podiatry, Howard County General Hospital, Podiatry Staff: Provident Hospital and Spring Grove Hospital Center.

### Paul L. Sheitel, D.P.M., A.A.C.F.S.
Associate American College of Foot Surgeons; Surgical Instructor, Maryland Podiatry Residency Program; Chief of Podiatry, Provident Hospital; Podiatry Staff: Howard County General Hospital, Spring Grove and Rosewood Hospital Centers.

# Table of Contents

## List of Color Plates

# Section I

# Soft Somatic Tumors:
# An Introduction

## Introduction

Soft tissue tumors of the foot represent both a serious and distressing malady to the patient and a complex problem in both diagnosis and management in the everyday practice of podiatry. It is the purpose of this monograph to offer a general discussion of both benign and malignant neoplasms and their diagnosis, and surgical management of tumors relating to the foot. This monograph will not deal specifically with the skin, but, primarily, with other soft somatic structures. Our definition of neoplasms in this monograph will be any new growth, whether it be classified as a cyst, granuloma, or tumor.

Tumors may arise from all three germinal layers of the body. The ectoderm gives rise to tumors involving both the skin and nerves. The endoderm gives rise to glandular tumors that are infrequently encountered in the pedal extremity. The mesoderm gives rise to various connective tissue neoplasms, as well as to muscular, vascular, and bone tumors.

## Etiology

The etiology of neoplasms is essentially unknown. However, the most common etiologic factors for some common tumors are bacterial, viral, and parasitic organisms. These agents may stimulate various forms of granulomatous types of masses and some very common benign neoplasms such as the plantar wart. Chemical and thermal injuries and toxic substances may also cause various types of neoplastic growths. Keloids and hypertrophic scars are most frequently seen as benign lesions, whereas skin malignancies such as squamous cell carcinoma and even Bowen's Disease are more common malignancies which may develop from previously benign lesions. Chronic inflammatory or metabolic processes may cause tissue inflammation which can lead to various conditions such as rheumatoid nodules. Other inflammatory diseases such as osteoarthritis, tuberculosis, gout, and syphilis may cause tumor-like conditions of the foot. Diabetes mellitus, one of the most frequent metabolic diseases seen may cause various forms of xanthomas involving the foot.

Trauma is probably one of the most common, related factors in the formation of new growths. Traumatic injuries have been known to stimulate a lesion that already exists or to even stimulate a new growth by irregular biological means. The most common tumors to which trauma has been attributed, are inclusion cysts, foreign body granulomas, and pseudo-sarcomas; vascular trauma may also be implicated in some tumors of vascular and neurologic origin.

Congenital and hereditary factors have also been shown to be contributing etiologic elements seen in patients who may develop tumorous conditions. The most frequent neoplasms seen are in patients with hemangiomas and in congenital diseases, such as tuberous sclerosis and von Recklinghausen's.

## Incidence

Unfortunately, precise incidence with regard to benign and malignant neoplasms of the foot is not known. This may be because benign neoplasms create very little morbidity or insufficient hazards to the patient's health to warrant such information. Malignant tumors, on the other hand, are so rare on the foot that the incidence would be difficult to establish. The literature reviews that are available are somewhat inconsistent.

One of the earliest statistical reviews in the literature was a study by Pack (1939) of 184 tumors of the foot, of which 137 were malignant. The most frequent malignancies encountered in his study were those of the skin and malignancies affecting tendon and synovial tissues were the second most frequently encountered.[1]

Perhaps the best and most recent effort in determining the incidence of cancer of the foot has been published in the *Third National Cancer Survey* by the National Institute of Health in their 1969 survey of a ten percent sampling of the U.S. population. This survey revealed a total of 61,409 malignancies.[9] Only 20 of these cases, however, affected the foot. It was interesting to note in this survey that caucasians were much more frequently affected compared to black patients, with an incidence almost ten times greater. The sex incidence shows that females had slightly more tumors than males.

A 1971-72 survey of skin cancer by the National Institute of Health revealed 9,512 tumors, representing a five percent sampling of the U.S. population.[9] Of this number, 161 skin tumors were found on the lower extremity, but only 15 tumors were found on the foot.

It should be mentioned that the American College of Foot Surgeons is presently trying to develop statistical information to assist both the practitioner and the researcher in their efforts to determine the etiology, diagnosis, and proper management of neoplasms affecting the foot.

## Clinical Picture

The clinical diagnosis of any soft tissue tumor can be extremely difficult. The foot is a relatively thin portion of the body and very often any soft tissue swelling is easily noticed. However, there are certain tumors which, due to their small size, rarely, if ever, show any soft tissue swelling. Therefore, palpation and examination for the possibility of neoplasms should be carefully performed. Perhaps the easiest method of careful palpation is that of two point palpation using the finger and thumb of the adjacent hand and gently rotating the fingers superficially to see if any unusual neoplasms respond to pressure. Never squeeze the foot in deep palpation initially; this technique may cause any benign lesion in this area to be forcefully pushed aside. Light stroking of the skin for structures involved should be employed in the most superficial evaluation.

Palpation of the patient's popliteal and inguinal lymph nodes should be performed whenever one is evaluating for soft tissue neoplasms. Any irregularity of the lymph nodes upon palpation should be highly suspect.

The patient's history is also an extremely important guide in one's diagnosis and evaluation of any soft tissue tumor, in addition to careful examination of the part involved.

Some tumors on the dorsal aspect of the foot are similar to those on the plantar aspect. Ganglion cysts are the most common lesions creating a soft tissue swelling on the foot. These cysts are most frequently seen overlying joints; however, giant cell tumors and related neoplasms are also encountered in this location on the foot.

Some frequently seen tumors involving the nail bed area are fibromas, glomus tumors, pyogenic granulomas, and while malignancies are rare, they have been reported. The most common malignancies are melanoma and squamous cell carcinoma.

Neoplasms most commonly seen on the plantar aspect of the foot are fibromas, giant cell tumors, lipomas, plantar fibromatosis, epidermal inclusion cysts, ganglion cysts, and neuromas. The metatarsal and heel regions of the foot are frequently traumatized. Malignancies in these areas are not uncommon.

### Signs and Symptoms

Pain and paresthesia are the most frequent symptoms that will cause one to seek help. It is not uncommon to see a ganglion on the dorsal surface of the foot creating such symptoms. On the other hand, ganglions or other tumors on the leg or thigh may reveal as neuro-muscular impairment, first seen in the pedal extremity.

Swelling is another common symptom that the patient may present to the podiatrist. Swelling or edema can often be misleading and careful evaluation and examination is indicated to rule out the many and varied causes of edema. Many soft tissue neoplasms may create what appears to be edema, but this may only represent the presence of a large lesion.

Skin color can be a very useful diagnostic sign, particularly in cases of vascular lesions. Certain vascular tumors may present themselves with either a bluish or reddish hue. Superficial skin changes with irregular borders may represent Bowen's Disease or a Kaposi's sarcoma.

The texture or density of soft tissue neoplasms may also present as very firm hard masses yielding to little or no

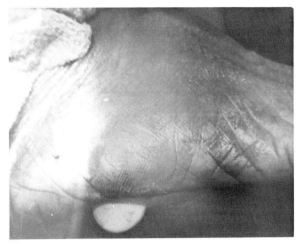

**Figure 1-1**

Rheumatoid Nodule. Unusual swelling over the base of the fifth metatarsal. Extremely tender on direct palpation. Clinically these lesions could almost represent any solidified mass. This might be considered a pseudo type of tumor.

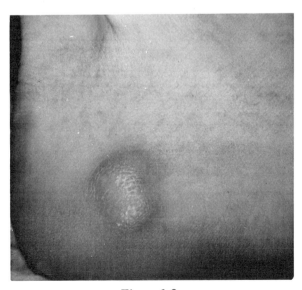

**Figure 1-2**

Vascular Leiomyoma. Lesion overlying the heel. Extremely firm on palpation and quite noticeable on examination. Diagnosis, again, can be almost any form of solid type of neoplasm.

digital pressure. Yet other soft tissue lesions may be very compressible and soft, such as neurofibromas and lipomas. However, even these lesions may have other presentations.

Most soft tissue neoplasms may take any shape or size. Skin lesions such as the dermatofibroma are classically seen as button-type lesions, whereas pyogenic granuloma often exudes a purulent material. Other forms of skin lesions may exhibit ulcerating areas such as those seen in squamous or basal cell carcinomas of the foot. Unfortunately, both the size and shape of the lesion seldom give many clues to their diagnosis. However, this sign may relate an important aspect in one's surgical criteria and the ability to preserve normal and vital structures. As a rule of thumb, radical excision is often the procedure of choice if it is a small malignancy. For large malignancies, amputation is usually more efficacious.

Limitation of function usually occurs in tumors overlying specific vessels, nerves, tendons, or other vital structures. Neurological diseases must also be ruled out since other tumors on the lower extremities may create such foot symptoms.

Deformity may present itself as one of the most gross signs that the clinician may see. It is not uncommon for massive hamartomas to render an appendage useless, as will other lesions pressing on major nerves. Many tumors can present similar signs and symptoms which often create a puzzling differential diagnosis.

### Diagnosis

Other than histologic examination of tissue and the cytologic examination of scrapings, punch biopsy, and/or fine needle aspirations of tumors of the foot, there are few, if any, laboratory studies which render a specific diagnosis. There are, however, certain laboratory studies which can preoperatively suggest the nature of the tumor. The definitive diagnosis still depends upon histologic examination. The following is an outline of those conditions in which laboratory studies might be useful in rendering a preoperative diagnosis.

*Blood*

   A. Benign:         Rheumotoid Nodules
(RA Factor, Antinuclear Antibodies (ANA), Sed Rate)

                   Xanthomas
(Glucose, Thyroid profile, serum lipid profile

   B. Malignant:    CBC, Bone marrow

*Urine*

   A. Malignant:    Multiple Myeloma
(Bence Jones Protein)

                   Melanoma
(Melanuria)

Conventional radiographic techniques will often fail to reveal a soft tissue tumor which does not secondarily invade or destroy adjacent bone or cause significant derangement to the internal parts of the foot. If the lesion contains calcium (such as a hemangioma) the radiographic diagnosis becomes somewhat easier.

Conventional radiographic techniques are rather inadequate to show the fine detail of soft tissue parts. Although the soft tissues themselves contain inherently greater contrast, traditional techniques and filming materials are not sensitive enough to reveal this contrast to the observer. Therefore, specialized techniques have been introduced which aid immeasurably in the detection, not only of intrinsic abnormalities of the soft tissues, but also the presence of foreign materials.

One such technique is the use of industrial x-ray film, which is very fine grained and allows considerable contrast and detail. Coupled with the use of low kilovoltage and relatively high radiation intensity, it helps to reveal fine soft tissue detail.

9

The Xeroradiographic technique with its edge-enhancement characteristic, considerably facilitates the visualization of soft tissue contrast and tends to make small tumors of the soft tissues more visible radiographically.

A new, but potentially useful, technique is computerized axial tomography. This is a newly developed technique, which couples a computer to an axial tomography machine. A radiation detector receives the radiation that has exited the part being studied and transfers information received to the computer which then makes a somewhat diagrammatic picture of that part. The advantage is that the detector and computer together are far more sensitive to even minute changes in the amount of radiation penetration than other conventional x-ray or even the xeroradiographic process, and will demonstrate extremely fine soft tissue details where other techniques may fail.

Computerized axial tomography, because of its far superior ability to detect slight differences in the inherent contrast of soft tissues, is best suited for detection of small soft tissue tumors in any part of the body. However, computerized axial tomography is currently limited to evaluation of the brain. A recent advance has been made in applying this technique to whole body radiography, but whether or not the foot will become a fit subject for this technique, in view of the instrumentation and expense involved, is at this time uncertain.

In certain situations, such as in hemangiomas or the more vascular tumors of the foot, arteriography or venography may be of value, not only in diagnosis, but in planning the surgical approach.

Diagnostic sonography may be of some value in lesions which are thought to be cystic, as this method of diagnosis is most excellent for differentiating solid from cystic lesions. If sonography reveals a lesion to be cystic, then cyst puncture, aspiration, and the injection of contrast material followed by radiographic filming to reveal the internal nature of the cyst may be a diagnostic aid.

**Surgical Management**

Various factors may determine the choice of surgical pro-

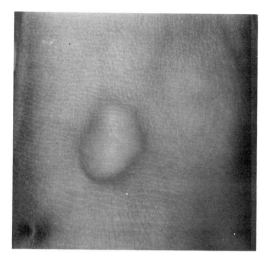

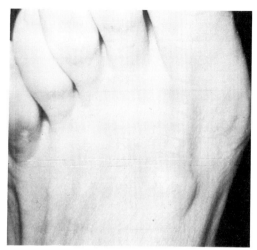

**Figure 1-3**

Ganglion Cyst. Soft tissue neoplasm overlies the anterior aspect of the foot and ankle. Diagnosis is more readily made due to its fluctuation and depressibility. However, these masses can be extremely firm causing some difficulty in clinical diagnosis.

**Figure 1-4**

Ganglion Cyst. Cystic mass overlying the extensor tendon of the first metatarsal. Swelling is the most common sign or sumptom from a neoplasm. Perhaps less that 25% of a correct diagnosis is made from clinical appearance.

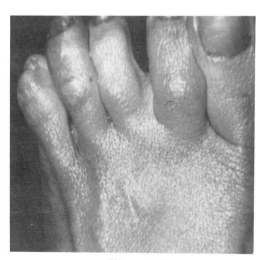

**Figure 1-5**

Traumatic neuroma with vascular malformations. Dorsally there is no sign of any edema or soft tissue swelling. Clinical appearance reveals separation of digits due to the pressure of an intermetatarsal lesion. This is a sign one should look for when evaluating metatarsal pain.

11

cedure depending upon the lesion involved. These factors include: histogenesis of the tumor, fixity or mobility, location, primary or recurring status of the lesion, degree of malignancy and level of invasion, the presence of regional or distant metastasis, and experience and judgment of the surgeon.

The surgical management of tumors as they involve the skin is often an easy procedure to perform. A problem exists when the lesion exceeds a certain size, then plastic repair may be necessary to correct the defect.

Skin incisions vary depending on the type of neoplasm that one is encountering. If the skin is immovable over a soft tissue mass, two semi-elliptical incisions should be employed. Too often the specific neoplasm involved has a close attachment to the epidermal structure. If one is dealing with a cyst, incision through the central portion of the lesion can cause a rupture and create some difficulty in the surgical extirpation of the lesion. If such a case exists, one may slide the skin medially or laterally and make the incision at that point. When the skin is released, the incision sits over the central portion of the neoplasm and will enable the surgeon to have better surgical exposure. The skin may be very thin and/or the surgeon's hand may be somewhat heavy and this might cause the surgical blade to pierce the neoplasm, thereby transferring tumor cells to adjacent and uninvolved structures, leading to a possible recurrence. One should avoid, if possible, close surgical dissection to the skin, since disruption of the blood supply can easily take place. Further complications, such as skin necrosis from inadequate skin dissection, can occur.

Skin lesions which overlie a joint may create another type of problem in which a joint contracture might occur unless proper steps are taken prior to surgery. If a keloid or hypertrophic scar develops, a waiting period of approximately 18 months should be considered before any additional surgical therapy is employed to treat that complication, particularly since many of the hypertrophic scars shrink over that period of time. If a keloid formation develops, intralesional injections of cortico-steroids might be performed

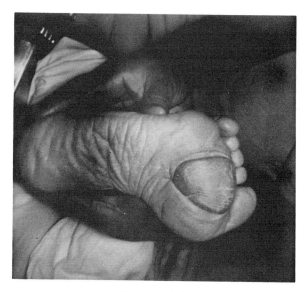

**Figure 1-6A**

Giant Rheumatoid Nodule. Extremely large swelling on the plantar aspect of the foot reveals a lesion of long standing. Close examination reveals stretching of the skin with plantar hypertrophy of the epidermis. Surgical management of the lesion usually requires two linear incisions in order to excise redundant skin.

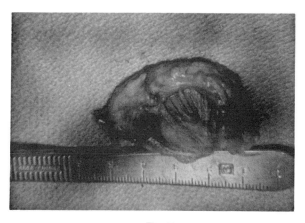

**Figure 1-6B**

This figure reveals a larger rheumatoid nodule on gross examination.

13

since the possibility exists that a larger keloid may result after surgical excision of such a lesion.

Tumors involving the plantar skin may possibly create even greater hazards. Plantar skin excisions should also require the removal of a very small portion of the subcutaneous tissue, since the pressure of weight bearing has a tendency to force this neoplasm toward the skin and other vital structures. If the excision is extensive, skin grafting in this area may also present even greater difficulties. Plantar skin is such a specialized organ that one should try to utilize it in rotation flaps, as the procedure of choice if at all possible toward weight bearing surfaces. Other tissue should be used to graft in the defect that the rotation flaps leave. Care should be taken in rotating the flaps, since the vascular supply should be kept intact and should usually lie proximal to the site.

One of the more difficult benign plantar tumors that one encounters on the foot are those of plantar fibromatosis and even though they are benign skin lesions thay may have a recurrence rate as high as 70 percent. These lesions are confused with fibrosarcomas. The surgical management of this specific tumor should involve a large excision of the plantar fascia, because of the high recurrence rate of the tumor. In surgical aftercare involving any tumor on the plantar surfaces of the foot, the patient should be non-weight bearing for approximately three weeks in order to reduce the possibility of severe plantar scarring.

Cystic tumors should also be carefully dissected, and one should look for possible off-shoots of such cysts which should be removed. Similar to cystic lesions, fatty tumors or lipomas may also have off-shoots which should be evaluated upon surgical exposure and be removed if they exist.

The surgical handling of a neoplasm should be mentioned. During surgical exposure and dissection, direct grasping of the tumor ought to be avoided; handling of non-vital tissue adjacent to the lesion should be the procedure of choice since grasping of such a lesion with the surgical instrument can cause it to disrupt or to tear. Surgical management in excising such neoplasms should consist of both blunt

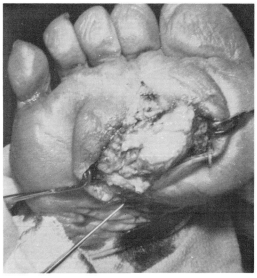

**Figure 1-7A**

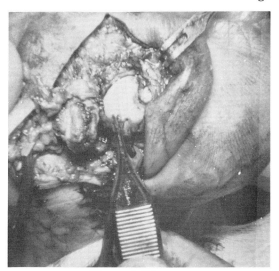

**Figure 1-7B**

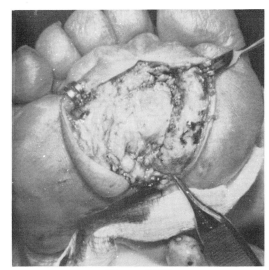

**Figure 1-7C**

These three figures represent the surgical dissection of a rheumatoid nodule of a plantar surface of the foot. One should be prepared to surgically close the defect after excision of the lesion. The greatest complication from defects is that of hematoma formation and wound breakdown. A drain should be inserted into the defect to facilitate healing.

15

and sharp dissection. The rule of thumb, however, is that the sharper the dissection, the less trauma one causes.

If one is excising a ganglion cyst or inclusion cyst, the surgical removal of any abnormality of the bone should also be performed because very often it is the bony projection which is creating much of the irritation underlying that benign tumor or ganglion cyst.

The closure of such tumor defects is important. One should have good hemostasis to prevent hematoma formation and poor wound healing. This can be performed by closing the subcutaneous tissue on a deep level and by tying off any bleeders that may be encountered. The subcutaneous tissue should be closed alternating layers, binding the medial side deep and the lateral side more superficially. One should be careful in underscoring such fatty or subcutaneous tissue because of the disruption of blood supply and further necrosis within the area itself. Small drains may also be used to reduce hematoma formation.

Needless to say, once the subcutaneous defect has been properly closed, skin closure should be even and without strangulation of the tissues. Poor skin closure or subcutaneous tissue closure can result in hypertrophic scars as well as keloid formation. In some instances, this formation can be much worse than the tumor being excised.

Probably the most difficult benign tumors to excise from the foot, are those of vascular origin, particularly deep cavernous forms of hemangioma. Too often, large vessels are involved and the surgical excision and ligation of vascular areas must be employed with care since loss of vascular supply to any area of the foot can create a deformity. Nerve tumors, on the other hand, may result in paresthesias or surgical neuromas as a postoperative complication. Unfortunately, there is no way to prevent such a neuroma from forming. If nerve repair is not feasible, one should try and bury the nerve stump in fat or osseous tissue, which may reduce pressure and motion, relieving neuroma type pain.

If tumors involve bone, a surgical bone resection should be performed and a biopsy carried out. Probably the most common tumors that may involve bone are those of giant cell

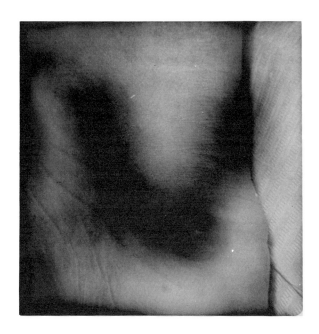

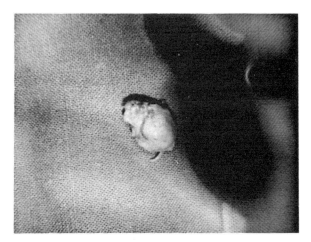

**Figure 1-8B**

Epidermal Inclusion Cyst. An unusual location is the posterior aspect of the heel for any cystic lesion. The most common lesion in this area might possibly be that of a ganglion cyst. Figure 1-8B reveals a gross specimen after surgical excision.

lesions and cavernous hemangioma. Malignancies of the deeper structures can very easily involve the bony architecture. If bone is involved with a malignancy, then amputation of the foot should be performed.

The surgical management of malignant skin lesions of the foot present a different situation than those of the benign. Malignant melanomas are probably the most common skin malignancy that one will encounter on the foot. The treatment often depends on what level of invasion this tumor may have. However, when malignant melanomas do involve the digits, the surgical amputation of the digits is the procedure of choice. Large malignant melanomas involving the plantar surfaces of the foot presents such a high incidence of metastasis that surgical amputation of the foot is the procedure of choice. The smaller melanoma, on the other hand, may only require a three to five centimeter range of normal tissue to be excised surrounding that lesion, followed by a skin graft.

The surgeon should employ wide excision, including the lymph node biopsy and evaluation. Do not enucleate tumors, instead utilize radical dissection. Routine ligation and/or excision of superficial or deep veins should be performed as a matter of expediency and safety since gross and microscopic studies of vascular structures may reveal tumor thrombi. Edema of the extremity may be a very minor penalty to pay with this technique as compared to amputation of the extremity. For unknown reasons, the arteries appear to be less permeable to tumor invasion than do veins. Therefore, the excision of peripheral arteries is often less necessary. If metastasis does occur through the blood stream to other vital organs, then the hope of a surgical cure can be abandoned. If metastasis, on the other hand, is by the lymphathic system through regional lymph nodes, a successful surgical procedure may then be performed.

If vital structures are involved, such as muscle, then amputation one level above the muscle should be performed. In sarcomas involving fascial attachments (fibrosarcoma) to bone, amputation should be performed at the joint above the involved bone area.

Different levels of amputation of the foot are as follows:

1. Digital
2. Les Franks
3. Shopart's amputation
4. Pirogoff amputation
5. Symes amputation
6. Below the knee amputation
7. Above the knee amputation

## Surgical Adjuncts

One of the simplest methods of surgical excision is curettage. This procedure can easily be performed on warts. Our personal experience has also shown that chemotherapy, especially using phenol, following the blunt form of surgical dissection has reduced recurrence. In tumors which affect the nail and nail bed areas, other precautions are necessary since many lesions may involve the nail bed as well as the epidermal areas of the toe. The surgical removal of any nail should be performed prior to further surgical evaluation. Such a precaution would prevent the possibility of postoperative infection since the nail bed area itself is generally non-sterile.

Excision of portions of the nail bed and nail matrix might be necessary to further eradicate such a neoplastic problem. Another specific example of these would be periungual fibromas which often involve the matrix areas of the nail. If such procedures are not performed, the recurrence rate may be as high as 90 percent.

Electrocautery may also be used around the nail and nail bed area, but one must be extremely careful with this modality because of the high destructive capacity which it possesses. Furthermore, utilization of electrosurgery should be limited to non-vital skin surfaces, because of the tremendous amount of scarring which may occur. Such scarring could interfere with tendon movement, as well as with other vital structures. Therefore, when electrosurgery is utilized, it is best performed in multiple stages so that one can actually see the progress of the tissue destruction.

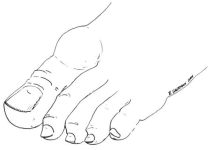

**Figure 1-9**

Soft tissue neoplasm showing bulging of the skin. If skin is non-moveable over mass, two semi elliptical skin incisions should be employed. When incising directly over a neoplasm, care should be taken not to pierce the lesions.

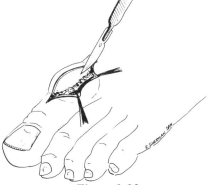

**Figure 1-10**

Drawing demonstrates encapsulated neoplasm and its relation to the epidermis and superficial fascial structures. The surgical blade should not penetrate the neoplasm since this may cause transfer of tumor cells.

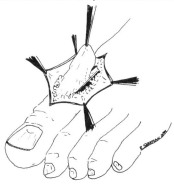

**Figure 1-11**

Demonstration of surgical excision of encapsulated neoplasm overlying first MP joint. Instruments should not grasp the neoplasm as shown, but should be holding non-vital tissue structures.

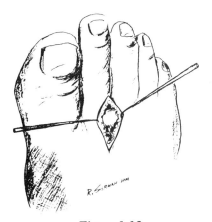

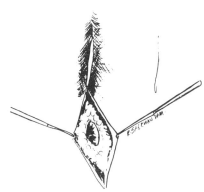

**Figure 1-12**

This figure represents a benign encapsulated tumor sitting in the intermetatarsal space. Underlying the neoplasm is a soft tissue nest of non-vital connective tissue.

**Figure 1-13**

This figure reveals the soft tissue nest supporting the benign neoplasm. This area of non-vital tissue should be removed in order to prevent recurrence of the tumor due to possible impregnation of tumor cells which may penetrate through the capsule.

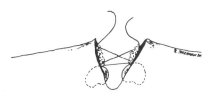

**Figure 1-14**

Representative drawing, showing closure of deep tumor defects to prevent hematoma formation and slow healing. Surgical drains may be necessary in large voids where hematoma formation can occur.

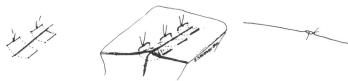

**Figure 1-15**

Representative drawing showing different views of deep and skin closure. Good skin apposition without tension is necessary.

Radiation therapy has also been utlized for various skin neoplasms, but on the foot it can be extremely dangerous since the foot presents such a bony surface that over utilization can cause severe scarring.

## Repair of Vital Structures

Nerve tissue is frequently encountered when large neoplasms affect the foot, whether they be malignant or benign. The involved portions of the nerve must be repaired if at all possible. Generally, neoplasms which cause nerve injury by compression will usually heal themselves after the excision of the lesion. The nerve should still be evaluated at the time of surgery. If nerve fibers are divided, local swelling usually follows, and there is a degeneration proximally of the myelin sheath and axon fibrils. Nerve regeneration generally occurs within a few days if the nerve ends are in good apposition. If there is a lack of apposition and no repair takes place, then local escape of axon fibrils and other cellular elements takes place. This causes a local mass or a neuroma to form. The extent of nerve tissue damage can be shown by the application of dilute methelene blue applied to the nerve ends. The methelene blue has a tendency to stain fibrous tissue and nerve fibrils differently. This aids in determining the extent of necessary dissection and the placement of sutures without injury to the nerve fibrils when instruments of higher magnification are utilized.

The following are the basic principles of nerve suture and repair:

1. Evaluate the amount of nerve to be excised.
2. Nerve should be cut at right angles.
3. Surgical sutures should be placed at the proximal and distal areas of the portion of nerve to be excised. This prevents rotation of the nerve and allows for better realignment of the nerve itself.
4. The nerve vesiculi or bundles should be adequately lined up as carefully as possible.
5. Lengthening of the nerve in the extremity may be performed by underscoring or re-routing the nerve.

6. Additional slack in the nerve can be created by:

A. Plantar flexion of the foot which helps increase the length if the posterior tibial nerve is involved.

B. Dorsiflexion of the foot which may reduce the gap in the peroneal nerve if it is involved.

7. Use small calibre suture material and atraumatic needles.

8. Utilization of the minimum amount of trauma inserting the sutures.

9. Use suture material of little or no reactive qualities.

10. The surface area of suture in contact with neural tissues should be reduced to a minimum.

11. The sutures should be placed in the epineurium since more reaction results if the perineurium is involved.

12. The nerve ends should be approximated without tension and/or torsion.

13. There should be good hemostasis so that the repair can be done in a dry operative field. Hematoma formation at the junction of nerve repair should be prevented.

14. In the closing of large nerve gaps, autogenous nerve grafts may be performed.

After repair of nerves, the extremity is fixed into a position that provides suitable relaxation for nerve healing and wound closure. Isolation of the deep repair from the skin closure by a loose inter-position of superficial fascia or fat should be employed. The foot is then placed in plaster casting, usually with both the knee and foot in the flexed position. Plaster immobilization should be left on for a minimum of four weeks, then re-applied for two subsequent four week periods, for a total of 12 weeks of immobilization. Following the removal of plaster immobilization, a vigorous form of physical therapy should be developed, starting out gradually and then with more intensity in order to prevent atrophy of the muscles involved and, most important, a permanent disability.

Tendon repair is usually not a difficult procedure to manage in the foot. The tendon should, however, be brought together and held while healing takes place without producing a scar at the site of the repair. This at times can be an ex-

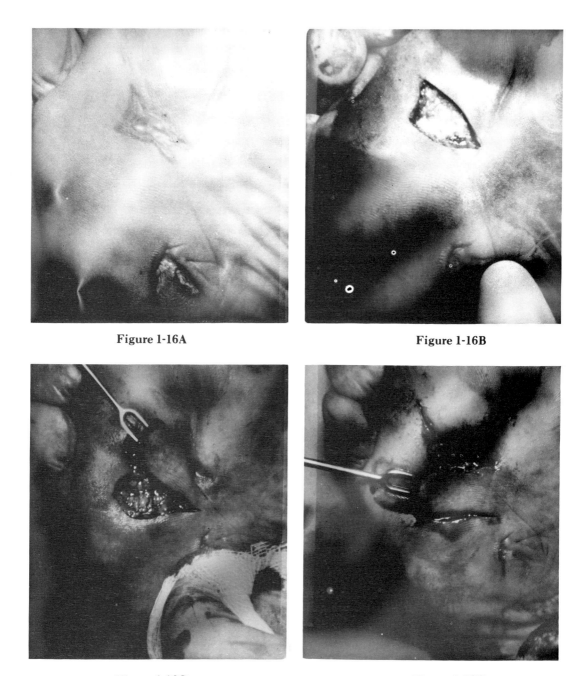

Figure 1-16A

Figure 1-16B

Figure 1-16C

Figure 1-16D

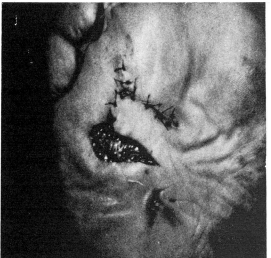

**Figure 1-16E**

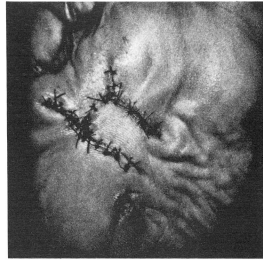

**Figure 1-16F**

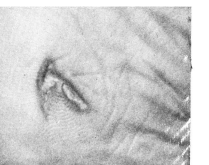

**Figure 1-16G**

Hypertrophic Scar. Clinically Figure 16 reveals two painful hypertrophic scars on the plantar surface of the foot outlined in blue. Careful surgical management should be developed prior to excision particularly in regard to proper closure on the plantar surface of the foot. The lesions are excised and using a rotation graft the first defect is covered. After the defect is closed on the distal lesion, the proximal lesion is then excised and with the use of a modified Z-plasty, skin closure is made easier.

*(Courtesy Joseph Orlando, M.D., Towson, Maryland.)*

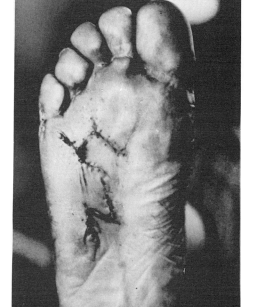

**Figure 1-16H**

tremely difficult procedure, yet it is very important. Any scarring of the tendon at the site of surgical repair can reduce the amount of movement that normally glides the tendon through its tendon sheath. Tendons, fortunately, have a great power of regeneration and can completely heal themselves within several weeks. Non-reactive suture material should be used if at all possible. Since tendon fibers are made up of longitudinal fibers, simple sutures have a tendency to pull out. Therefore, mattress sutures may be better employed while suturing tendons. Suture material should be brought out to the proximal cut end of the tendon, inserted into the distal cut end of the tendon, and then tied. Various pull-out suture techniques may also be employed. This often results in preventing a certain amount of tendon scarring which is created from the reaction of any foreign material. One must try and restore adequate tension to as near normal as possible so that the excursion of a muscle contracture is adequate to produce full range of motion in the joint. One can best judge the proper tension by bringing the joint severed by the tendon to the normal position of rest for that digit. Often this can be gauged by adjacent tendon actions. One may also place tension on the proximal end of the tendon to obtain the limit of excursion distally and then unite the tendon to bring the digit into the normal position of rest. If grafting is necessary, one should always try to graft a tendon of smaller size and thickness to allow for an easier glide pattern in the tendon sheath. Tendons of larger size often result in a less successful procedure. If tendon transfers or substitutions of tendons are made, then the re-routing of these tendons should pass as directly as possible to their new location, and should pass through soft subcutaneous fat to allow for an easier gliding mechanism.

## Surgical Complications

Complications from tumor surgery vary just as in other types of surgery that one performs on the foot. Some of these have already been mentioned. However, it should be pointed out that tumor surgery leaves a much greater recurrence rate than one would expect to see in other bone or joint surgical

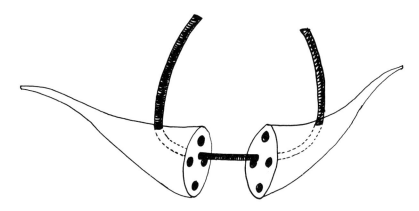

**Figure 1-17**

Fine surgical suture material is necessary to coaptate nerve. Nerve bundles must be aligned properly in order to enhance proper nerve transmission.

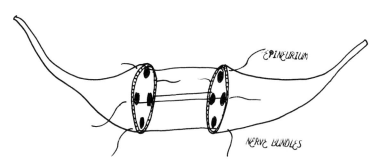

**Figure 1-18**

Representative drawing of nerve repair by placing four equally spaced 7-0 silk sutures to coaptate a severed nerve.

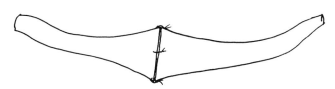

**Figure 1-19**

Neurorrhaphy. Closing of nerve ends in repair. Additional sutures may be necessary to create an airtight closure.

procedures that a podiatrist performs. It should be remembered that tumor tissue may invade or involve other types of tissue, whether it be that of bone, tendon, nerves, vessels, or skin. If neoplastic cells have invaded surrounding vital structures, the podiatric surgeon should not be overly conservative in his surgical dissection. It is probable that one of the greatest errors in surgical judgment, in treatment of soft tissue neoplasms, is the conservatism of the surgeon himself.

However, if the tendons or nerves must be severed and excised, repair of such structures should be instituted as best possible. Tumors of large proportions often leave quite a defect in the foot. Proper closing of these defects is important to wound healing, and it is often one of the largest complications of tumor surgery. With proper closure of such defects, poor healing will be put at a minimum and heavy scarring will also be reduced. Vascular complications which one may encounter are gangrene, particularly of a digit, and, perhaps even more frequently, thrombo-phlebitis. It is not uncommon for only vascular impairment or blockage to occur.

The greatest surgical error is that of enucleation, or shelling out of the lesion, and not excising it and its adjacent subcutaneous tissue, (which may be surrounding it), since this often leads to recurrence. Most soft tissue neoplasms have a tendency to create what might look like a birds nest or tissue sac, which essentially retains these tumors or may keep them confined to a small area. These soft tissue sacs should also be excised after the removal of a tumor.

It should be pointed out that even benign neoplasms, which are often encapsulated, have a tendency for the various tissue cells of that tumor to penetrate that tissue encapsulation and involve the adjacent tissue structure. This is the primary reason for the excision of adjacent non-vital tissue. Too often encapsulation of a lesion is taken for granted.

Deformity usually results when massive surgical intervention is pursued and poor tissue repair of vital structures has been performed. Amputation creates the most noticeable deformity, but at the same time rehabilitation of the area may be more useful to the patient and most important, prevent undesirable pain and death.

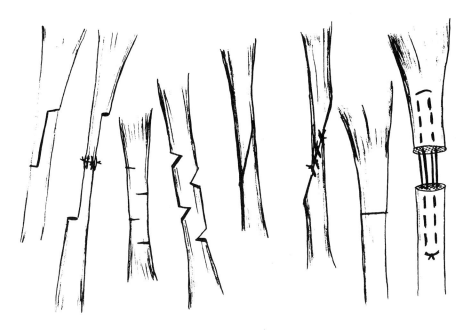

**Figure 1-20**

These drawings represent various methods of tendon repair and tendon lengthening.

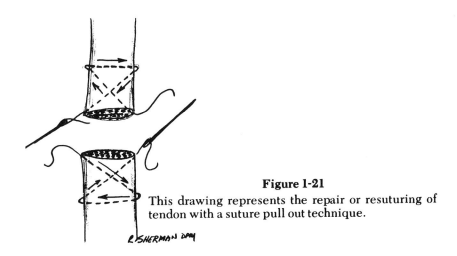

**Figure 1-21**

This drawing represents the repair or resuturing of tendon with a suture pull out technique.

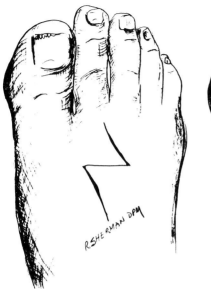 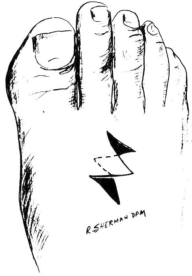

**Figure 1-22**

The following illustrations show Z-plasty procedure utilized to change the directions of skin tension and scar lines and to offer the surgeon the opportunity prevent contraction.

**Figure 1-23**

Z-plasties, depending on degree of angles utilized, can offer the surgeon the length desired of a particular wound area.

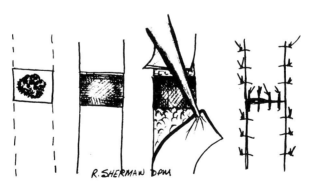

**Figure 1-24**

The drawings represent a skin neoplasm excised by block excision and repair of skin defect by sliding the skin margins proximally and distally to close the defect.

Metastasis is the worse complication of any malignant tumor. Adequate lymph node dissection in any malignancy should be evaluated. If there is definite lymph node invasion, then further surgical treatment must be undertaken.

Infection is the second most common postoperative complication from surgery. The most frequent infections encountered on the foot are those caused by staph or strep organisms. Specific infections are not frequently encountered. These infections are usually due to foreign body type reactions, particularly such as one may see from a rupturing cyst and in which the contents act as a foreign body. The excision of large lesions may leave a large dead space area which would increase the chance of hematoma development. Careful attention to hemostasis and a contoured pressure dressing will help prevent this hematoma formation and further prevent infection.

The application of gelfoam in deep tissue cavities or voids will help retard hematoma formation. However, this is another foreign body being placed into the wound and can also increase the possibility of an infection. It should also be noted that nail infections may not be as they appear. Podiatrists should rule out the possibility of a squamous cell carcinoma if a chronic paronychia is present. Also, Bowen's disease of the nail may be present and even possibly a keratoacanthoma. Black fungating borders suggest the presence of a malignant melanoma.

Cosmetic deformities are often seen when skin is involved. Large tumors often require excision of involved skin surfaces and skin grafting, or other means of surgical and plastic repair. Fortunately, the patient is able to hide the foot in a shoe or sock, but, at the same time, the individual must walk on that structure. If tumors involve large areas of the plantar skin, chronic trauma may cause breakdown and ulceration due to weight bearing pressures. Therefore, the surgeon should evaluate his surgical approach very closely in this area.

Local anesthesia is probably used in about 90 percent of podiatric surgery today. Anesthestic blocks in dealing with neoplasms should be given as regional blocks. One should avoid, if at all possible, infiltration forms of anesthesia in this type of surgery since the penetration of the hypodermic needle into a tumor can cause disruption, or possible transfer of tumor cell to adjacent tissue. Large neoplasms often need a general form of anesthesia.

## Summary

The podiatrist's surgical evaluation should depend on his patient, as well as his patient's history. Having a general knowledge of neoplasms and locations of foot involvement has significant bearing upon one's surgical technique. Prior to surgical employment, all diagnostic aids possible should be utilized. Depending on the existence of the neoplasm, the surgeon should make his patient aware of the possibility that the neoplasm, though excised, could still recur. Systemic diseases should also be evaluated for their possible relationship to that neoplasm. The success of the podiatrist's surgical intervention greatly depends on his surgical judgment, anatomical knowledge, his ability to prevent deformity, and last but not least, his rapport with the patient.

Fortunately, a multitude of therapies exist, whether they be chemotherapy, radiation therapy, electrocautery, or various forms of surgical excision, including amputation. In the very near future, there will probably be various forms of laser surgery employed in the area of podiatric oncology.

## Bibliography

1. Berlin, S.J.: ACFS neoplasm survey of the foot: a preliminary study. *Jour. Foot Surg.*, **Vol. 13**, No. 1, 1974.
2. Berlin, S.J.: Soft tissue surgery (tumors, tendons, and plastic surgery). *Jour. Foot Surg.*, **Vol. 14**, No. 1, 1975.
3. Berlin, S.J.: ACFS neoplasm survey of the foot–1974: a continuing study. *Jour. Foot Surg.*, **Vol. 14**, No. 3, 1975.
4. Crenshaw, A.H. (Editor): *Campbell's Operative Orthopedics*, Vol. I and II, 5th Ed., C.V. Mosby Co., St. Louis, 1971.
5. Krufky, E.: Personal Communication. Dept. of Radiology, George Washington University School of Medicine, Washington, D.C.
6. McGregor, I.A.: *Fundamental Techniques of Plastic Surgery and Their Surgical Applications*, 5th Ed. Williams and Wilkins Co., Balt., Md., 1972.

7.  Pack, G.T.: Tumors of the hands and feet. *Surgery*, **1**: 1–26, 1939.
8.  Passen, S.: Personal Communications. Dept. of Pathology, Maryland General Hospital, Balt., Md.
9.  *Preliminary Report Third National Cancer Survey*, 1969 Incidence. National Institute of Health, Bethesda, Maryland.
10. Scatto, J.: Personal Communications. Statistical Branch, Dept. HEW, Washington, D.C.
11. Stout, A.P. and Lattes, R.: *Tumors of the Soft Tissues.* AFIP Second Series, Washington, D.C., 1967.
12. Wiley, A.M.: Ganglion and hemangioma as a cause of plantar neuritis. *Post-Graduate Medical Jour.*, **34**: 489–490, 1958.

# Section II

# Fibrous and Fat Tumors

**Introduction**

The following chapter on fibrous and fat tumors of the foot will not be dealing specifically with fibromas and the reader is referred to Volume Three of Podiatric Medicine and Surgery, entitled *Skin Tumors of the Foot: Diagnosis and Treatment.* This chapter will include the other fibrous tumors which were excluded from Volume Three. Tuberous sclerosis is a frequently encountered systemic condition revealing many fibrous tumors on the foot and is included in this chapter.

**Tuberous Sclerosis**

*Definition*

Tuberous Sclerosis is a complex, protean, neuroectodermal, dysplastic disease belonging to a group of diseases known as the neurocutaneous disorders. The disease is characterized classically by the triad of adenoma sebaceum, epilepsy, and mental retardation. It is included along with von Recklinghausen's disease, von Hippel-Lindau syndrome, Sturge-Weber syndrome and ataxia telangiectasia in those diseases broadly classed as the phakomatoses.

*Synonyms*

Epiloia, Burneville's Disease, Pringle's Disease

*History*

Bourneville (1880) described a three year old child with "acne rosacea," epilepsy, arrested physical development, hemiplegia, and idiocy. Pringle (1890) is credited with first describing the facial lesions and accepting the term "adenoma sebaceum," coined five years earlier by Balzer and Menetrier. Hallopeau and Leredde (1895) first described the shagreen patch on the back. Kothe (1903) described subungual fibromas and adenoma sebaceum as being related and described a case. Vogt (1908) associated the cerebral lesions of the disease with the classical triad. Sherlock (1911), coined

36

the term "epiloia" which is a combination of "epi-" for epilepsy and "-anoia" for mindlessness. Berg (1913) hypothesized the familial incidence of the disease.

## Incidence

Not all individuals with tuberous sclerosis are mentally retarded, nor do they require confinement to mental institutions. Consequently, no figures are currently available that estimate the incidence of the disease in the general population. Individuals with the incomplete form of the disease go unrecognized and consequently are missed in any statistical evaluation of the disease. However, Lagos and Gomez estimate that one in 300,000 people present the classic triad of tuberous sclerosis, and one in 150,000 exhibit the incomplete form.[76] In mental institutions, the incidence ranges between 0.1 percent to 0.9 percent of the resident population. The following is a chart of three studies conducted during a period from 1960 to 1972 which substantiates this incidence in mental facilities:

| Date | Cases | Total Population | Percent |
|------|-------|------------------|---------|
| 1963 | 103 | 11,000 | 0.9%[87] |
| 1969 | 32 | 3,400 | 0.9%[4] |
| 1972 | 23 | 3,000 | 0.7%[1] |

Both sexes are reported as being equally affected, as are all races. However, in the study by Feinstein (1972) the ratio of males to females was two to one and caucasians to blacks was three to one.[47]

## Etiology

Tuberous Sclerosis is primarily a defect in the organization of connective tissue inherited as an autosomal dominant with variable expressivity. However, as many as 50 percent of the cases appear to result from a mutation. The disease also tends to be familial. Interestingly, at one time the disease was considered a variant of von Recklinghausen's disease. However, according to Nickel (1961) and Zeligman

(1974) any neurofibroma that might be found in a patient with tuberous sclerosis is merely an incidental finding, which has been perpetuated in the literature.[87,133] Most researchers believe that the basic defect is in the collagen tissue and that "collagenosis" might be a better term to describe the disease.

## Clinical Picture

A facial lesion known as *adenoma sebaceum* is considered pathognomonic of the disease. It is the most common skin lesion and its diagnostic value is second only to the characteristic tuberous lesions in the brain. These lesions, which make their first appearance between the ages of four to six, are described as small, discrete, yellowish-red or pink, maculo-papular eruptions distributed over the nose, nasolabial folds, cheeks, forehead, and chin, with the upper lip noticeably excluded. The lesions are almost always bilaterally symmetrical. In the early stages, the lesions may go unnoticed by parents or examiners but growth is progressive until puberty. At this time, the fully developed lesion appears as smooth, glistening nodules with overlying telangiectatic vessels and yellow puncta. These fully developed lesions are compatible with those originally described by Pringle (1890)[93] On occasion, these lesions may become verrucous, pedunculated, or coalesce to form irregular aggregates.

The *shagreen* patch is the most diagnostic lesion occurring on the trunk (*peau chagrine*, untanned leather, collagen plaque).[87] These lesions are slightly elevated, flat, flesh colored areas of variable size with an orange peel (peau d'orange) appearance where the skin appendages cause an indentation of the skin. The lesions, which range in size from one centimeter to ten centimeters, are classically located in the lumbosacral area and are considered to be connective tissue nevi.[38] Dawson states that shagreen patches and periungual fibromas alone are peculiar to the disease.[33]

Tuberous sclerosis is readily diagnosed when the classical triad of adenoma sebaceum, mental retardation, and epilepsy are present. In the absence of the last two features, the diagnosis may be difficult and rest upon the presence or absence of other cutaneous lesions, radiographic changes, or electroencephalographic studies. Van der Hoeve states that flat retinal tumors (phakomas) are diagnostic.[125] Their great rarity, however, limits their usefulness. The family history is positive in a high percentage of cases, and, in any given family, the manifestations are rather constant. Many cases, however, are not familial. Cerebral calcifications in a cotton ball configuration are highly suggestive, and, in fact, it is these potato-like lesions on x-ray from which the syndrome derives its name.

Periungual fibromas (Koenen's tumors) represent the most consistent lesion associated with tuberous sclerosis found on the foot. They usually appear later in life, usually after puberty, and continue to develop with age. Nickel, in a study of 103 cases noted the presence of these tumors in 35 cases, with the following age distribution and sex occurrence.[87]

| Age (Years) | Number | Males | Females |
|---|---|---|---|
| 0–9 | 1 | 1 | 0 |
| 10–19 | 12 | 5 | 7 |
| 20–29 | 9 | 5 | 4 |
| 30–39 | 7 | 2 | 5 |
| 40–49 | 3 | 0 | 3 |
| Over 50 | 3 | 0 | 3 |
| | 35 | 13 | 22 |

The lesions are usually described as digital, firm, flesh-colored tumors which are asymptomatic and protrude from under the nail folds or subungually. Early lesions may appear as a ridge in the nail or as a "budding seed" accompanied by a ridging distal to the bud.[87] The lesions may achieve considerable size and disrupt the nail bed; frequently they are large enough to produce pain as a result of pressure from footgear. According to Nickel and Reed, periungual fibromas outnumber subungual ones three to one.[87]

Depigmented lesions (white spots, white leaf-shaped macules) are the only other skin lesions that seem to appear

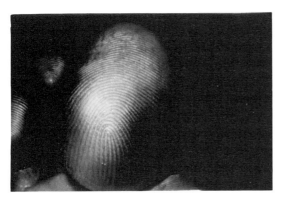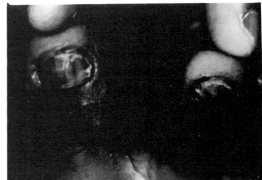

Fibroma. A large subcutaneous fibroma involving the hallux, the toe measuring approximately 4½ inches in diameter. The photographs reveal both plantar (A) and dorsal (B) views of the hallux digit.

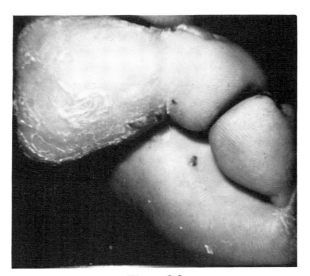

**Figure 2-2**

A large pedunculated fibroma involving the fourth toe. *(Courtesy of Louis Shapiro, D.P.M., Albuquerque, N.M.)*

with any significant regularity in individuals with the disease. Fitzpatrick (1968) described these hypomelanotic macules fully and stated that these lesions are present at birth and may represent the only cutaneous sign of tuberous sclerosis.[48] Frequently, they go unnoticed or are regarded as unimportant since they are quite inconspicuous in fair-skinned infants, but can readily be detected if illuminated with Wood's light. These lesions may occur on any part of the body but to date none has been reported to occur on the foot.

Cafe-au-lait macules, ichthyosis, vitiligo, hypertrichosis, leukoderma, fibroepithelial tags, port-wine hemangiomas, keratodermas, soft tissue calcifications and lipomata are other skin or soft tissue lesions that occur with variable frequency. None of these are considered pathognomonic.[49]

*Nervous System*

Variable degrees of mental deficiency and epilepsy are characteristic of the disease. Both entities, if present, appear early in life and vary over a wide latitude in their manifestations. Not all patients with tuberous sclerosis are mentally retarded and, in fact, some are quite intelligent. It is estimated that 50 percent of people with the disease are able to live outside of institutions and, consequently, may be seen in practitioner's offices or clinics.[87]

Glial tissue represents the supportive connective tissue of the central and peripheral nervous tissue. Since the disease is basically one of over production of collagen, it is not uncommon to see proliferative changes about the cranial and peripheral nerves. When these changes involve the peripheral nerves, the latter may resemble neurofibromata but are unrelated to von Recklinghausen's disease.[61]

In general, individuals with tuberous sclerosis have a propensity to tumor formation. It is estimated that 50 percent of all rhabdomyomas of the heart are associated with the disease,[12] 60 percent of tuberous sclerosis patients have renal hamartomas,[77] and 85 percent of the patients have associated osseous manifestations.[96]

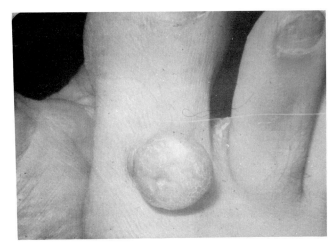

**Figure 2-3A**

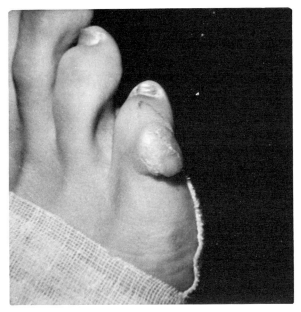

**Figure 2-3B**

Dermatofibromas of the digits are not uncommon findings; they are usually very firm button-like type of lesions. Figure 3A is a large lesion involving the hallux. *(Courtesy of Herbert Rosen, D.P.M., Owings Mills, Md.)* Figure 3B represents a large dermatofibroma of the fifth toe closely resembling that of a corn. *(Courtesy Jerry Krieger, D.P.M., Manassas, Va.)*

## Differential Diagnosis

The differential diagnosis of tuberous sclerosis primarily rests upon the recognition of the adenoma sebaceum. This facial lesion, as the most constant cutaneous lesion, may very well be the only visible lesion of the disease, and yet this "forme fruste" variety of the disease may be extremely difficult to diagnose, except by biopsy. The lesion must be differentiated from multiple cystic benign epitheliomas, syringocystadenomas, basal cell nevus syndrome, acne rosacea, acne vulgaris, verruca plana, and drug eruptions.

Periungual fibromas are rarely difficult to diagnose, but, nevertheless, must be differentiated from subungual corns, subungual verrucae, and juvenile fibromatosis.

## Pathology

The histopathology of adenoma sebaceum has been the only confusing aspect of the disease. Original descriptions ascribed the fundamental process as a hypertrophy of the pilosebaceus glands. It is currently accepted that the facial lesions are not sebaceous adenomas, but rather a part of an overall hamartomatous change of the connective and vascular tissue in the skin. The sebaceous glands play only a passive roll. According to Nickel and Reed, the lesions are angiofibromas.[87] Yokovlev and Guthrie stated that the adenoma sebaceum as well as the periungual fibromas often arise from elements of the peripheral glia or Schwann cells and are thus analogues to the neurofibromas of von Recklinghausen's disease.[132] Nickel and Reed confirmed this observation and reported that, in a histologic evaluation of four patients with periungual fibromas, the lesions had a neural appearance with stellate and small giant cells.

The periungual fibroma is characterized by proliferation of spindle-shaped fibroblasts and minute capillary vessels. The fibroblasts are surrounded by intersecting bundles of collagen and occasional elastic fibers. The lesion is basically located in the dermis extending from just beneath the stratum basalis into the subcutaneous tissue. According to Mehregan, a characteristic finding in these tumors is the pre-

43

sence of intracytoplasmic inclusion bodies in the fibroblast.[83]

The shagreen patch consists of dense bands of collagen involving the entire dermis and closely resembles a connective tissue nevus.

### Foot Involvement

As stated earlier, periungual fibromas remain the most consistent foot lesion associated with tuberous sclerosis. Feinstein reported on four patients of 22 studied who demonstrated periungual fibromas. A total of seven tumors were present: three on the fifth toe, two on the third toe, and one each on the second and fourth toes. All of the lesions were small with the largest being approximately one centimeter in diameter. All the lesions were asymptomatic.[47] Butterworth reported a case of multiple, dull red, firm proliferations emerging from the nail grooves of five or six toes in one patient.[26] The majority of the lesions were slightly larger than a pinhead, but one on the great toe was the size of a pea. The smaller lesions had a tendency to be roughly triangular with the apex directed distally. In another case, Butterworth described fibromas that appeared as longitudinal striations and transverse white bands on the nails.[26] Nickel and Reed, in a study of 33 cases of periungual fibromas, found four lesions which they described as quite extensive. Some of these lesions were arranged in the form of an arch around the base of the nail. They found that early lesions may appear as ridges in the nail or as a "budding seed" accompanied by a ridge distal to the bud.[87] Skeer presented a case with multiple fibromas on the hallux nails with similar lesions at the posterior nail fold of the lesser toes.[109] He described the process as beginning at the root of the nail and protruding between the matrix and nail wall lying on the nail plate. Busch found that these lesions are more common on the toes than fingers and postulated shoe pressure as a possible etiologic factor.[24] The following chart itemizes this occurrence:

| Researcher | Cases | Toes | Fingers |
|---|---|---|---|
| Butterworth[26] | 10 | 5 | 2 |

| | | | |
|---|---|---|---|
| Feinstein[47] | 13 | 4 | 0 |
| Nickel[87] | 103 | 33 | ? |
| Lagos[76] | 12 | 10 | 2 |
| | 138 | 52 | 4 |

In addition to periungual fibromas, numerous orthopedic and radiologic observations have been made as they relate to tuberous sclerosis and the foot. Reed estimated that 85 percent of patients with the disease have some bone manifestation.[96] Feinstein, in a study of 22 patients, reported the most common foot deformities as the following:[47]

| | |
|---|---|
| Digital contractures | —20% |
| Equinus | —15% |
| Pes planus | —15% |

Hallux abducto valgus, pes cavus, talipes equino varus, calcaneo valgus, and metatarsus adductus were also noted but, in all probability, were just incidental findings. Smith, in a study of 32 cases, also found equinus and pes planus as a common deformity.[110] Radiographically, the most common bone lesions that appear are pseudocysts and cortical thickening which Nickel states as being much more common in the metatarsals and phalanges than in the hand.[87] According to Holt and Dickerson, the vaguely marginated cystic lesions tend to be more common in the younger patient while cortical thickening and periosteal new bone is more common in the older patient.[63] Osteoporosis and a history of multiple pathologic fractures have also been reported. In addition, according to Feinstein, approximately 90 percent of the patients with positive radiographic findings also present with adenoma sebaceum.[47]

*Treatment*

From the above, it is apparent that the only soft tissue lesion with which the podiatrist may find himself confronted is the periungual fibroma. However, these fibromas may attain sufficient size to produce pain from shoe pressure necessitating surgical removal. Actual destruction of lesions

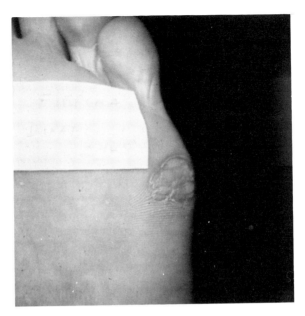

**Figure 2-4**

Mosiac fibroma. A relatively large mosiac pattern type of fibroma with various connective tissue septums separating fibrous bundles is located under the fifth metatarsal head. Surgical excision in this area would require the removal of the 5th metatarsal head because of the weight bearing area and to necessitate proper skin closure.

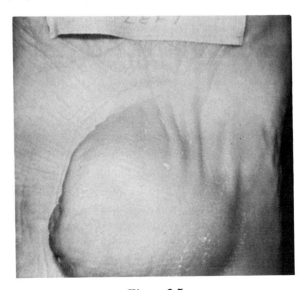

**Figure 2-5**

Plantar fibromatosis. Represents a severely enlarged plantar fibromatosis in a diabetic patient. The surrounding skin areas become somewhat hyperkeratotic due to pressure.

is the best mode of therapy, and this may be accomplished by electrodesiccation, electrolysis, curettage, cauterization, cyrotherapy, planing, or excision. Butterworth prefers electrodesiccation since, if properly employed, it results in little scarring.[25] Despite all attempts at surgical resolution, there is a noticeable tendency for the lesions to recur. Skeer presents a case with multiple periungual fibromas on the hallux and lesser toes which were removed surgically; all of the lesions later recurred.[109] Berlin stated that since these lesions have such a high recurrence rate, radical excision of the tumor and surrounding nail bed and matrix should be performed.[14] It is worthy of mention that, for many of the lesions, local anesthetic is unnecessary.[83]

## Prognosis

The eventual outcome for patients with tuberous sclerosis varies with the severity of the disease and the extent of visceral involvement. Individuals with only cutaneous lesions generally live a normal life span without further cutaneous or visceral involvement. There have been no reports of any malignant transformations on any of the skin lesions. The lesions tend to progress to adult life and then become static.

The more severely involved patients are committed to institutions where the five year survival rate is 30 percent, the 15 year survival rate 15 percent, and the 30 year survival rate 5 percent from the time of birth. The most common causes of death are status epilepticus, cardiac or renal failure, or secondary infection.

## Plantar Fibromatosis

### Definition

Plantar fibromatoses are a benign proliferation of fibrous tissue, which replace varying portions of the plantar aponeurosis with eventual "invasion" of the overlying skin.

*History*

Lederhose (1897) was the first to describe plantar fibromatosis, but until Pickrin (1951) described 18 cases,[91] not much more had been written about this entity. Warthan and Rudolph pointed out, in their report of isolated cases of plantar fibromatosis, that the lesions tend to recur and ulcerate, and, therefore, must be differentiated from sarcomas.[127] El-Banhawy discussed the desirability of excision of the entire plantar fascia, if the fibromatosis was widespread.[42] Aviles reported over 22 cases and also indicated the need for differentiating these lesions from malignant lesions.[8]

*Etiology*

According to Meyerding, the etiology seems to be a combination of chronic inflammation aggravated by trauma, with function, heredity, age, and occupation being predisposing factors.[84] Other conditions associated with plantar fibromatosis (and considered to be of possible etiological significance) are epilepsy, Peyronie's disease, coronary occlusion, and syringomyelia. Trauma due to fractures of the lower extremity has also been recorded as a possible etiologic factor.

*Clinical Picture*

The lesions usually appear before the age of 30, but may be asymptomatic or unrecognized until later in life. They are usually bilateral, asymptomatic nodular abnormalities that are located to the medial portion of the plantar aponeurosis. They occur in the male in a ratio of nine to one, according to Gelfarb, yet other studies have not proved male predominance.

Examination of the lesion may reveal a single nodule or multiple nodules. The diameter of these lesions ranges from three to ten centimeters. The skin is usually freely moveable over individual nodules. Unlike Dupuytren's contracture of the hand, contractures of the plantar structures or toes are rare. The majority of nodules are usually located in the an-

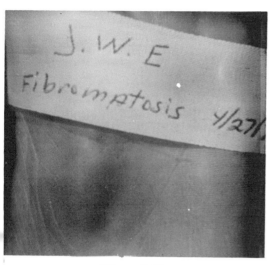

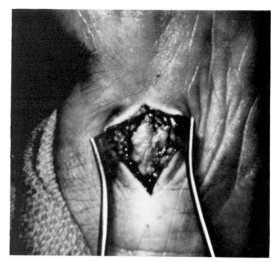

**Figure 2-6A**  **Figure 2-6B**

Plantar fibromatosis. This is a large multi-lobulated plantar fibromatosis lesion lying more medially, plantarly located in the foot. Figure 6A reveals size and skin bulging and Figure 6B shows surgical exposure.

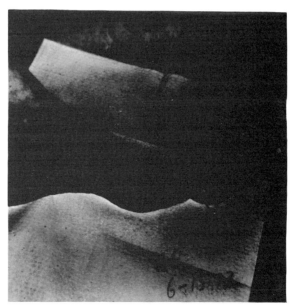

**Figure 2-7**

Plantar fibromatosis. Photograph reveals an extremely unusual location for plantar fibromatosis involving the hallux. *(Courtesy of Joseph Reynolds, D.P.M., Salt Lake City, Utah.)*

terior one third of the plantar fascia. Pickrin reported that most of the nodules in the antero-medial margin of the plantar surface of the calcaneus shared the same compartment as the flexor digitorum brevis muscle.

The clinical appearance of plantar fibromatoses may be confused with giant cell tumor of tendon sheath, leiomyoma (painful), lipoma (radiolucent), benign and malignant synoviomas, fibrosarcoma, neurofibroma of von Recklinghausen's, and granuloma annulare.

## Pathology

The gross pathology is that of an irregular, non-circumscribed, matted mass of dense gray-white connective tissue. Microscopically, there are young fibroblasts arranged in strands and whorls. Inflammatory reaction is uncommon. The surrounding tissues are infiltrated by this fibrous tissue. Bizarre histological changes may occur, including loss of cell polarity, nuclei variability in size and shape, and, at times, atypical mitoses. It is because of these variations that plantar fibromatoses may be mistaken for fibrosarcoma. Usually, however, the fibroblasts are well differentiated, uniform in size and shape, and devoid of mitotic activity.

## Treatment

The conservative approach is the recommended form of treatment, and may include injection therapy, padding, and shoe therapy. Surgery is not recommended until the nodules become painful or large enough to produce disability. Another reason for the conservative approach is that the nodules have a tendency to recur after surgery.

In a surgical approach Curtin emphasizes that the incision should be placed so as not to leave a scar on a weight-bearing surface, and that it should also give good exposure and not jeopardize the skin flaps.[32] Skin grafting in this area has not caused irritation or interfered with ambulation. It has been reported, however, that a medial approach on the side of the arch tends to cause tissue breakdown of the area with necrosis. Curtin's incision is a lazy "S" type, starting from just behind the first metatarsal head and extending over the lateral side of the calcaneus.[32] Care should be taken not to damage the medial plantar nerves and vessels. After dissecting the fascia, the skin edges should be approximated with interrupted sutures of 4-0 monofilament nylon. Postoperatively, the patient should not bear weight for approximately 21 days and should keep the leg elevated.

*Prognosis*

The prognosis is only fair, since a high percentage can recur.

## Juvenile Fibromatosis

*Introduction*

Keasby (1953) first described a distinctive tumor which appeared in the palms and soles of small children and was of fibroblastic origin.[69] It was described as a benign tumor of self-limited growth with a propensity to recur. Keasby termed this tumor, found in three girls and one boy, "calcifying juvenile aponeurotic fibroma."[69] One appeared in the plantar fat pad directly under the calcaneus and presented as a painless, poorly circumscribed, fixed, firm mass, not adherent to the skin and not associated with contracture deformities. X-ray showed a relatively radio-opaque, soft tissue mass with no associated lesion of the bone. The fine stippling of focal calcifications, which is characteristic of these tumors, could be visualized. Keasby felt that the cellularity, wide infiltration, and multicentricity of the juvenile fibroma may explain why the young child is the most likely "host" for this tumor.

Many descriptions of plantar and palmar fibromatosis have been reported. Shapiro reported a case of juvenile aponeurotic fibroma in the shoulder of an eleven year old female.[106] Lichtenstein and Goldman (1964) reported six cases but related their findings to a cartilaginous origin rather than skeletal muscle or adipose tissue origin.[78] Stout described fibromatosis in children but termed it a "pseudo-sarcomatous fasciitis"[118] since it simulated the appearance of a sarcoma, but not its natural history. He reported only one case on the foot, in a total of 123 cases in his 12 year study, from 1948 to 1960, in which the majority of occurrences were in the upper extremity. However, he did report a tumor with a foci of calcification large enough to be detected on x-ray in the intramuscular region of the thigh of a 13 year old male.

Kapiloff and Prior reported the excision of a small, circumscribed, indurated mass on the plantar aspect of the foot of an 8 year old boy which recurred several times.[67] Microscopic examination revealed a benign tumor, though highly cellular, characteristic of juvenile aponeurotic fibroma.

In another paper, Stout reported five cases of juvenile fibromatosis in the feet and three cases in the toes of infants and children, ranging in ages from birth to 13 years.[117] He compared a tumor that clinically and grossly resembled a juvenile aponeurotic fibroma involving the thenar eminence, but proved, microscopically, to be a well differentiated fibrosarcoma.

Fibroblasts are cells abundantly mobilized in the reparative processes of the body not only in granulation tissue and scar formation, but also in desmoplasias (or productive fibroses) accompanying neoplastic growths. Proliferating fibroblasts take an active but variable part in the formation of the "tumors" produced by malignancies and the "hardness" of some tumors and also proliferate as part of other neoplasms, as in conjunction with lipoblasts and primitive muscle cells in myosarcomas.

### Synonym

Aponeurotic calcifying fibroma.

### Etiology

This tumor appears to arise from a diffuse, multicentric proliferation of fibroblasts, developing into a compact and circumscribed solitary tumor. Keasby purposely described this tumor as an evolutionary lesion based upon a tumor in a 2-1/2 year old child, that had a diffuse pattern, while the circumscribed nodular lesion was found in older children,

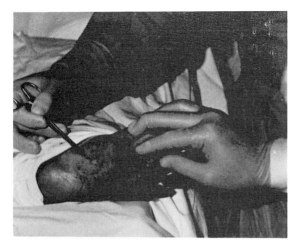

Figure 2-8A

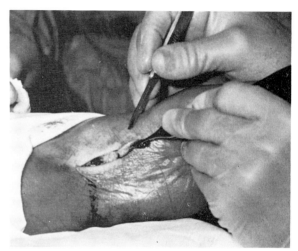

Figure 2-8B

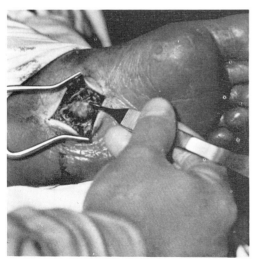

Figure 2-8C

Plantar fibromatosis. The following seven surgical exposures represent a plantar fibromatosis in a 14 year old male. (A) reveals swelling of the lesion on the plantar surface of the left foot. (B) two semi-elliptical incisions are made because of close skin adherence with the neoplasm. (C) represents wide surgical exposure isolating the lesion completely and its surrounding tissue.

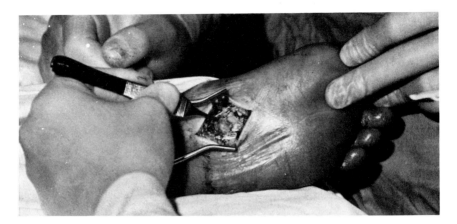

**Figure 2-8D**

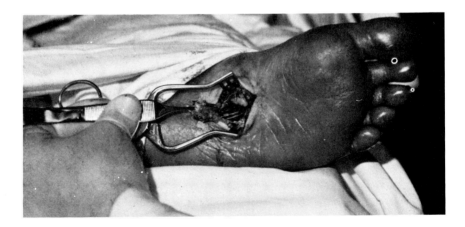

**Figure 2-8E**

(D) shows the grasping of the neoplasm and excising the surrounding tissue with the neoplasm. (E) reveals the neoplasm prior to complete excision exposing some of the plantar fascial threads as it closely adheres to the muscle belly.

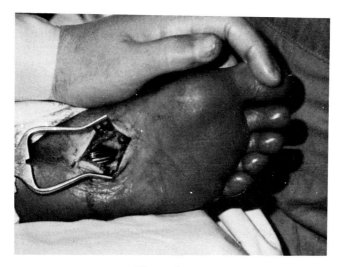

**Figure 2-8F**

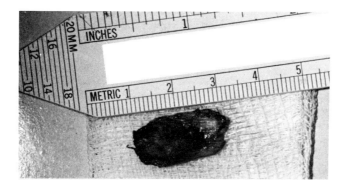

**Figure 2-8G**

(F) reveals the neoplasm completely excised and surrounding plantar fascia. (G) The final picture represents the neoplasm completely excised with surrounding plantar fascia.

ranging in age from 7 to 9 years. Yet the tumor in both age groups appears to be composed of either fibroblasts diffusely infiltrating fat and voluntary muscle, or a compact neoplasm invading the same tissue. According to Steinberg, juvenile fibromatosis is a form of fibrositis, which he felt could be diagnosed by finding creatinuria of more than 150 mg in a 24-hour period.[112] However, in Kapiloff's case involving the foot, the 24-hour urine creatine was only 140 mg.[67]

*Pathology*

The distinctive nature of the juvenile aponeurotic fibroma is the "peculiar" cell type of which this tumor is composed. Unlike the usual fibroma, in which one sees greatly elongated, fusiform nuclei enclosed in long cell bodies, the aponeurotic fibroma is dominated by numerous large darkly staining, plump, oval nuclei. These nuclei appear vesicular since a narrow margin of chromatin is always found beneath the nuclear membrane. The second distinctive feature of the calcifying juvenile fibroma is the polarization of the cells in one direction in sharp contrast to most fibromas wherein cells are haphazard in arrangement or arranged in intertwining bundles. These characteristic nuclei and their striking parallel orientation are probably the distinguishing microscopic features of this tumor.

Keasby's fibroma is infrequent but clearly differentiated from other fibroma-like tumors by its peculiar histopathology. In the differential diagnosis of an ossifying fibroma (which occurs only in bone), the juvenile aponeurotic fibroma must be considered. The dermal fibromas, encompassing such tumors as sclerosing angiomas and xanthofibromas, must be considered also, although they are probably more likely to be related to trauma and to occur more frequently in the elderly patient. Neurofibromas may occur in childhood and clinically resemble the juvenile aponeurotic fibroma. Hemangioma is also found frequently in children and must also be considered. Plantar fibromatosis is a distinctive clinical entity that is related, but it is more likely to appear in the third and fourth decades of life. However, Pickren described plantar fibromatosis as occurring

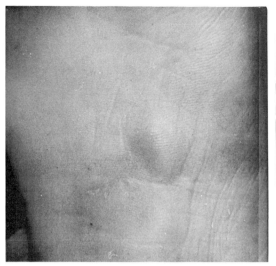

**Figure 2-9A**

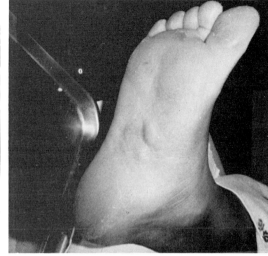

**Figure 2-9B**

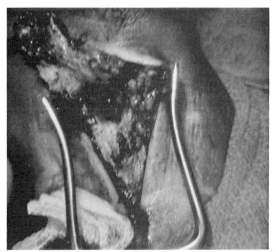

**Figure 2-9C**

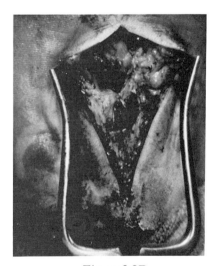

**Figure 2-9D**

Plantar fibromatosis. History of recurrent lesion in an 18 year old female, the lesion first being excised at age 14. The initial surgery was performed with a transverse incision. Recurrence revealed two separate fibromatosis bundles, with scar tissue within the center. A linear excision was made on the plantar surface of the foot revealing radical surgical dissection of the plantar fibromatosis and surrounding fascia.

much earlier.[91] Stout also reports one instance of plantar fibromatosis in a 5 year old child.[117]

Fibromas, with origin in a tendon sheath, are encapsulated, attached to a particular tendon sheath, and show no evidence of calcification or ossification. The giant cell tumors of tendon sheath origin are firm and sharply marginated.

Lipomas must also be considered since juvenile aponeurotic fibromas may occur within fatty areas; however, radiographically, lipomas are radiolucent rather than showing the dense, calcium-stippled, soft tissue opacity characteristic of the juvenile aponeurotic fibroma.

Angiomatous tumors may clinically resemble the juvenile aponeurotic fibroma.

## Clinical Picture

The juvenile aponeurotic, calcifying fibroma may appear indistinguishable from various other soft tissue or bony tumors. In recurrent tumors that have been removed previously, deposition of scattered, irregular areas of poor, cellular, collagenous tissue have been found, along with palisaded areas of calcium deposition. These foci of calcification are peculiar since they give no evidence of occurring in areas of degeneration. The calcification occurs in a regular linear formation. In fact, the combination of calcification, multinucleated giant cells, and closely crowded, darkly staining, tumor nuclei in many areas resembles the microscopic appearance of Codman's chondroblastoma of bone.

## Treatment

Complete excision of the tumor is recommended but difficult to achieve since the tumor lacks any type of capsule. Recurrence is likely if any of the original lesion remains. The features that make this particular tumor unique and differentiate it from other fibromatous tumors include its cellularity; local infiltration into and replacement of muscle, fat, vessels, nerves, and skin; its tendency to recur if incompletely excised; and its characteristic x-ray picture of a relatively opaque, unattached, soft tissue mass with faint calcific stippling.

*Prognosis*

Favorable with complete surgical removal.

## Nodular Fasciitis

*Definition*

Nodular fasciitis is a self-limited, fibroblastic proliferation of tissue which usually develops in deep fascial structures. These are non-encapsulated type lesions which usually occur in areas that are subject to trauma. They are infrequently seen in the foot and may be confused with plantar fibromatoses or, possibly, malignancy.

*Synonyms*

The terminology used to describe this lesion has been controversial. Konwaler first introduced the term "subcutaneous pseudosarcomatous fibromatosis (fasciitis)"; now, avoiding the term pseudosarcomatous because of the connotations of the word, other terms, such as nodular fasciitis, infiltrative fasciitis, and proliferative fasciitis have all come to designate a non-neoplastic proliferative reaction in the fascia.

*History*

Price described and presented 65 cases of nodular fasciitis as a single clinical entity that was histiologically benign.[92] The intention was to so identify this lesion that reference to a sarcoma would be precluded when the lesion was first seen clinically.

Mehregan reported that, after analysis of over 350 cases, most lesions were found in the fascia of the upper extremity.[82] Kleinstiver confirmed this statistic but also indicated the need to differentiate this lesion from a sarcoma.[72] Before 1955, most pathologists often classified this lesion as either liposarcoma, fibrosarcoma, or rhabdomyosarcoma. Now most pathologists recognize the lesions benignancy and use nodular fasciitis as the proper term for this clinical entity.

## Incidence

According to Mehregan, the following chart summarized the findings of several researchers as to age, sex, and location of 314 cases reported.

### AGE, SEX, AND LOCATION OF 314 CASES

|  | Price[92] | Soule[111] | Stout[119] | Hutter[65] | Total % |
|---|---|---|---|---|---|
| Total Cases | 65 | 56 | 123 | 70 |  |
| *Age Group Year* |  |  |  |  |  |
| 0–9 | 3 | 2 | 6 | 1 | 4.0 |
| 10–19 | 6 | 3 | 17 | 8 | 11.3 |
| 20–29 | 21 | 7 | 21 | 8 | 19.0 |
| 30–39 | 16 | 15 | 30 | 18 | 26.3 |
| 40–49 | 12 | 13 | 18 | 13 | 18.6 |
| 50–up | 4 | 14 | 26 | 16 | 20.0 |
| Unknown | 3 | 2 | 5 | 6 | — |
| *Sex* |  |  |  |  |  |
| Male | 45 | 27 | 65 | 29 | 54.0 |
| Female | 19 | 28 | 57 | 38 | 46.0 |
| Unknown | 1 | 1 | 1 | 3 | — |
| *Location* |  |  |  |  |  |
| Upper extremity | 33 | 35 | 56 | 33 | 50.8 |
| Lower extremity | 7 | 10 | 25 | 14 | 18.1 |
| Trunk | 21 | 8 | 30 | 15 | 24.0 |
| Head and Neck | 4 | 2 | 12 | 4 | 7.1 |
| Unknown | — | 1 | — | 4 | — |

## Clinical Picture

Nodular fasciitis is usually a freely movable, subcutaneous mass, which is not fixed to the skin. The average age of the patient with this tumor is usually in the mid-thirties, with the majority of lesions appearing between the third and sixth decades of life. There is no sex prevalence. One half of the lesions were located in the arm and forearm, with the head and neck being the least common sites of occurrence. Of 200 cases, 115 were associated with tenderness

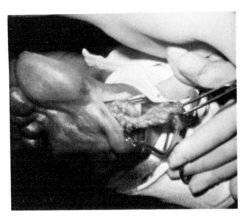

**Figure 2-10**

Nodular fasciitis. Surgical exposure revealing a
nodular ill-defined mass underlying the first
metatarsal head. This lesion was very painul during
ambulation.

or pain, and 85 lesions were asymptomatic. Duration of the lesions was listed as less than one month in 57 percent, between one and three months in 28 percent, and more than three months in 15 percent.

## Differential Diagnosis

The differential diagnosis of nodular fasciitis is essentially that of a solitary, subcutaneous nodule without evidence of a systemic disease process. These nodules consist of a loosely organized proliferation of cells and fibers in an abundant matrix, but must be distinguished from myxomatous lesions of the soft tissues. Fasciitis can be distinguished from myxoma by gross examination, for fasciitis forms a firm, circumscribed mass, rather than the mucoid amorphous mass that characterizes myxoma. Histologically, also, fasciitis is more cellular with a much denser reticulin stroma. The cells are usually adult fibroblasts, and fasciitis usually contains a prominent vascular component with foci of cellular inflammatory reaction; most nodules contain multinucleated giant cells. Myxomatoid tumors lack all of these above characteristics.

Myxoid liposarcoma is a rather large, deep-seated, mucoid mass, containing large areas of necrosis, which is not manifested in fasciitis. Neurofibroma and neurilemoma may, at times, contain foci of edema and subsequently simulate fasciitis histologically. More than half of the cases of nodular fasciitis reported were classified as fibroma, fibromatosis, or fibrosarcoma.

Fibromatosis must be differentiated from fasciitis. Clinically, the tumor of fibromatosis is larger, firmer, more deeply seated, and more fixed to the deeper tissues than is the nodule of fasciitis. The fibromatoses arise in deep fascia and tend to infiltrate progressively into adjacent fascia and muscle. Histologically, the stroma of fasciitis is reticular, whereas that of fibromatosis is collagenous. Finally, clinically, fibromatoses are very prone to local infiltrative growth and to local recurrence following excision, a factor not characteristic of fasciitis.

The neoplasm with which fasciitis is most often confused is fibrosarcoma. Two types are recognized, one is histologically similar to or even identical with a desmoid and is referred to as well differentiated fibrosarcoma or low-grade, non-metastasizing fibrosarcoma. The difference is the type of stroma seen histologically. Differentiation between fasciitis and the potentially metastasizing fibrosarcoma is primarily based on the degree of cellularity and the cell arrangement, morphology, and evidence of involvement. Fibrosarcoma is more cellular, being usually composed of densely packed spindly cells with little or no intracellular material and evidence of cellular atypia having a variable amount of stroma. The most important feature distinguishing fasciitis from fibrosarcoma is the appearance of the cells. The cells of fasciitis are normal fibroblasts that are actively proliferating, whereas the cells of a fibrosarcoma are malignant cells, variable in size and shape, and with coarse and irregularly distributed nuclear chromatin. Fasciitis is not likely to be confused with other conditions characterized by subcutaneous nodules. The subcutaneous nodules of rheumatic fever and rheumatoid arthritis are histologically different from nodular fasciitis. Other possibilities to be considered are sclerosing lipogranuloma, panniculitis of the Weber-Christian type, erythema nodosum, and erythema induratum (nodular vasculitis).

## Pathology

Gross examination shows nodular fasciitis to usually be a firm, well demarcated, often rapidly growing tumor, usually one to two centimeters in diameter by the time it is seen and located in the subcutaneous tissue or fascia anywhere in the body.

Microscopically, it is characterized by proliferating young fibroblasts in an irregular pattern. The distribution of cells varies from areas of closely packed cells to a more characteristic pattern with a myxoid stroma. The cells are spindle-shaped or stellate and often resemble those growing in tissue culture. They have large, atypical, vesicular nuclei. Various numbers of inflammatory cells may be present, mainly lymphocytes or plasma cells. Proliferating endothelial cells forming small vessels are a prominent part of the histological pattern and are often arranged in a radiating pattern around the periphery of the lesion. Occasionally calcification of some lesions of nodular fasciitis may be seen, but this seems to be rare.

*Treatment*

The treatment of choice is usually wide surgical excision, especially on the plantar aspect of the foot, in which weight-bearing contributes to the pain associated with these nodules.

*Prognosis*

With careful surgical excision, recurrence is not likely, and the prognosis is good. However, examination of the pathologic specimen must be good to differentiate these benign lesions from malignant ones.

**Fibrosarcoma**

*Definition*

A fibrosarcoma is a malignant tumor of fibroblastic or fibrocystic origin.

*History*

The first sarcomatous tumor of the sole was reported by Treves (1887).[122] A number of cases of congenital fibrosarcomas have been reported. Dreyfuss described a congenital spindle cell fibrosarcoma of the dorsum of the foot,[39] and Hudson also (1936) reported a congenital fibrosarcoma on the foot.[64] Wells (1940) reported on 31 cases of congenital malignant tumors; three on the foot, one of these being fibrosarcoma.[130] Bollinger (1953) stated that congenital sarcoma was rare and found only 35 proven cases in the world literature, half of which occurred in an extremity. The predominant type in the extremities is fibrosarcoma. He reported a case of congenital fibrosarcoma of the instep of the foot and stated there had been only two previously reported cases.[19]

*Incidence*

Fibrosarcomas may arise at any age, but the highest incidence appears to be in the third, fourth, and fifth decades. Ariel, in a report of 39 cases, reported an average age of 39.4 years, with 53 percent of the cases arising between 30 and 50.[7] Stout reported on 144 cases in which 56.2 percent arose between the ages of 30 and 50 and 90.3 percent between ages 20 and 50.[115] In 78 cases, Dockerty found the average age of onset to be 44.7 years, with two-thirds of the cases arising in the third, fourth, and fifth decades.[37] In Brindley's study (1955), no relationship between the age of the patient and the degree of malignancy of the tumor could be established.[21]

Jensen described six cases of neurofibrosarcoma involving the dorsal and lateral surfaces of the fingers and toes with the average age of onset of two and one-half months. He stated that multiple tumors were frequent.[66] Neye also reported well-differentiated, soft tissue fibrosarcomas of the fingers and toes, sometimes multiple, found only in infants and young children. The sex incidence was equal.[98]

The distribution of fibrosarcoma according to sex appears to be about equal. Reporting on 232 cases, Brindley stated that there was probably no sex difference. Ariel, in 39 cases, found 38.5 percent arising in males, whereas Dockerty, in 78 cases, reported twice that frequency in males.

Fibrosarcomas may arise in the body, although they show a definite predilection for the connective tissue sheaths of nerves, the sheaths and fascia of muscles, the periosteum of bones, and the dermal connective tissues. They also seem to have a predilection for the extremities, particularly the lower extremity, and commonly arise in the fibrous tissues of bone. Turek stated that the most frequent site of fibrosarcoma of bone was the long bones, especially the femur. Other common sites are the ribs, skull, vertebrae, and mandible.[124]

Shanks classified fibrosarcomas as either periosteal or endosteal, or of soft tissue origin. The periosteal form bears no relationship to periosteal osteogenic sarcoma since it originates in the fibrous, non-osteogenic layer of the periosteum. The endosteal form in about 80 percent of the cases is found near the knee. The other bones commonly affected are the humerus and pelvis. The extraosseous fibrosarcoma, he stated, may originate in the skin, subcutaneous tissue, tendons, fascia, and muscle.[105] McKenna reported 552 cases of sarcomata of the "osteogenic series," (osteosarcoma, fibrosarcoma, chondrosarcoma, parosteal osteogenic sarcoma, and sarcoma arising in abnormal bone), of which 60 were intramedullary fibrosarcomas. Two of these arose in bones of the foot, one in the calcaneous and one in a metatarsal.

Brindley reported an incidence of fibrosarcoma of 0.19 percent, or approximately two cases per 10,000 patients,[21] while Broders found an incidence of one in 4,000 patients or 0.25 percent.[22] Ariel reported the incidence of fibrosarcoma was 5.4 percent of all malignant neoplasms of the soft somatic tissues. Of the 39 cases reported by Ariel, ten were on the lower extremity (25.6%), six on the thigh (15%), two on the knee (5.1%), and two on the foot (5.1%).[7]

Stout, in a study of 144 fibrosarcomas, found 42 (29.2%) on the lower extremity.[115] Brindley, in a study of 45 cases of fibrosarcoma of the extremities, found 62 percent on the lower extremity, 23 in the thigh (51%), three in the leg (6.6%), and two on the foot (4.4%). He found no difference in degree of malignancy between tumors of the upper as opposed to the lower extremity.[21]

Dockerty, in 78 cases of fibrosarcoma of the extremities, found that 72 percent occurred in the lower extremity, which he ascribed simply to the larger volume of soft tissue.[37] Broders found that 65.5 percent (152) of 232 cases of primary sarcomas of the extremities were fibrosarcoma, and that 104 or 69 percent of these extremity sarcomas were on the lower extremity—eight of these occurring on the foot.[22] Bich, in a study of 24 cases of fibrosarcoma of the extremities, found 8.35 percent (two) on the foot.[16] The results of Ariel's and Stout's statistics show that of 183 cases of fibrosarcoma, 52 or 28.4 percent occurred on the lower extremity.

*Etiology*

The etiology of fibrosarcoma has been established as being that of most neoplasms. In addition, fibrosarcomas are occasionally associated with other diseases of bone. The relationship of Paget's disease and fibrosarcoma is well known, and fibrosarcomas have developed after irradiation therapy. Robbins stated that although fibrosarcomas may originate in benign fibromas, they usually arise as *de novo*.[100] Waugh, Kirshbaum, and others reported fibrosarcomas arising in cases of chronic osteomyelitis.[71,128]

A number of people noted the possible relationship of trauma to the development of fibrosarcoma. Ariel reported several cases developing in burn scars, abdominal incisions, areas of myositis ossificans, and irradiated tissues.[7] Broders noted a relationship to trauma in 11.2 percent of his cases.[22] Kulchar has noted that the frequent and repeated trauma to which the foot is subjected may produce pain in lesions ordinarily asymptomatic or may provide the stimulus for, or accelerate the rate of, transformation of a comparatively benign, or only potentially malignant lesion, to one actually malignant.[75] Silverstone states that sarcomata too often appear following injury, which, while not always severe, is associated with persistent swelling. The early, poorly differentiated, fibroblasts which appear in great numbers after tissue injury, resemble the basic cell of the sarcoma.[108] Goldenberg reported a fibrosarcoma of the calcaneus which developed following trauma.[57] Dockerty stated, however, that, although in 19 of 78 cases (approximately 25%) patients gave a history of trauma to the area, only in one case was it probably the etiologic factor.[37] Brindley summarized the problem by identifying the possible etiologic factors which have to be considered in any given case:

a) Trauma is a theory with little supportive evidence. Three patients in our series of 45 (6.7%) gave a definite history of localized trauma, followed by tumor formation.

b) Radiation is a special type of injury, and there is mounting evidence of the relationship of the development of malignant neoplasms following x-ray therapy. In our study, one patient developed fibrosarcoma after roentgen therapy to an apparently benign bone cyst.

c) Malignant transformation of previously benign lesions, e.g., fibroma, osteitis fibrosa cystica, and myositis ossificans, have occured at times, following trauma.

d) Heredity seems to be of little or no importance in the development of fibrosarcoma.[21]

*Clinical Picture*

The most common initial symptom or chief complaint of patients with a fibrosarcoma is the presence of a mass or "swelling". In Dockerty's study of 78 cases, the presence of a mass was the chief complaint in all of the patients. Pain was not a prominent symptom. In 29 of the 78 cases (38%), pain was listed as a symptom, but in only one case was it severe.[37] In the study of 45 cases by Brindley, it was noted that most of the patients were aware of the presence of a mass many months before consulting a doctor; only 24 percent complained of pain.[21] Turek stated that fibrosarcoma of bone associated with the gradual onset of pain, usually continuous, and worse at night. These were followed by the gradual appearance of a smooth, firm, rubbery swelling, firmly fixed to the underlying bone. Occasionally, the tumor is infiltrative and fixes overlying tissues, thereby restricting joint motion. At times, pathological fractures arise.[124] Dockerty found that constant constitutional symptoms were not present. Only two of 78 patients had lost a significant amount of weight. Laboratory examinations of blood and urine did not disclose any abnormality. Edema was present in varying amounts, evidently depending on the extent of obstruction of circulation by the mass. On palpation, the tumor is not as hard as a carcinoma nor as soft as a lipoma.[37]

Kulchar stated that fibrosarcoma of the foot first appears as a small, well circumscribed tumor that grows slowly to become a reddish, nodular tumor. Ulceration is uncommon, but the tumor is locally invasive and destructive and may metastasize.[75]

Fibrosarcoma must be considered as a possible diagnosis in evaluation of any soft tissue mass on the extremities. Unfortunately, microscopic examination is the only definite means of establishing the diagnosis.

Roentgenologic examination of the area, however, may

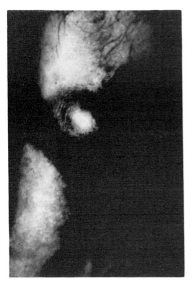 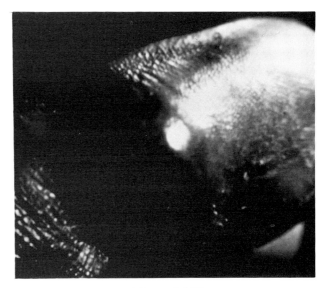

**Figure 2-11A**                    **Figure 2-11B**

Figure 11A represents a large subcutaneous fibroma at the anterior aspect of the foot and ankle. Figure 11B shows a subcutaneous fibroma involving the plantar aspect of the hallux.

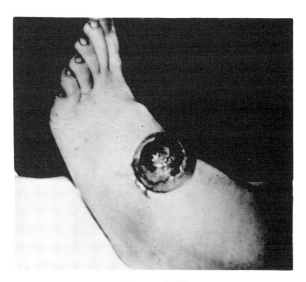

**Figure 2-12**

Fibrosarcoma. A slowly growing malignant tumor. This individual is a young male with a history of this neoplasm being excised on two separate occasions prior to this examination and being benign. *(Courtesy Earl G. Kaplan, D.P.M., Detroit, Mich.)*

prove useful, for extraosseous (soft tissue) fibrosarcomas may be visualized with a soft tissue x-ray technique; they appear to be rounded or lobulated, but seldom contain calcific deposits or invade bone.[105] Dockerty reported that in 55 percent of their 78 cases, roentgenograms showed a soft tissue mass.[37] Periosteal fibrosarcomas show up as soft tissue shadows, slightly denser than muscle, using soft tissue x-ray technique. The shadow is usually a single lesion and is immediately adjacent to the cortex of a long bone. Directly beneath the tumor shadow, is a saucer-shaped cortical defect of varying depth and, with the upper and lower corners of the periosteal shadow, triangles of reactive periosteal new bone may be found (Codman's triangles), particularly in the more slowly growing tumors. Slight calcific densities are sometimes seen within the shadows. The tumor is generally large, in contrast to the amount of bone destruction. If the tumor is very infiltrative, the sharp borders of the shadow are lost. When the tumor has penetrated the cortex, the latter is riddled with small lytic areas. The medulla then becomes involved and shows vague areas of rarefaction.[124] When the tumor originates in the medulla as an endosteal fibrosarcoma, a central, irregular, moth-eaten area of rarefaction is present, but without the clear definition of a cyst. At times, however, it may present the appearance of a sclerosing lesion, resembling Paget's Disease.[105,124] However, the bulk of the tumor is composed of myxoid fibroblastic proliferation with many capillaries and some lymphoid and histiocytic cells. Mitoses may be numerous, and there is a lack of encapsulation and irregular extension into adjacent tissues.[1] Apfelberg reported a case in a 37 year old male who had a tumor on the left heel for 18 years which was slowly increasing in size. Eventually, it was successfully excised locally. In this particular lesion, accurate histopathological diagnosis is necessary to prevent mutilation and morbidity resulting from misdiagnosis of fibrosarcoma or other malignancy.[6]

*Differential Diagnosis*

Because fibrosarcomas may remain localized for months, they may be confused with benign fibromas. The latter, however, have a greater tendency to involve the tendon and tendon sheath than the joint capsule; whereas fibrosarcomas are described more frequently in the joint capsule than elsewhere. However, clinically and, occasionally, histologically, the two lesions may be difficult to differentiate. The usual tumors in this area are not malignant and are derived from precartilagenous connective tissues, namely osteochondromas, ganglia, and giant cell tumors. Other tumors occurring at this site are angiomas, lymphangiomas, lipomas, and fibromas. Pseudosarcomatous fasciitis (or fibromatosis) is a benign growth which also often closely simulates sarcomas, grows rapidly, usually in the subcutaneous tissues, and affects children as well as adults.

The outstanding features of fibrosarcomas are slow growth and late metastasis. Early cyst-like changes in several bones and rapid regrowth of the tumor after marked improvement in response to radiation seem to be characteristic of malignancy and should outweigh a confusing histologic picture.[5]

Jensen stated that most cases of digital neurofibrosarcoma in infancy are mistaken for a benign blister or wart and consequently were inadequately treated.[66] He added that dermatofibrosarcoma protuberans is closely related to digital neurofibrosarcoma, but the former has a predilection for the anterior surface of the body and rarely occurs on the digits. Another difficult differential diagnosis, according to Jensen, is sclerosing hemangiomas, but these are gray, yellow, or pink and usually occur in adults.

## Pathology

On section, malignant fibromatous tumors show the characteristics of all sarcomas, being soft, gray-white, tissue masses which have the consistency of raw flesh. The tissue may be "pulpy" in the areas of necrosis and hemorrhage. The margins are poorly defined and extension into the surrounding tissues may be evident.

Histologic examination discloses all degrees of differentiation from slowly growing, well differentiated neoplasms to markedly anaplastic, rapidly growing tumors. The more malignant fibrosarcomas sometimes are so anaplastic that it is difficult to identify the cell or origin.[100] The degree of malignancy tends to be proportional to the frequency of mitotic figures, the number of tumor giant cells, and the scarcity of collagen fibers. The most malignant types are very cellular tissue, composed of small cells resembling mesenchymal cells. These cells have scanty cytoplasm and small, dark, rounded nuclei with frequent mitoses and are packed so tightly that little intercellular substance is seen. They are considered to be the least differentiated form of fibroblasts.

In the better differentiated tumors the preponderant cell is the spindle cell, which is larger and contains more cytoplasm, and has a nucleus that is ovoid and vesicular. These cells, too, are packed tightly, but more intercellular fibers are apparent in the cells. These fibers are arranged in fascicles or bundles, typically in whorls, but open with a palisading or criss-crossing effect ("storiform" pattern). The least malignant tumor is composed chiefly of fibroblasts, contains more intercellular collagenous materials, and resembles a nerve sheath sarcoma. In individual tumors, frequently all three types of cells are present. The degree of malignancy is suggested by the preponderant cells, but not absolutely so. There is no evidence of new bone formation.[44]

Broders (1936) described a microscopic grading system for malignant tumors as an index of the degree of malignancy.[22] Four grades were used with Grade I indicating the lowest grade and Grade IV the highest degree of malignancy. The amount of fibrogenesis, the relative proportion of fibers and cells, and the degree of differentiation of the tumor cells from the foundation were selected for the grading of fibrosarcomas. Using these criteria, three descriptive types of fibrosarcoma may be distinguished: fibrous, fibrocellular, and cellular.

The fibrous fibrosarcoma in Grade I is a slowly growing tumor, composed of cells closely approaching fibroblasts in appearance and producing an abundance of collagen fibers. In Grades II and III, there is an increasing degree of cellularity and progressively less fiber protuberance. The Grade IV tumor is a highly malignant tumor, which is very cellular, exhibits numerous mitotic figures, and contains a few collagen fibers.[22]

Brindley, in his study of fibrosarcoma of the extremities, classified them according to grades, as follows:

| | |
|---|---|
| Grade I | 15 (33.3%) |
| Grade II | 12 (26.7%) |
| Grade III | 7 (15.6%) |
| Grade IV | 11 (24.4%) |

Dockerty[37] classified his 78 cases of fibrosarcoma of the extremities, as follows:

| | |
|---|---|
| Grade I | 17 (22%) |
| Grade II | 19 (24%) |
| Grade III | 29 (37%) |
| Grade IV | 13 (17%) |

Combining these two studies gives an average representation of the incidence of each grade:

| | |
|---|---|
| Grade I | 32/123 or 26.0% |
| Grade II | 31/123 or 25.2% |
| Grade III | 36/123 or 29.3% |
| Grade IV | 24/123 or 19.5% |

Extension into the lumen of blood vessels of fibrosarcomas is common. Hence, the majority of these neoplasms metastasize rather early in their development. Brindley stated that most patients who die of fibrosarcoma have metastases to the lungs. It may, however, metastasize to numerous other areas.[4] Kulchar, however, stated that fibrosarcoma of the foot is usually locally destructive and invasive, but seldom metastasizes.

## Foot Involvement

Anspack stated that fibrosarcoma of the plantar tissues was characterized by slow, early growth, with a tendency to remain localized for months and years. Symptoms often seem to be due chiefly to trauma or mechanical interference by the tumor rather than to inflammatory swelling. He reported a case of a 19 year old white male with the chief complaint of discomfort over the mid-portion of the plantar surface of the right foot with gradual swelling. The patient refused treatment and died from metastases from the fibrosarcoma four and one-half years after the first symptons appeared in the foot.[5]

Silverstone reported a case of a 36 year old female with a chief complaint of pain and swelling of the great toe, which developed gradually, after being stepped on nine months previously. Physical examination showed a cyst-like swelling on the lateral side of the great toe, just distal to the first metatarsophalangeal joint. The range of motion was limited by pain. X-rays showed cystic spaces in the first metatarsal head. A ganglion was removed and a Mayo procedure for resection of the first metatarsal head performed. A year later, the patient returned with severe pain and swelling of the first metatarsophalangeal joint. Re-exploration showed a white, tense cystic mass extending from the fibular aspect of the first metatarsal stump deeply into the foot. Part of the phalanx was removed and biopsy of the mass taken. The pathology showed a fibrosarcoma. X-rays showed no evidence of metastasis. An amputation of the leg, seven inches below the knee was performed. The patient was found to be in good health, 45 months following surgery.[108]

Goldenberg reported a case of a 45 year old male with a chief complaint of left heel pain. He had a history of having struck his heel, two years previously, on a steel beam. After the accident, pain developed gradually until nine months later when the pain was constant. X-rays showed involvement of the calcaneus only. The patient was treated by excising the calcaneus, *in toto*. The Achilles tendon was sutured to the proximal end of the plantar fascia. The pathology report was a well differentiated fibrosarcoma. After five years the patient had no evidence of recurrent tumor or metastasis.[57]

Schreiner has reported two cases. One involved a 37 year

old male with a fibrosarcoma of the inner surface of the heel, approximately four centimeters in diameter, associated with inguinal node metastases. The tumor had been present for one year prior to his visit, following an injury to the foot, and had been previously excised. The patient was then treated with x-ray therapy, but died six months later from metastases. The second case involved a 28 year old man with a chief complaint of "sore on top of foot for one year." Examination revealed an ulcerated tumor approximately five centimeters in diameter. He was treated with roentgen therapy but died two years later.[104]

Weis reported a case of a 51 year old female who gave an interesting, but tragic history. At age 45, she had noted swelling on the dorsum of both feet, just proximal to the toe webs. There had been no previous history of trauma. The masses enlarged symmetrically and were painful. She had consulted a physician, who gave her "vaccine treatments" daily for two weeks, but with no relief. She refused biopsy or exploratory surgery. After five years, the masses had extended midway to the knee, with the contours of the feet and ankles lost in the tumor mass. She died at age 51, emaciated and in pain. Post mortem examination showed bilateral fibrosarcoma.[129]

Bich reported two cases. One involved a 75 year old male with fibrosarcoma of the heel which had recurred three times after excision. The patient died four years after the initial surgery. The second case involved a 50 year old woman with a spindle cell fibrosarcoma of the foot, involving the subcutaneous tissue and tendon sheaths, present for ten months prior to admission. A biopsy established the diagnosis. Following negative chest x-rays, an above-the-knee amputation was performed; but she died two months later from metastases to the liver.[16]

Bollinger reported the case of a three month old child with a large mass on the inner aspect of its foot. The mass had grown from a smaller one, the size of a finger tip, noticed on the second day after birth. The tumor was locally excised and was diagnosed as a fibrosarcoma. Despite a below-the-knee amputation, the baby died nine months later.[19]

Dreyfuss reported the case of a white male infant, who,

one week after delivery, had a lump the "size of a split hazel-nut" on the dorsum of the right foot. The family physician had thought it was a ganglion and attempted to crush it without success. Instead, it rapidly became larger. A biopsy showed a spindle cell sarcoma. A mid-thigh amputation was performed, and one year later the baby was still alive and well.[12]

Jensen reported a digital neurofibrosarcoma which first appears, generally in infancy, as a small, pea-sized nodule growing slowly over a period of weeks or months. The tumor is a non-tender, firm, glistening, skin-colored mass, fixed to the overlying skin but may be moveable beneath, and is usually located on the dorsal or lateral surface of a finger or toe.[66]

The incidence of fibrosarcoma of the foot compared to the lower extremity based on Ariel's, Brindley's, and Broders's studies is illustrated in Table I:

## TABLE I

### Incidence of fibrosarcoma on the foot compared to the entire lower extremity:

| Reporter | Cases on Lower Extremity | Cases on Foot | Percentage |
|---|---|---|---|
| Ariel[7] | 10 | 2 | 20.00% |
| Brindley[21] | 28 | 2 | 7.15% |
| Broders[22] | 88 | 8 | 9.1 % |
| Total | 126 | 12 | 9.53% |

This shows that 9.53 percent of 126 cases of fibrosarcoma of the lower extremity occur on the foot. The total number of cases of fibrosarcoma of the foot, however, is small. The distribution of these cases is computed in Table II.

## TABLE II

### Fibrosarcoma of the foot reported in the literature:

| Location | Number | Author |
|---|---|---|
| 1) Calcaneus | 1 | McKenna[80] |
| Metatarsal | 1 | McKenna[80] |
| 2) Dorsum of toes (two on a hallux; one on a third toe) | 3 (2 patients) | Reye[98] |
| 3) Tendons (one Achilles; one in front of ankle; one on dorsum of toe) | 3 | Copeland[29] |
| 4) Soft tissue (plantar) | 1 | Anspack[5] |
| 5) Soft tissue (foot) | 2 | Ariel[4] |
| 6) Soft tissue (foot) | 8 | Broders[22] |
| 7) Foot | 2 | Brindley[21] |
| 8) Soft tissue (plantar) | 1 | |
| Subcutaneous and tendon | 1 | Bich[16] |
| 9) Hallux | 1 | Silverstone[108] |
| 10) Calcaneus | 1 | Goldenberg[57] |
| 11) Foot (dorsum) | 1 | Dreyfuss[39] |
| 12) Instep | 1 | Bollinger[19] |
| 13) Foot | 1 | Wells[130] |
| 14) Foot | 2 | Schreiner[104] |
| 15) Foot (bilateral) | 2 (1 patient) | Weis[129] |
| 16) Foot | 1 | Hudson[64] |

(33 tumors) (31 patients)

In addition, Jensen reported six neurofibrosarcomas on the digits, over the distal phalanx of the fingers and toes, in early infancy but did not break down the distribution as to how many were on the toes.

Copeland's study included 30 typical fibrous tissue neoplasms in which the origin could be assigned with reasonable accuracy to the tendons or tendon sheaths. Of these 30, ten were on the flexor surface of the hand or foot and five of the ten were spindle cell fibrosarcomas, with three of these on the foot, as illustrated in Table II.[29] Anspack stated that fibrosarcomas were the most frequent malignant tumors originating in the joint capsule.[5] Kulchar stated that the most common sarcoma of the foot was the fibrosarcoma.[75] Goldenberg reported a fibrosarcoma of the calcaneus and stated there was no previously reported case of this type in the literature.[57] Finally, Schreiner reported 37 cases of malignant tumors of the foot, of which two were fibrosarcomas.[104]

## Treatment

The type of treatment employed for fibrosarcoma depends on several factors, such as: degree of malignancy, location of the tumor, size of the mass, whether metastasis has occurred, and whether or not it is a primary or a recurrent tumor. In general, fibrosarcoma of the extremities gives the physician a choice of wide excision or amputation although irradiation may be used as adjunctive therapy. Well differentiated, slowly growing, solitary lesions are amenable to wide local excision and may effect a cure. In larger tumors, however, the treatment of choice consists of wide excision or amputation. The final result is dependent more upon the inherent degree of malignancy of the tumor, rather than on the type of surgical procedure.[22]

Stout cautions against local wide excision and states that the high recurrence rate of 60 percent for soft tissue tumors shows that excision is too often inadequate, chiefly because many surgeons do not appreciate that fibrosarcoma is a tumor that infiltrates beyond its palpable confines.[115] Ariel feels that radical surgical excision is the only suitable method for ablating fibrosarcomas. Radiation therapy, he feels, may be used to supplement surgical treatment for palliation.[7] Kulchar states that extensive and rapidly growing tumors, even in the absence of regional and pulmonary metastases, require amputation, the resection usually being made at the junction of the upper third and lower two-thirds of the leg.[75] McKenna feels that fibrosarcoma of bone involving the foot should be treated by below-the-knee amputation.[80] However, Goldenberg has reported treating a well differentiated fibrosarcoma of the calcaneus by resection of the calcaneus only; the patient was doing well after five years.[57]

Dreyfuss and Bollinger recommend amputation for congenital fibrosarcoma of the foot.[19,39] Robbins advised that when deep fibrosarcomas occur on the extremities, radical excision or amputation with local lymph node resections should be attempted.[100] Brindley states that most authors agree that irradiation is of doubtful value in the treatment of fibrosarcoma. When surgery is not feasible, however, the patient should have the benefit of roentgen therapy. He adds that occasionally a patient is cured by this method. Windeyer states that wide surgical removal is generally advocated as the treatment of choice, but adds that he has found that radiotherapy can play an important part in the management of fibrosarcoma in the following situations:

1) If an operable tumor is large and rapidly growing, preoperative radiotherapy should be given to cause complete or partial regression, since this will facilitate surgery and decrease the chance of metastasis at the time of operation.

2) Radiotherapy alone or followed by local excision may be justified in a few instances in an operable tumor on the grounds that the deformity or disability resulting from radical surgery might be avoided.

3) Postoperative radiotherapy may be necessary under certain conditions but, on the whole, does not give the same control as wide surgical removal alone or in conjunction with preoperative radiotherapy.

4) Palliative radiotherapy can give considerable relief to patients with a more advanced disease.[131]

*Prognosis*

Local recurrence of well differentiated, slowly growing fibrosarcoma may occur if the lesion has not been totally removed, but re-excision may still produce a cure.[100] In general, fibrosarcomas which arise in superficial tissues, such as the subcutaneous tissue, have a better prognosis than tumors arising in the deeper structures. In determining the prognosis, the surgeon must consider the site, size, duration, rapidity of growth, invasion of important structures, such as nerves and vessels, and previous treatment. Next to the degree of differentiation, location is the most important single consideration. Tumors of the lower extremity are more serious than in the upper extremity, with tumors of the buttocks and thigh having an especially poor prognosis.[22]

Fibrosarcoma is noted for its tendency to recur following surgical excision. Brindley reported a recurrence rate of 54.5 percent in the extremities.[21] Stout reported a 60 percent recurrence rate, with a slightly poorer prognosis for lower extremity tumors;[115] Ariel reported 56 percent.[7] Copeland reported recurrence in each of three cases of fibrosarcoma of the tendon sheaths in the foot following local excision;[29] Dockerty reported the percent recurrence rate by grade of tumor, stating that the prognosis was more favorable with Grade I and II tumors than III and IV:

| | |
|---|---|
| Grade I | 17 – 13 recurrences (76.5%) |
| Grade II | 19 – 13 recurrences (68.5%) |
| Grade III | 29 – 19 recurrences (65.5%) |
| Grade IV | 10 – 9 recurrences (90.0%) |

or a total recurrence rate of 72 percent.[11]

In their series of 132 patients with fibrosarcoma of the extremities, Broders reported the following survival statistics:[22]
Three years, 28 patients (21.0%); five to twenty years, 24 patients (17.5%); five to ten years, 18 patients (14.4%); and ten to twenty years, 6 patients (4.5%).

Ariel reported an 81.3 percent five year survival rate for fibrosarcoma of soft tissues.[7] Bich reported that 11 of 20 patients (55%) with fibrosarcoma of the extremities were alive after five years.[16] Crenshaw stated that, after proper treatment, patients with fibrosarcoma of bone had a five-year survival rate of about 20 percent.[31]

Brindley stated that five-year survival rates vary widely from 30 to 50 percent. In a study of fibrosarcoma of the extremities, he reported a five-year survival rate of 63 percent, with a slightly better prognosis for female patients of 72 percent, as opposed to 53 percent for males. Brindley further stated that patients with lower extremity tumors had a higher five-year survival rate of 68 percent in comparison to upper extremity tumors of 54 percent. He has also reported his survival statistics broken down according to the grade of malignancy:[21]

| Grade | 0–years | 2–5 years | 5–10 years | 10 years plus |
|---|---|---|---|---|
| I | 2 | 2 | 3 | 6 |
| II | 3 | 1 | 3 | 2 |
| III | 1 | 2 | 3 | 1 |
| IV | 2 | 0 | 3 | 1 |

Dockerty reported a five-year survival rate for patients with fibrosarcoma of the soft tissues of the extremities, regardless of grade, of 38 percent. He added that, without regard to treatment employed, the patients in their series having Grade I tumors had about three times as good a chance of surviving five years after surgery than patients with Grade IV tumors.

Their statistics are as follows:[37]

| Grade | Five Years Plus | | Ten Years Plus | |
|---|---|---|---|---|
| | Cases | % Survival | Cases | % Survival |
| I | 8 | 57 | 4 | 28 |
| II | 5 | 38 | 2 | 15 |
| III | 8 | 31 | 4 | 15 |
| IV | 2 | 20 | 2 | 20 |

## Lipoma

### Definition

Lipomas are common, idiopathic, benign neoplasms, composed of mature fat cells and often occur in conjunction with other tissue structures. Several different types are: (1) angiolipomas which have a prominent vascular pattern; (2) angiomyolipoma which is a type found in the kidney composed of smooth muscles and increased blood vessels within the lipoma; (3) the fibrolipoma which is an admixture of fat and fibrous tissue; (4) the rare hibernoma, or fetal fat cell lipoma, which simulates the hibernating organs of some animals and consists of brown multilocular fat; (5) a myelo-

81

lipoma containing bone marrow elements within the lipoma which may occur within the adrenal medulla; and (6) lipomas which occasionally affect the synovium and are called lipoma arborecens, due to their multiple limbs.

The size of lipomas varies from very small to huge; frequently they are multiple. If not encapsulated, their fine structure cannot be distinguished from adipose tissue. Swelling is ordinarily the only clinical finding for they usually do not cause pain or dysfunction.

Adiposis dolorosa (Dercum's Disease) is a variant of multiple lipomatosis and is characterized by painful fatty infiltrations (covered in more detail elsewhere). In rare instances, multiple fatty tissue growths are present in the subcutaneous fat as well as in the visceral fat. This condition is known as systemic multicentric lipoblastosis. The lesions have a tendency to recur after excision, but there is no evidence of malignant growth or metastasis.

### History

Cornil (1884) reported what was probably the first case of intramedullary lipoma of bone.[23] The first recorded lipoma of the foot was apparently described by Bland-Sutton (1897) who reported a fibrolipoma of the plantar surface of the foot.[17]

### Incidence

Benign lipomas are common tumors, particularly in adults, although they are also seen in infants and older children.[74] Females, according to Adair, have a greater tendency to accumulate fat tissue, and findings show that in a study of lipomata in 134 patients, 73 percent were women.[1]

Lipomas may occur in any location but are most commonly found in the subcutaneous tissue, particularly that which contains abundant fat. Lipomas are also common in the retroperitoneal, mediastinal, and omental fat. Aldredge observed that although the distribution of adipose tissue is widespread, neoplasms composed of adipose tissue alone rarely occur in some locations, especially on the palm and on

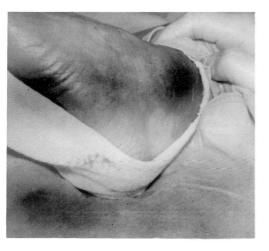

**Figure 2-13A**

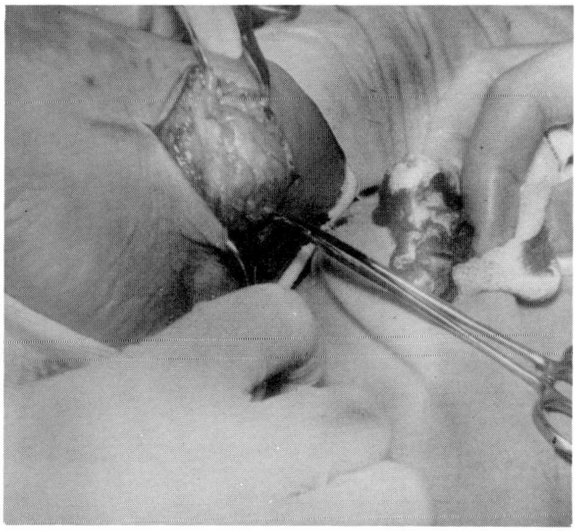

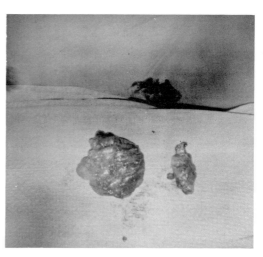

**Figure 2-13B**

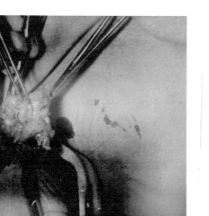

**Figure 2-13C**

**Figure 2-13D**

Lipoma. A relatively large lipoma along the medial aspect of the foot and ankle. This lesion was located in a geriatic patient and caused severe discomfort. Additional photographs reveal large surgical exposure of the mass and surgical dissection. The tumor was completely excised in two sections.

the foot.[2] Intramuscular lipomas occur less frequently. Lipomata in flat bones, particularly the vertebrae, according to Ayres, are not frequent.[9] Primary intramedullary lipomas of bone, however, are rare according to Child, with only three cases in the literature prior to 1955.[20]

There are three basic lipomas involving bone: intramedullary, periosteal, and those associated with secondary lipomatosis. Tumors of the last group involve bone only secondarily, the entity being primarily a diffuse lipomatosis of the soft tissues, with a lipoma apparently becoming adherent to the periosteum and eventually penetrating through it by chronic pressure entering the medullary area. Although this type of neoplasm is rare, the most frequent site of involvement, according to Child, is the foot. Periosteal lipomas are more frequent than the other types and may involve the long bones of the extremities.[20]

## Etiology

In some cases, lipomas are multiple, grow to a large size, and have a familial factor in their causation.[4] Eibel's cases of painful juxtamalleolar lipomata in four females between the ages of 45 and 50, three of whom were undergoing menopause, suggests the possibility of hormonal factors being involved in this particular type of lipoma.[41] Mueller's case of an intramedullary lipoma of the tibia, in the same area where a fracture occurred and healed two years previously, raises the question of trauma as being an inciting factor.[85]

## Clinical Picture

Clinically, the benign lipoma is usually totally asymptomatic, save for its presence as a non-tender soft tissue mass. Lipomas typically grow slowly, but some attain massive size. For example, DeLamater reported a classic case of a 275 pound retroperitoneal lipoma in a patient who weighed only 90 pounds after its removal! Any soft tissue tumor eventually may cause pain by encroaching against nerves or periosteum; deep-seated lipomas may cause concern by producing pressure distortion of surrounding struc-

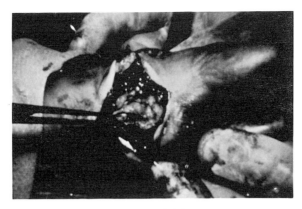

**Figure 2-14**

Fibrolipoma. Surgical exposure revealing fibro fatty mass underlying the first metatarsal head.

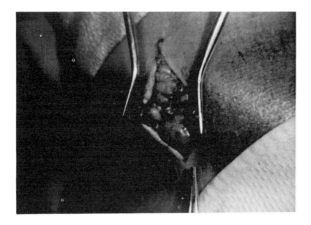

**Figure 2-15**

Lipoma. A small multi-lobulated lipoma at the lateral anterior aspect of the foot and ankle. History of pain on and off for approximately two years prior to diagnosis being made of a neoplasm present. Symptoms completely alleviated after surgical excision.

tures as determined on x-ray. Kenin reported a deep periosteal lipoma in a four year old girl whose chief complaint was swelling of the right calf. X-rays showed anterior bowing of the tibia and widening of the space between the tibia and the fibula. There was also sclerosis of the adjacent cortices of both bones. Two years after excision, the bowing had decreased and the sclerosis was gone.[70]

Nerve compression with pain and hypesthesia is frequently associated with deep intramuscular lipomas; several cases have been reported in the upper extremity. Gold reported a case of a 45 year old female with a benign lipoma causing pain in the right forearm radiating into the hand, pain over the elbow on joint motion, paresthesia in the fourth and fifth fingers, and hypesthesia along the course of the ulnar nerve.[56] Richmond reported a case of a deep intramuscular lipoma which caused paralysis of the posterior intra-osseous nerve.[99] In a study of 32 patients with partial paralysis of an extremity due to nerve compression from a benign soft tissue mass, Barber found five involved the peroneal nerve and four the sciatic nerve.[10]

Lipomatous involvement of bone is more consistently associated with pain. Mueller's case of an intra-medullary lipoma of bone following a fracture was associated with increasing pain.[85] Ayres reported an intra-osseous lipoma of the lower tibia in a 30 year old male, who had slight pain in the ankle for 14 years; the involved ankle was slightly larger, but there was no evidence of inflammation.[9]

Clinically, a superficial lipoma appears as a soft moveable mass with a characteristic rubbery consistency and indistinction of boundaries. Lipomas are often difficult to delineate pathologically since many types of local overgrowths of fat or abnormal collections of fatty tissue exist that are frequently referred to as lipomas but are not truly new growths.

Gold suggested that the diagnosis can often be made radiographically when we see a lobulated, sharply demarcated, radiotranslucent area which is almost pathognomonic.[56] Fairbank reported a periosteal lipoma, which on x-ray showed a bilobed translucent area in muscles beside a normal radius.[46] Central calcification has been re-

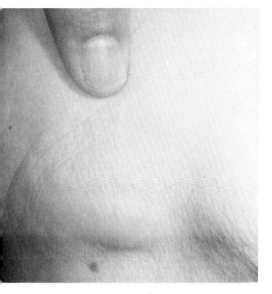

**Figure 2-16A**

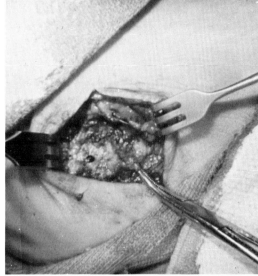

**Figure 2-16B**

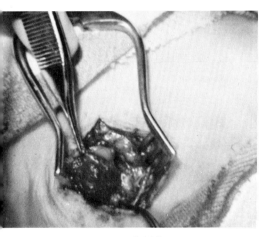

**Figure 2-16C**

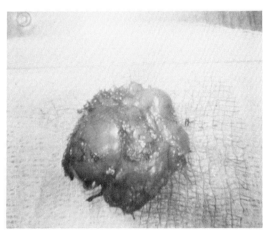

**Figure 2-16D**

Lipoma. Photographs reveal the location of the lipoma being just plantar to the perioneal tendons of the foot and ankle. This involved a 16 year old male who had moderate discomfort, not only from shoe pressure, but also from just the swelling of the lesion. Other photographs show surgical exposure and complete surgical excision of the tumorous mass.

ported by Greenfield.[60] Kenin reported a periosteal lipoma adjacent to the femur, in which bone excrescences projected into the adjacent area of soft, translucent tissue, which disappeared within a year following excision of the tumor.[70] The intramedullary lipoma of the tibia reported by Mueller showed translucency in the medullary canal.[85] Ayres reported an intra-osseous lipoma of the lower end of the tibia that caused slight expansion of the shaft.[9] Strauss observed that deep lipomas of the hand and foot are very seldom identified before operation. Out of 34 such cases prior to 1931, only one was recognized as such before excision.[120]

*Differential Diagnosis*

The differential diagnosis of a lipoma includes fibroma, cyst, hemangioma, abscess, muscle herniation, other soft tissue masses, and synovitis with effusion. The tumors are sometimes tense enough to suggest a cyst. Stevenson states that examination may be confusing since, with an extensive lipoma, pressure on one area can increase the fullness elsewhere suggesting a fluid-filled cyst or sac-like synovitis with effusion. He noted that peritendinitis crepitans is notably absent with lipomata.[113]

Lipomas and neurofibromas have certain similarities. Transillumination has been of some aid in their differentiation, as the lipomas are translucent and the neurofibromas are opaque to transmitted light. An interesting characteristic of lipomas is that under conditions of starvation and glyconeogenesis a loss of body fat will ensue, but a lipoma will not decrease in size.

*Pathology*

Grossly, a lipoma is characterized by a poorly delineated, thinly encapsulated, soft, multilobular mass of typical adult adipose tissue. Demarcation of the tumor may be difficult because of poor encapsulation and the tendency for the lobules to project into surrounding fatty tissue. These tumors are commonly composed of multiple discrete masses of fat separated only by thin septa of fibrous tissue. On cross-section, the characteristic yellow translucence of adult fat is present. Hemorrhage and necrosis are uncommon.

On microscopic examination, typical vacuolated adult fat cells are present, demonstrable only by a thin rim of cell membrane separating them from adjacent cells. Intracellular connective tissue stroma is usually scant, and vascularization is not prominent. Admixture of fibrous tissue may be present in certain lipomas which has suggested the term fibrolipoma. Intra-osseous lipomas in flat bones may contain hemangiomatous elements. The character of the intra-osseous lipoma is the same as the subcutaneous lipoma, except that it traverses focally by bone trabeculae.[9]

## Foot Involvement

Abnormal deposits of adipose tissue are occasionally encountered in the foot and ankle. However, these are not specifically diagnosable and are usually not neoplasms. The true encapsulated and asymptomatic lipoma is rarely encountered on the foot.[51] The most common type of localized "fat hyperplasia" is that found in close relation to the external malleoli which generally occurs in obese females, most commonly after the age of forty.[34] Tachdijian feels that lipomas are one of the more common tumors of the foot and are seen in infants as well as in older children. He states that lipomas of the foot usually occur in the subcutaneous tissues of the instep or deep into the plantar fascia. Occasionally, he adds, they may be found on the dorsum of the foot involving the tendon sheaths or digital nerves.[121] Strauss found that lipomas of the tendon sheaths of the hands and feet occur more frequently inside than outside the sheaths.[120] Bryan, including the series of Strauss, described 45 lipomata originating in tendon sheaths, nine of which were in the foot and ankle.

Adair found no lipomas in the feet and only two on the dorsum of the hands in 352 lipomata removed from 134 patients.[1] Among 390 subcutaneous lipomata, Geschickter found six in the hand and only one on the foot.[53] Bich, in a study of 300 soft tissue tumors of the extremities, found that 162 were lipomas, suggesting that lipomas account for over

50 percent of soft tissue tumors of the extremities. He also found that about one third of soft tissue tumors of the extremities are malignant, or potentially so, and stressed the need for accurate diagnosis.[15] Booker, in a review of the literature prior to 1961, found that of 155 lipomatous tumors of the extremities, 31 were on the hands, but only two were on the foot (1.3%). In his own studies, he found three lipomas of the foot and one liposarcoma.[20]

In our search of the literature for lipomas involving the foot, a total of 30 tumors were found. Their location and references are found in Table I. Of these 30 tumors, nine involved tendon sheaths, one involved only bone, two involved bone and soft tissue in the same foot, one involved the plantar fascia, and 18 involved soft tissues alone.

## TABLE I

### Reported Cases of Lipomas Involving the Foot

| Location | No. of Tumors | Author |
|---|---|---|
| 1. Tendon sheaths | 9 | Bryan[23] |
| 2. Soft tissue (lateral to achilles tendon) | 1 | Giannestras[54] |
| 3. Soft tissue (subcutaneous) | 1 | Geschickter[53] |
| 4. Juxta-malleolar | 4 | Eibel[41] |
| 5. Os Calcis | 1 | Child[27] |
| 6. Entire foot | 2 | Barretson[11] |
| 7. Soft tissue (instep) | 2 | Tubby[123] |
| 8. Plantar Fascia | 1 | Bland-Sutton[17] |
| 9. Instep | 1 | Galinski[51] |
| 10. Instep (sole) | 3 | Booker[20] |
| 11. Heels, bilateral | 1 | Bloom[18] |
| 12. Extensor surface of foot and ankle -2, heel -1, toe -1 | 4 | Berlin[14] |
| Total | 30 | |

Lipomas involving the foot appear to be more symptomatic, probably because of weight bearing and the wearing of shoes. Booker reported three such cases: (1) A 22 year old female had a painful mass on the right sole, present

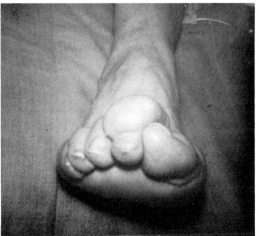

**Figure 2-17A**

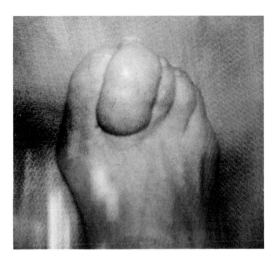

**Figure 2-17B**

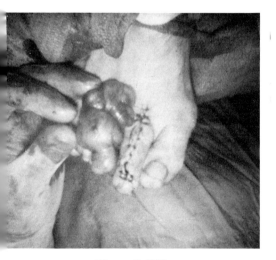

**Figure 2-17C**

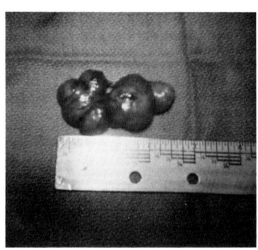

**Figure 2-17D**

Lipoma. Large and strange lipoma mass involving the second toe. Figures represent clinical enlargement of the second toe, and surgical excision of the mass. *(Courtesy of Richard Lootens, D.P.M., Detroit, Mich.)*

for six months but painful for only three months. X-rays showed a radiolucent area extending into the web space between the fourth and fifth toes. Excision revealed a benign lipoma. (2) An 8 year old boy who had a mass on the foot just below the medial malleolus, extending into the instep, whose parents stated a "ganglion" had been excised at the age of two and one half years. The mass, however, returned and grew rapidly and was re-excised and found to be a benign lipoma. (3) a 45 year old female with a mass in the right sole which appeared cystic. The overlying skin was bluish, but the color disappeared on pressure, suggesting an angioma. When excised, the lesion was found to be a lipoma.[20]

Galinski reported an interesting case of a complication of a lipoma in a 44 year old male with pain on the inside of the right heel that had begun one year previously with a dull aching pain, but more recently magnified to sharp shooting pains that occurred on walking. Palpation revealed a soft, fleshy mass in the instep of the foot. The mass, three centimeters in diameter, was found to be over a herniation in the belly of the abductor hallucis muscle. The mass was excised and the defect closed; the patient experienced complete relief. Galinski feels the pressure from the lipoma caused atrophy of the muscle sheath with normal activity, causing the herniation which corresponded to the onset of the sharp shooting pains.[51]

Tubby reported two cases of a lipoma of the instep accompanied by swelling and pain on walking or palpation.[123] Giannestras reported a case of a patient with a lipoma arising lateral to the Achilles tendon, which had increased in size over a number of years.[54] Eibel's cases of painful juxta-malleolar lipomata were all oval masses, approximately two and one half inches in their greater diameter, located anteriorly and inferiorly to the lateral malleolus.[41] They were rubbery in consistency, but not warmer nor more congested than the adjacent soft tissue. Surgical excision afforded complete relief of pain in a three year follow-up after conservative treatment of dieting, arch supports, and physical therapy had failed.[41]

Child reported a case of a 22 year old white male, who, two years prior to admission, had developed a dull aching pain in the right heel, aggravated by standing, walking, or running long distances. X-rays revealed an area of radiolucency 1.5 x 2.5 centimeters in size in the os calcis. The lesion was excised and the defect packed with bone chips. The pathology report was benign lipoma.[27]

Barretson reported two adult male patients who were treated for enormous enlargement of the right foot. This was shown to be due to lipomatosis, causing expansion and destruction of the bones and joints, which had begun early in life.[11]

Bloom described a patient with bilateral lipomas of the heels associated with "congenital erythema" of the area.[18] Kogoj stated that, in the Hanhart syndrome, there is a diffuse keratosis of the palms and soles which eventually occurs elsewhere and that, associated with these keratoses, there are subcutaneous lipomas.[74]

### Treatment

The treatment of choice for the symptomatic lipoma is excision with careful dissection to insure complete removal since recurrence always follows incomplete removal. Deep intramuscular lipomas are well encapsulated and are usually shelled out quite easily. Intramedullary lipomas should be excised and the bone defect packed with bone chips. Extraneural lipomas causing nerve compression require surgical excision. Barber suggests using a double tourniquet under general anesthesia with frozen section diagnosis to distinguish the uncommon liposarcoma or other malignancy.[10] Neurolysis or translocation may be necessary. Booker indicates that a bloodless field is essential and also advocates a tourniquet.[20]

### Prognosis

The prognosis is excellent following complete removal.

## Adiposis Dolorosa

*Definition*

Adiposis dolorosa is a rare systemic disturbance characterized by localized overgrowth of subcutaneous fat by painful, tender, tumor-like masses.[100] It is a variant of multiple lipomatosis, but the cause of pain is poorly understood.

*Synonyms*

Dercum's Disease.

*History*

The syndrome was first described by Dercum (1882), and therefore is also known as Dercum's Disease.[35]

*Incidence*

Kling stated that juxta-malleolar adiposis dolorosa occurs mainly in obese women past middle age. He reported 112 cases, only two of which involved the ankles. (1.8%).[73]

*Etiology*

The cause of adiposis dolorosa is unknown. Harlan, however, reports a study of two families in which there appears to be a hereditary factor. In one family there were four cases in three generations, and in the other family there were four cases in two generations.[62]

*Clinical Picture*

The chief clinical manifestations are obesity and painful subcutaneous lipomata.[62] Pastor stated that the four cardinal signs of adiposis dolorosa were adiposity, asthenia, pain, and psychic disturbances. Asthenia is usually marked and can be incapacitating. He reported one case in which there were pads of fat around the metatarsal bones of each foot which were painful on walking and palpation.[90]

Kling reported 112 cases of juxta-malleolar adiposis dolorosa. He stated that this was characterized by accumulations of subcutaneous fat around joints which are markedly tender to touch or pressure. The condition is usually bilateral, with the most frequent occurrence being on the medial sides of the knees, less commonly around the elbows, and rarely on the sides of the ankle. In a significant percentage of cases, there is associated muscular contraction with a limited range of motion of the affected joint. There is usually pain and stiffness in the joint and some crepitus, which may cause an erroneous diagnosis of osteoarthritis.[73]

## Differential Diagnosis

Many cases of adiposis dolorosa go unrecognized, being mistaken for endocrine obesity, associated with arthritis, or menopausal psychosis.[90] Adherence to the four cardinal signs and symptoms, however, is usually helpful.

## Treatment

All means of treatment, including diet, need to be used, combined with physical therapy. Surgery is not usually advisable.[73]

## Piezogenic Pedal Papules

## Definition

The prefix piezo comes from the Greek and means "pressure"; hence, these lesions may be papules caused by pressure.

## History

When first described by Shelly and Rawnsley (1968), these cystic lesions, which they called piezogenic pedal papules, were considered very common but were seldom diagnosed and were usually asymptomatic. Since they appear visible on weight-bearing (and most patients are examined in a non-weight bearing position) they have been commonly overlooked. In his reported case, Shelly stated that the papules were viewed as true dermatoceles,[107] that is, the herniations of fatty subcutaneous tissue into connective tissue defects in the dermis. The extrusion of fat, with its vasculature and associated nerves, could very well be responsible for the complaint of many patients that their feet hurt while standing.

Galinski reported a case of these typical fatty cutaneous herniations involving a muscle in the foot.[50] Our personal experiences have revealed this condition to be present in people suffering from acutely painful heel spurs. Yet, at this time, no definite relationship or correlation has been established.

Schlappner reports that there is no apparent sex, age, or family predominance.[103] They found that a large percentage of patients examined in the weight-bearing position had clinical evidence of non-painful piezogenic papules, but did not differentiate between the above factors. However, the presentation of several cases showed that the histopathology of, and differentiation between, non-painful and painful piezogenic papules is different, in terms of size and consistency.[103]

Cohen reported four cases of piezogenic pedal papules.[28] One patient complained of discomfort only when weight-bearing, and evidence of these papules was clinically demonstrated when in that position; but, as soon as the patient was placed in a non-weight bearing position, the papules and the pain disappeared. In another case, a young girl was not aware of these papules, and, upon weight-bearing, was completely asymptomatic. These observations lead us to conclude that it is the pain which brings the papules to the patient's attention. It is, therefore, very likely that papules may be very common although undetected. Careful examination of the patient in both on- and off-weight-bearing positions should be considered in dermatological and orthopedic screening and history.

*Incidence*

There have been no studies to indicate how common this finding is. However, it is more noticeable in obese individuals and is frequently seen in patients who complain of heel pain with associated heel spurs.

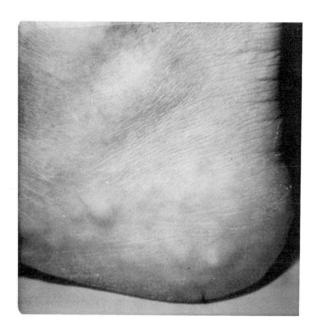

**Figure 2-18**

Piezogenic pedal papules. Piezogenic pedal papules are essentially fat herniations involving the heel pad area which may be noticed on the medial or lateral surfaces of the foot. These are most frequently seen on obese individuals and heel spurs are not an uncommon finding when these lesions are noticed. Fat herniations may also be seen in the metatarsal area.

## Clinical Picture

Piezogenic pedal papules present a cobblestone appearance on the medial and lateral aspects of the heel on weight-bearing. These multiple cystic lesions are semi-firm, but disappear with digital pressure. In patients with painful lesions, standing or walking produces an aching pain in the heels that can become progressively more painful as standing or walking is prolonged. Elevation of, or avoidance of pressure on, the heels relieved the pain almost immediately. The onset of pain is usually sudden when standing for prolonged periods of time. The lesions are usually skin-colored, and may vary from one or two papules to as many as eight or nine dispersed over one area of the heel.

## Pathology

Grossly, the nodules are tiny fragments of fat. They are primarily due to herniations of subcutaneous fat into the dermis with fibrosis of the overlying dermis. According to Grant, the heel of his patient showed non-specific degeneration of the dermal collagen, with some hyalinization and blurring of architectural detail.[58] Comparison studies by Schlappner, who examined sections of pedal papules excised from ten patients, showed variations in appearance and consistency between the painful and non-painful papules.[103] Sections of a non-painful papule of a normal heel revealed the normal anatomical relationship of fat and fibrous tissue, forming a well-supported cushion between the bone and the skin. In sections taken from painful papules, three prominent changes were revealed: the dermis was thickened and dense with only a few irregular islands of fat cells; there was a loss of compartmentalization of the small fat lobules in the deep portions of the dermis and at the dermal-subcutaneous junction; and the trabeculae of the subcutaneous tissue were lost or thinned out, and the subcutaneous fat hung down from the dermis as a poorly supported, tear-shaped globule.

Microscopically, in the painful papules of greater than two years duration, the dermal tissue was dense, increased in thickness, and almost devoid of fat tissue, with homogenization of collagen; some specimens showed evidence of tissue necrosis and hemorrhage at the dermal-subcutaneous junction, extending into the trabeculae between the fat lobules.

Painful piezogenic pedal papules are generally larger than the non-painful papules. The larger fatty lobules form, by fusion or smaller fat chambers, as the normally separating trabeculae become degenerated or destroyed. Tissue degeneration in the overlying dermis and the associated pain implicate pressure as one of the components in the cause of these lesions.

## Differential Diagnosis

This can generally be made clinically because no other cystic or neoplastic diseases of the foot present non-progressive, multiple, regressive lesions of this type seen only on weight-bearing. Biopsy will be the conclusive evidence.

## Treatment

Usually conservative treatment with supportive orthotic devices or cushioning of the shoe is used to relieve pressure on the heel.

Surgical excision of the fatty protrusions in some cases may be necessary.

## Prognosis

This benign "cystic" lesion will occasionally cause discomfort and pain over long periods of weight-bearing, but the prognosis is very good with symptomatic therapy.

## Liposarcoma

## Definition

Lipsarcomas are malignant neoplasms which arise from fat cells. They are extremely uncommon tumors, which tend to occur in older persons and to favor the retroperitoneal and mediastinal fat deposits, but may occur wherever fat is present.

*History*

Virchow (1857) reported the first malignant tumor of fat tissue.[126] Ewing (1928) described a liposarcoma developing in the bone marrow.[43]

*Incidence*

Liposarcomas tend to occur in older persons although cases in children have been reported. Anderson stated that liposarcoma is a relatively common type of soft tissue malignancy in infancy and childhood.[4] In 134 cases reported in the literature, Stout found that 60 percent of all patients were above 40 years of age.[114] Sawyer stated that the age range is generally 20–80, with a medium in the 50's.[101] Reszel found the mean age to be 50.2 years in a study of 222 cases of liposarcoma.[97] Bollinger (1953) reported that a literature search showed only one congenital liposarcoma occurring in the extremities.[19]

Liposarcomas tend to occur slightly more often in males. Pack reported that, of 105 cases of liposarcoma, 59 were male (56.2%).[89] Stout, in a series of 39 cases, reported 59 percent were males.[114] Reszel found that 61.5 percent were males in his study of 222 cases.

Liposarcoma, though rare, is the most frequent malignant tumor of soft tissue.[31] In Pack's study of 717 malignant tumors of soft somatic tissues, 104 (14.6%) were liposarcomas.[89] Anderson reported that liposarcomas comprise some 20 percent of all soft tissue malignancies.[3]

While benign lipomas are more common in the subcutaneous tissues, liposarcomas seem to have a predilection for the deeper soft tissues. Liposarcomas occur most often around the buttocks, in the lower limbs and in the retroperitoneal spaces.[4] Pack's study of 105 cases of liposarcoma showed 49.4 percent occurred in the lower extremities, with 40 percent in the thigh, 6.7 percent in the leg, and 2.7 percent in the foot. He stated that, in the extremities, liposarcomas seem to be intimately associated with the intermuscular, deep fascial, and periarticular tissues.[89] In a review of 499 liposarcomas of the soft tissues, Stout found 41 percent to be in the lower extremities.[116] In 222 cases of liposarcoma involving the extremities and limb girdles, Reszel found that the lower extremity was involved three times more than the upper extremity and that the proximal portions of the limbs were affected more than the distal.[97] Liposarcoma of bone is rare.[124]

Liposarcoma involving the foot is apparently rare since very few cases have been reported in the literature. Pack reported only three cases out of 105 involving the foot.[89] Booker reported a case of myxoliposarcoma on the dorsum of a foot in a 46 year old female.[20] Murphy reported a liposarcoma on the plantar surface of the heel of a 46 year old white male.[86] Kauffman (1959) reported two congenital liposarcomas of the foot.[68]

## Etiology

The etiology of liposarcoma is unknown. Some arise in pre-existing lipomas, but the majority do not.[89-116] Some authors feel that trauma plays a role in the development of liposarcoma. Pack (1939) stated that some liposarcomas were unquestionably caused by a single acute injury, which caused traumatic fat necrosis, healing with or without calcification. By stimulation of adult fat cells it can grow diffusely as a sarcoma possessing many grades of anaplasia and malignancy.[88] However, by 1954, he had changed his conclusion and believed that trauma plays only a minor role in the etiology of liposarcoma.[89] Sawyer stated that there is little evidence that trauma is a contributory factor in the development of liposarcoma.[101]

## Clinical Picture

Liposarcoma usually starts as an inconspicuous swelling of the soft tissues with steady progressive growth until it reaches such proportions as to demand the attention of the patient. The patient's usual complaint is the gradual enlargement of a tumor. Pressure symptoms may ensue when the neoplasm reaches a certain size, but pain is quite rare at the outset. The rate of growth of liposarcomas shows great variability.[89] Some attain massive proportions. Stout, for example, reported a number of cases in which the tumor weighed over 1000 grams.[116]

As a general rule, liposarcomas are firmer, less easily compressed, and more fixed to underlying tissues than lipomas. The first sign or evidence of a deeply situated liposarcoma may be only a uniform swelling of a leg or arm.

Liposarcoma of bone is characterized by osteolytic destruction, predilection for the extremities and for long bones, and destruction of the cortex with spread into contiguous soft parts. It is characterized by a slow course with eventual spread to other bones, and, finally, visceral metastases.[124]

*Pathology*

On gross examination, liposarcomas have a somewhat more opaque, gray-white to yellow appearance than lipomas, and are usually poorly delimited and not encapsulated. Some liposarcomas are highly pigmented, varying from yellow to orange-yellow, and even brown, with or without evidence of hemorrhage.[89] Some liposarcomas achieve massive size. Most invade surrounding structures.

Microscopically, the liposarcoma shows great variation as does the fibrosarcoma. In the better differentiated liposarcomas there may be almost normal looking fat cells interspersed among large anaplastic cells. The latter have abundant, commonly vacuolated cytoplasm, and large, atypical nuclei. These cells tend to resemble anaplastic fibroblasts but can be identified as lipoblasts by their vacuolation and fat content (often requiring special stains for demonstration). As a general rule, cells tend to revert toward anaplastic fibroblasts in the more malignant forms of liposarcoma; it is not uncommon to find areas, in these malignant growths, which may deserve the designation of fibroliposarcoma.[100]

Stout proposed the following classification of liposarcomas:

1. **Well differentiated Myxoid Type**: This tumor, resembling embryonal fat, is composed of adult fat cells, stellate em-

bryonal cells, or spindle-shaped lipoblasts. The lipoblasts are usually small, but mitotic figures are seldom seen. These tumors may assume bulky proportions.

2. Poorly Differentiated Myxoid Type: Here, the characteristic cells are bizarre lipoblasts, sometimes monstrous, containing misshapen, pyknotic, or hyperchromic nuclei.

3. Round Cell or Adenoid Type: These tumor cells are spherical, with a central nucleus and abundant, foamy, liquid-containing cytoplasm.[114]

Reszel proposed a system for classification of liposarcomas, into three types: myxoid, lipogenic, and pleomorphic. In their study of 222 cases, 46.6 percent were myxoid, 20.3 percent lipogenic, and 33.3 percent pleomorphic. Expressing the degree of differentiation, the tumors were graded I through IV. Based on this system, 23 percent of the tumors were Grade I, 26.6 percent Grade II, 39.2 percent Grade III, and 11.3 percent Grade IV.[97]

### Differential Diagnosis

Diagnoses of liposarcoma, as in other malignancies, depends on microscopic examination of the tumor. Soft tissue x-ray technique is helpful but not reliable. Deep lipomas appear as translucent lobular masses. Liposarcomas have more fibrous and mysomatous tissue and are relatively more opaque.

The poorly differentiated liposarcomas have the same capacity to metastasize and invade as fibrosarcomas. The well differentiated ones rarely metastasize,[100] but undifferentiated liposarcomas usually metastasize, via the blood stream rather than the lymphatics.[116]

### Foot Involvement

Murphy reported a case of a 40 year old white male, who, following a fall, noticed pain and a mass in the plantar tissues of the left heel. X-rays were negative for bone pathology. At surgery, a yellowish, fatty tumor was found beneath the plantar fascia, extending from the os calcis to the metatarsal heads. It shelled out easily and appeared encapsulated. The pathology report was liposarcoma. The patient got along well for one year, then experienced more pain and return of the

**103**

mass. A below-the-knee amputation was performed. Two years later, the patient experienced pain in the lower chest, and x-rays showed unexcisable vertebrae metastases. Cobalt therapy was instituted, but the patient died shortly thereafter, three years after the original surgery.[86]

Booker reported a case of a 46 year old female with a mass on the dorsum of her foot. At surgery, the mass appeared encapsulated and was locally excised. The pathological report was myxoliposarcoma. It recurred within three months, and a below-the-knee amputation was performed. Death from pulmonary metastasis occurred a year and a half following the initial surgery.[20]

## Treatment

As opposed to fibrosarcoma, liposarcomas are, in general, quite radiosensitive; but, like fibrosarcoma, most authors suggest wide excision or amputation with or without radiation therapy.

Giannestras stated that, conceivably, a small, histologically low-grade fibrosarcoma or liposarcoma of the foot could be amenable to wide local excision. Amputation, however, would be indicated in the majority of these patients with the level of amputation dictated by the specific situation under consideration.[54]

Stout advises that undifferentiated liposarcomas are tumors of the greatest malignancy and call for the most drastic surgical treatment. Only superficial tumors, four centimeters or less in diameter, could be expected to respond favorably to x-ray therapy, and excision or amputation is the only therapy for larger growths.[116]

Pack gives the following advice concerning treatment. The pseudoencapsulation of the average liposarcoma suggests its benignancy and tempts the surgeon to perform a simple enucleation. The choice between radical surgical excision and amputation depends on innumerable factors that include the degree of malignancy which requires microscopic confirmation, the location, the degree of fixation, whether primary or recurrent, and the presence of metastasis.

If the tumor is on an extremity, and the attempt at local

removal fails, either because of technical difficulties or because the surgeon realized the futility of the effort, an immediate amputation may be performed above the level of the tourniquet. If local excision is performed, the one imperative requirement is a wide, all-encompassing elliptical excision of the skin and surrounding tissue and the scar, if a previous biopsy or attempted excision was performed. Recurrent liposarcomas may fungate through an operative scar, become infected and necrotic and even cause death by sepsis.

The entire group of muscles, involved with or encompassing the inter-intramuscular liposarcomas, should be removed from their origins to their insertions. If the liposarcoma is on an extremity, the order of dissection should be from above downward.

If preoperative irradiation has been given, five or six weeks should be allowed to elapse in order for maximal regression to occur and the radiation reaction to subside.

In the case of amputation, the upper level of severance must be high, if not extreme. The general rule of amputating above the level of origin of the muscle groups involved is a good principle to observe. Invasion of bone results in subperiosteal and intramedullary extension of the tumor superiorly and inferiorly. Therefore, amputation through or above the joint with which the bone articulated proximally is indicated.

The embryonal myxoliposarcomas are known to be very radiosensitive, but the recurring liposarcoma is less so. However, the radiosensitivity of liposarcomas is greater than their radiocurability. Of 12 patients treated, Pack states that only two (16.6%) were sterilized. Preoperative irradiation is never employed overlying bone, e.g., in the pretibial region of the foot, or for those invading bone. Pack believes that postoperative irradiation is indicated whenever the resected tumor is recurrent. The metastases are usually quite responsive to x-ray therapy.[89]

Edland states that, because of the high incidence of local recurrence after resectional or excisional surgery, routine postoperative irradiation is recommended. In most cases, wide excision and postoperative radical radiotherapy can prevent amputation or mutilating surgery. Radiotherapy appears to be best employed as a surgical adjunct, rather than an elective initial substitute in accessible locations.[40]

McNeer tabulated some interesting statistics concerning radiation therapy for liposarcomas, stating the beneficial effect of adjunctive irradiation when employed pre- or postoperatively.

The five and ten year-survival rates of these patients are impressively superior to those treated by excision alone. The local recurrence rate of those treated by surgery alone was about the same as those treated by preoperative radiation (21% vs 25% respectively). In the patients given postoperative radiation, the recurrence rate was higher (43%), yet, in spite of this, the survival rate was not unfavorably affected.[81]

*Prognosis*

Survival rates for patients with liposarcoma appear to be a function of degree of malignancy and location. Pack stated that the end-results, based on the location of the tumors, do not show too great a variability, with the best rates occurring on the arm (55%) and foot (50%), and the lowest rates on the buttocks (25%) and groin (25%). He reported that in 64 cases, the highest survival rate, (87.5%), was obtained when wide local excision was followed by irradiation. Overall, he reported a 60 percent five-year survival rate.[89] Sawyer stated that from the evidence presently available, the rate of mortality in patients with liposarcoma appears to be fairly consistent at 50 percent.[101] Reszel stated that recurrences of liposarcomas are extremely common.[97] Of patients treated by local excision and observed for five years or more, 70 percent showed evidence of recurrence. The five-year survival rates were as follows:

| | |
|---|---|
| Lipogenic liposarcoma | 60.0% |
| Myxoid liposarcoma | 33.3% |
| Pleomorphic liposarcoma | 47.3% |

The five-year survival rates based on grade of malignancy were as follows:

| | |
|---|---|
| Grade I | 75.0% |
| Grade II | 40.0% |
| Grade III | 37.3% |
| Grade IV | 31.8% |

## Bibliography

1. Adair, F.E. et al: Lipomas. *Amer. Jour. Cancer,* **16**: 1104–1120, 1932.
2. Aldredge, W.M. et al: Lipoma of the Thenar. *Surgery,* **24**: 853–854, 1948.
3. Anderson, W.A.D.: *Pathology,* 5th ed. C.V. Mosby Co., St. Louis, 1966.
4. Anderson, W.A.D. et al: *Synopsis of Pathology,* 7th ed. C.V. Mosby Co., St. Louis, 1968.
5. Anspack, W.E. et al: Fibrosarcoma of plantar tissues. *Amer. Jour. Cancer,* **40**: 465, 1940.
6. Apfelberg, D.B. et al: Pseudosarcomatous fasciitis: a case report. *Plast. Recon. Surg.,* **42**: 275, 1968.
7. Ariel, I.M. et al: Fibrosarcoma of the soft somatic tissues: a clinical and pathologic study. *Surgery,* **31**: 443, 1952.
8. Aviles, E. et al: Plantar fibromatosis. *Surgery,* **69**, 1: 117–120, 1971.

9. Ayres, W.W. et al: Lipoma of bone of intra-osseous origin, *JBJS,* **33A**: 257–259, 1951.
10. Barber, K.W. et al: Benign extraneural soft tissue tumors of the extremities causing compression of nerves. *JBJS,* **44A**: 98–104, 1962.
11. Barretson, J. et al: Two cases of lipomatosis involving bone. *Brit. Jour. Radiol.,* **20**: 426–432, 1947.
12. Batchelor, T.M. and Maun, M.E.: Congenital glycogenic tumors of the heart. *Arch. Path.,* **39**: 67–87, 1945.
13. Beeson, P.B. et al: *Cecil-Loeb Textbook of Medicine,* 12th ed. W.B. Saunders Co., Philadelphia, 1967.
14. Berlin, S.J. et al: *Skin Tumors of the Foot: Diagnosis and Treatment.* Futura Publ. Co., N.Y., 1974, p. 200.
15. Bich, E.M.: Lipoma of the extremities. *Ann. Surg.,* **104**: 139–143, 1936.
16. Bich, E.M.: End results in cases of fibrosarcoma of the extremities. *Arch. Surg.,* **37**: 973, 1938.
17. Bland-Sutton: Lipoma of the plantar fascia. *Practitioner Lond.,* **XII**, 461, 1897.

18. Bloom, D.: A case for diagnosis: congenital erythema of the soles with a lipoma on each heel, presented before Manhattan Dermatological Society, 1958. *Arch. Derm.*, **79**: 726, 1959.

19. Bollinger, J.A. et al: Congenital sarcoma of the foot: case report and review of the literature. *Amer. Jour. Dis. Child.*, **86**: 23, 1953.

20. Booker, R.J.: Lipoblastic tumors of the hands and feet: review of literature and report of 33 cases. *JBJS*, **47A**: 727–740, 1965.

21. Brindley, H.H. et al: Fibrosarcoma of the extremities: review of 45 cases. *Amer. Jour. Dis. Child.*, **86**: 23, 1953.

22. Broders, A.C. et al: Clinical aspects of fibrosarcoma of the soft tissues of the extremities. *Surg. Gyn. and Obs.*, **62**: 1010, 1936.

23. Bryan, R.S. et al: Lipoma of the tendon sheath. *JBJS*, **38A**: 1275–1280, 1956.

24. Busch, J.: (Cited by Skeer) *Urol. Cutan. Rev.*, **42**: 110, 1938.

25. Butterworth, T. and Strean, L.P.: *Clinical Genodermatology.* Williams and Wilkins Co., Baltimore, 1962.

26. Butterworth, T. and Wilson, M.C.: Dermatologic aspects of tuberous sclerosis. *Arch. Derm. and Syph.*, **43**: 2–11, 1941.

27. Child, P.L.: Lipoma of the os calcis: report of a case. *Amer. Jour. Clin. Path.*, **25**: 1050–1052, 1955.

28. Cohen, H. and Gibbs, R.C.: Painful piezogenic pedal papules. *Arch. Derm.*, **Vol. 101**: 98–99, 1970.

29. Copeland, M.M. et al: Tumors of bone. *Amer. Jour. Cancer*, **25**: 496, 1936.

**30. Cornil, A.V. et al: Manuel d'histologic patholigique. 1: 393, Paris: F. Alcan, 1884.**

31. Crenshaw, A.H.: *Campbell's Operative Orthopedics*, 5th ed. C.V. Mosby C., St. Louis, 1971.

32. Curtin, J.W.: Fibromatosis of the plantar fascia. *JBJS*, **17**: 1605, 1965.

33. Dawson, J.: Pulmonary tuberous sclerosis and its relationship to other forms of the disease. *Quart. Jour. Med.*, **23**: 113–145, 1954.

34. DeLamater, J.: Mammouth tumor. *Cleveland Med. Jour.*, **1**: 31, 1959.

35. Dercum, F.X.: Three cases of hitherto unclassified affection resembling in its grosser aspects obesity, but associated with special nervous symptoms; adiposis dolorosa. *Amer. Jour. Med. Science*, **104**: 521, 1892.

36. Du Vries, H.L.: *Surgery of the Foot*. 3rd ed. C.V. Mosby Co., St. Louis, 1973.

37. Dockerty, M.B. et al: Fibrosarcoma of the soft tissues of the extremities: a review of 78 cases. *Surgery*, **28**: 495, 1950.

38. Domonkos, A.N.: *Andrew's Diseases of the Skin.* W.B. Saunders Co., Phila., 1971, p. 662.

39. Dreyfuss, M.L.: Congenital sarcoma. *Jour. Pediat.*, **34**: 583, 1949.

40. Edland, R.W.: Liposarcoma: a retrospective study of fifteen cases, a review of the literature and a discussion of radiosensitivity. *Amer. Jour. Roentgen.*, **103**: 778, 1968.

41. Eibel, P.: Juxtamalleolar lipomata. *Clin. Ortho.*, **49**: 191–194, 1966.
42. El-Banhawy, A.: Dupuytren's disease of the foot (fibromatosis of the plantar fascia). *Jour. Egyp. Medical Assoc.*, **43**: 378–384, 1960.
43. Ewing, J.: *Neoplastic Diseases*, 3rd ed. W.B. Saunders Co., Phila., 1928.
44. Ewing, J.: A review of the classification of bone tumors. *Surg. Gyn. and Obst.*, **68**: 971, 1939.
45. Fairbank, H.A.: Dupuytren's contraction of plantar fascia. Section of Orthopedics, 1932.
46. Fairbank, H.A.: A parosteal lipoma. *JBJS*, **35B**: 589, 1953.
47. Feinstein, M.H.: Foot pathology associated with tuberous sclerosis and neurofibromatosis. *JAPA*, **62**: 337, 1972.
48. Fitzpatrick, T.B., Szabo, G., Hori, Y., Simone, A.A., Reed, W.B., and Greenberg, M.H.: White leaf shaped macules. *Arch. Derm.*, **98**: 1–6, 1968.
49. Forfar, J.D. and Arneil, G.C.: *Textbook of Paediatrics*. Churchill-Livingstone, London, 1973, pp. 773–774.
50. Galinski, A.W.: Cutaneous herniations: a case report. *JAPA*, **60**: 128, 1970.
51. Galinski, A.W.: Unusual etiology of a foot hernia: a case report. *JAPA*, **62**: 26–28, 1972.
52. Gelfarb, M. et al: Plantar fibromatosis. *Arch. Derm.*, **85**: 158, 1962.
53. Geschickter, C.F.: The treatment of lipomas and liposarcomas. In *The Treatment of Cancer and Allied Diseases*, Vol. 3. G.T. Pack and E.M. Livingston, N.Y., Paul B. Hoeber, Inc., 1940, Chapter 125.
54. Giannestras, N.J.: *Foot Disorders*, 2nd ed. Lea & Febiger, Phila., 1973.
55. Gibbs, R. and Costello, M.J.: *Palms and Soles in Medicine*. C.C. Thomas, Inc., Springfield, Ill., 1967.
56. Gold, A.M. et al: Deep intermuscular lipoma of an extremity (case). *JBJS*, **36A**: 146–148, 1954.
57. goldenberg, R.R.: Well differentiated fibrosarcoma of the calcaneus. Report of a case treated by resection. *JBJS*, **42A**: 1151, 1960.
58. Grant, J.: Piezogenic pedal papules. Letters to the editor. *Arch. Derm.*, **101**: 619, 1970.
59. Greenberg, L.: Dupuytren's contracture of plantar and palmar fascia. *JBJS*, **21**, no. 3, 1939.
60. Greenfield, G.B.: *Radiology of Bone Diseases*. J.B. Lippincott Co., Phila., 1969.
61. Harkin, J.C. and Reed, R.J.: Tumors of the Peripheral Nervous System, Armed Forces Institute of Pathology, *Atlas of Tumor Pathology*, Fascicle 3, 93, 1968.
62. Harlan, W.L. et al: Hereditary factors in adipose dolorosa, (Dercum's disease). *Amer. Jour. Hum. Genet.*, **15**: 184, 1963.
63. Holt, J.F. and Dickerson, W.W.: The osseus lesions of tuberous sclerosis, *Radiology*, **58**: 1, 1952.

64. Hudson, O.C.: Intra-uterine fibrosarcoma of the foot: a case report. *Amer. Jour. Cancer*, **26**: 568, 1936.

65. Hutter, R.V.P. and Stewart, F.W.: Fasciitis: a report of 70 cases with follow-up proving the benignity of the lesion. *Cancer*, **15**: 992–1003, 1962.

66. Jensen, A.R. et al: Digital neurofibrosarcoma in infancy. *Jour. Pediat.*, **51**: 566, 1957.

67. Kapiloff, B. and Prior, J.T.: Fibromatosis in children. *Plast. Recon. Surgery*, **10**: 276–282, 1952.

68. Kauffman, S.L. et al: Lipoblastic tumors of children. *Cancer*, **12**: 912, 1959.

69. Keasby, L.: Juvenile aponeurotic fibroma (calcifying fibroma). A distinctive tumor arising in the palms and soles of children. *Cancer*, **6**: 338–346, 1953.

70. Kenin, A. et al: Periosteal lipoma: a report of two cases with associated bone changes. *JBJS*, **41A**: 1122, 1959.

71. Kirshbaum, J.D.: Fibrosarcoma of the tibia following chronic osteomyelitis. *JBJS*, **31A**: 413, 1949.

72. Kleinstiver, B.J. et al: A study of 45 cases and a review of the literature. Nodular fasciitis. *JBJS*, **Vol. 50A**, no. 6, 1968.

73. Kling, D.H.: Juxta-articular adiposis dolorosa. *Arch. Surg.*, **34**: 599, 1937.

74. Kogoj, F.: *Formenkreis der Ichthyosiformen und Keratotischen Hauterkrankungen. Lehrbuch der Haut-und Geschlechtskrankheiten.* Gustav-Fischer, Stuttgart, 1962.

75. Kulcher, G.V.: Benign and malignant tumors of the foot. *JAMA*, **124**: 761, 1944.

76. Lagos, J.C. and Gomez, M.R.: Tuberous sclerosis: reappraisal of a clinical entity. *Mayo Clin. Proc.*, **42**: 26, 1967.

77. LeBrun, H.I., Kellet, H.S., and Macalister, C.L.O.: Renal hamartoma. *Brit. Jour. Urol.*, **27**: 394–407, 1955.

78. Lichtenstein, L. and Goldman, R.L.: Cartilage analogue of fibromatosis. A reiteration of a condition called juvenile aponeurotic fibroma. *Cancer*, **17**: 810–816, 1964.

79. McEnery, E.T. et al: Palmer lipoma. *Arch. Surg.*, **79**: 699, 1959.

80. McKenna, R.J. et al: Sarcomata of the osteogenic series (osteosarcoma, fibrosarcoma, chondrosarcoma, parosteal osteogenic sarcoma and sarcomata arising in abnormal bone). An analysis of 552 cases. *JBJS*, **48A**: 1, 1966.

81. McNeer, G.P. et al: Effectiveness of radiation therapy in the management of sarcoma of the soft somatic tissues. *Cancer*, **22**: 391, 1968.

82. Mehregan, A.H. et al: Nodular fasciitis. *Arch. Derm.*, **93**: 204–210, 1966.

83. Mehrehan, A.H. et al: Recurring digital fibrous tumors of childhood. *Arch. Derm.*, **106**: 214, 1972.

84. Meyerding, H.W. and Shellito, J.G.: Dupuytren's contracture of the foot. *Jour. of Intern. Coll. Surg.*, **11**: 595, 1948.
85. Mueller, M.C. et al: Intramedullary lipoma of bone: report of a case. *JBJS*, **42A**: 517–520, 1960.
86. Murphy, B.M. et al: Liposarcoma of the foot, a case report. *Jour. Michigan Med. Soc.*, **54**: 468, 1955.
87. Nickel, W.R. and Reed, W.R.: Tuberous sclerosis. *Arch. Derm.*, **85**: 89–106, 1962.
88. Pack, G.T.: Symposium: tumors of the hands and feet. *Surg.*, **5**: 1, 1939.
89. Pack, G.T.: Liposarcoma: a study of 105 cases. *Surg.*, **36**: 687, 1954.
90. Pastor, N. et al: Adiposis dolorosa (Dercum's disease). *JAMA*, **110**: 1261, 1938.
91. Pickren, J.W. and Smith, A.G.: Fibromatosis of the plantar fascia. *Cancer*, **4**: 846, 1951.
92. Price, E.B. and Silliphant, W.: Nodular fasciitis: a clinicopathologic analysis of 65 cases. *Amer. Jour. Clin. Path.*, **35**: 122–136, 1961.
93. Pringle, J.J.: A case of congenital adenoma sebaceum. *Brit. Jour. Derm.*, **2**: 1–14, 1890.
94. Prior, J.T.: Fibromatosis in children. *Plas. Recon. Surg.*, **10**: 276–282, 1952.
95. Prior, J.T. and Sisson, B.J.: Dermal and fascial fibromatosis. *Annals of Surg.*, **Vol. 139**: no. 4, 1954.
96. Reed, W.B., Nickel, W.R., and Campion, G.: Internal manifestations of tuberous sclerosis. *Arch. Derm.*, **87**: 715–728, 1963.
97. Reszel, P.A. et al: Liposarcoma of the extremities and limb girdles: a study of 222 cases. *JBJS*, **48**: 229, 1966.
98. Reye, R.D.K.: Recurring digital fibrous tumors of childhood. *Arch. Path.*, **80**: 228, 1965.
99. Richmond, D.A.: Lipoma causing a posterior interosseous nerve lesion. *JBJS*, **35B**: 83, 1953.
100. Robbins, S.L.: *Pathology*, 3rd ed. W.B. Saunders Co., Phila., 1967.
101. Sawyer, K.C. et al: The unpredictable fatty tumor. *Arch. Surg.*, **96**: 773, 1968.
102. Schaffzin, E.A. and Chung, S.M.: Congenital generalized fibromatosis with complete spontaneous regression. *JBJS*, **3**: 657, 1972.
103. Schlappner, O.L. et al: Painful and non-painful piezogenic pedal papules. *Arch. Derm.*, **106**: 729–733, 1972.
104. Schreiner, B.F. et al: Primary malignant tumors of the foot: a report of 37 cases. *Radiol.*, **21**: 513, 1933.
105. Shanks, S.C. et al: *A Textbook of X-ray Diagnosis*, 4th ed. W.B. Saunders Co., Phila., 1971.
106. Shapiro, L.: Infantile digital fibromatosis and aponeurotic fibroma: a case report of two rare pseudosarcomatous lesions and review of the literature. *Arch. Derm.*, **99**: 37, 1969.

107. Shelly, W.B. and Rawnsley, H.M.: Painful feet due to herniations of fat. *JAMA*, **205**: 308–309, 1968.

108. Silverstone, E.: Trauma and fibrosarcoma of the foot. *Brit. Med. Jour.*, **1**: 958, 1952.

109. Skeer, J.: Adenoma sebaceum (Pringle), von Recklinghausen's disease, subungual fibromatosis associated with tuberous sclerosis—a symptom complex. *Urol. Cutan. Rev.*, **42**: 110, 1938.

110. Smith, T.K., Gregerson, G.G., and Samilson, R.L.: Orthopedic problems associated with tuberous sclerosis. *JBJS*, **51**: 97, 1969.

111. Soule, E.H.: Proliferative (nodular) fasciitis. *Arch. Path.*, **73**: 437–444, 1962.

112. Steinberg, C.: Fibrositis including Dupuytren's contracture: a new method of treatment. *New York State Jour. Med.*, **47**: 1679–1682, 1947.

113. Stevenson, T.W.: Synovitis of the wrist. *Plast. and Recon. Surg.*, **2**: 443–458, 1947.

114. Stout, A.P.: Liposarcoma, malignant tumor of lipoblasts. *Amer. Surg.*, **119**: 86, 1944.

115. Stout, A.P.: Fibrosarcoma, the malignant tumor of fibroblasts. *Cancer*, **1**: 30, 1948.

116. Stout, A.P.: Tumors of the Soft Tissues. *Atlas of Tumor Pathology*, Section 2, Part 5, Armed Forces Institute of Pathology, 1953.

117. Stout, A.P.: Juvenile fibromatosis. *Cancer*, **7**: 953, 1954.

118. Stout, A.P.: Pseudosarcomatous fasciitis in children. *Cancer*, **7**: 953, 1954.

119. Stout, A.P.: Fibrous tumors of soft tissues. *Minn. Med.*, **43**: 455–459, 1960.

120. Strauss, F.H.: Deep lipomas of the hand. *Ann. Surg.*, **94**: 269–273, 1931.

121. Tachdijian, M.O.: *Pediatric Orthopedics*. W.B. Saunders Co., Phila., 1972.

122. Treves, F.: *Trans. Path. Soc. Scand.*, **39**: 308, 1887.

123. Tubby, A.H.: Diffuse painful lipoma of the foot. *Amer. Jour. Orth. Surg.*, **Vol. VI**: 689, 1908.

124. Turek, S.L.: *Orthopaedics*, 2nd ed. J.B. Lippincott Co., Phila., 1967.

125. Van der Hoeve, J.: Eye symptoms in phakomatoses. *Tran. Opthal. Soc. UK*, **52**: 380–401, 1932.

126. Virchow, R.: Ein Fall von Bösartigen, zun Theil in der Form des Neuromas auftretenden Fellgeschwulsten. *Virchows Arch. F. Path. Anat.*, **11**: 281, 1857.

127. Warthan, T.L. and Rudolph, R.I.: Isolated plantar fibromatosis. *Arch. Derm.*, **108**: 823, 1973.

128. Waugh, W.: Fibrosarcoma occurring in a chronic bone sinus. *JBJS*, **34B**: 642, 1952.

129. Weis, C.R.: Bilateral fibrosarcoma of the lower extremities. *JAMA*, **93**: 1378, 1929.

130. Wells, H.G.: Occurrence and significance of congenital neoplasms. *Arch. Path.*, **30**: 535, 1940.
131. Windeyer, B. et al: Radiotherapy: the place of radiotherapy in the management of fibrosarcoma of the soft tissues. *Clin. Radiol.*, **17**: 32, 1966.
132. Yakovlev, P.I. and Guthrie, R.H.: Congenital ectodermatoses (neuro-cuteneous syndromes) in epileptic patients. *Arch. Neurol. Psychiat.*, **26**: 1145–1194, 1931.
133. Zeligman, I.: Personal Communication. 1974.

# Section III

# Tumors of Muscle, Tendon and Joints

## Ganglions (Synovial Cysts)

### Definition

A ganglion is a thin-walled, cystic, soft tissue mass. It is filled with a colorless to amber colored liquid of varying viscosity and is located in the subcutaneous tissue, almost invariably in contact with fibrous joint capsule or tendon sheath.

### History

The first documented evidence of a synovial cyst was by Hippocrates who described the lesion as an aggregate of mucoid flesh. Eller (1746) ascribed the lesion to a rupture of the tendon sheath, but Henle (1847) called it a mucinous tumor. Gosselin (1876) considered the lesion a retention cyst, while Hoeftman, during the same year, described it as a synovial dermoid. Volkmann (1882) felt it to be a herniation of the synovial membrane although Buxton (1923) considered it a true tumor of the tendon sheath. Carp and Stout (1928), as well as DeOrsey (1937), described the mass as a mucinous degeneration of connective tissue in close proximity to joint capsules or tendon sheaths.[26]

### Etiology

The etiology of ganglia is unknown although the literature is congested with speculative explanations. What is clear is that their site of origin is in the synovial tissue of diarthrotic joints and tendon sheaths. Jayson stated that increased intra-articular pressures, subsequent to arthritic changes in a joint, produces blowouts of the capsule at foci of decreased resistance.[77] Bowerman states that ganglia may be categorized depending upon whether they are associated with trauma, with the arthritides, or are of an idiopathic nature. It is their contention that any joint injury or disease associated with joint effusion can produce the cysts.[16] Taylor feels that the mass is a true herniation of the joint capsule, a slowly formed lesion allowing sufficient time for synovial hypertrophy of the inner cyst wall which is a consistent finding. They further state that if this were not the case, the patient's chief complaint would be pain and tenderness consistent with rupture of the synovium—an infrequent clinical finding.[134] Carp and Stout state that the cysts are a result of mucinous degeneration of connective tissue stemming from traumatic obliterative endarteritis causing nutritional deficiency of connective tissue.[26] Bunnell ascribes the mass to a basic defect in the capsule or tendon sheath, permitting protrusion of the synovial tissue. This theory is supported by the fact that, if one can excise the involved capsule and effect closure, the recurrence rate is minimal.[22]

The most commonly accepted theory was proposed by Jayson and Dixon who, via arthrography with radio-opaque dyes, state that through a valvular mechanism synovial fluid is able to exit the joint or tendon sheath into the mass and not return.[77] They were able to demonstrate a definite common stalk with the joint which allowed injected dye to pass from the joint into the main cyst while not regurgitating into the joint upon pressure on the cyst. Taylor supports this view by stating that the "valve" is a consistent finding when the inner aspect of the involved synovium is closely examined.[134] Grahame, in an extensive study of Baker's cysts, invariably was unable to compress the fluid contents back into the knee joint.[63] Clinically, the fact that the mass increases in size on joint motion and will resorb if the joint is immobilized for a long enough period of time, tends to support this theory.

## Incidence

Ganglionic cysts are not uncommon soft tissue lesions and have been reported as occurring at almost every morphological site. The extremities by far represent the most common location, while appearance on the torso, particularly the back, is rare. Although the terms "ganglion" and "synovial cyst" may be used interchangeably, the former is usually reserved for those masses found on the back of the wrist while the latter represents all other body locales except the popliteal space where the eponym of "Baker's cyst" is ascribed.

The literature is replete with reports of ganglionic cysts.

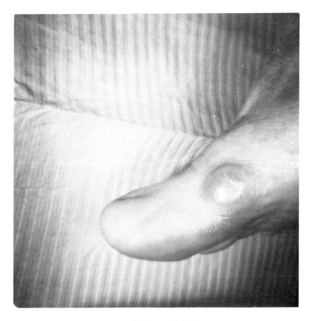

**Figure 3-1A**

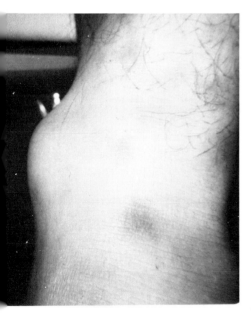

Ganglion Cyst. (A) an unusual location for a ganglion cyst on the hallux toe. However, there is a history of chronic irritation in this region. (B) reveals a large ganglion cyst on the medial aspect of the ankle, a relatively more frequent location for a ganglion cyst.

**Figure 3-1B**

The masses have been reported in patients ranging in age from 2 to 76 years, with the mean age being in the mid-thirties. Females outnumber males two to one with an equal racial distribution. Of the vast number of cases reported, relatively few have been described on the foot or ankle, the incidence ranging between three and five percent of reported cases. On the other hand, the incidence of synovial cysts on the lower extremity which produce foot symptomatology is considerably higher depending on the lesion site and its proximity to nerves and blood vessels. In a review of 760 ganglion cysts, 166 involved the lower extremity with only 32 located on the foot; yet 45 lesions presented foot symptoms.[11,20,26,35,38,68]

## Clinical Picture

Patients usually present with a chief complaint of a sudden or gradual appearance of a swelling, with or without discomfort, on the dorsum of the foot or infra-malleolar regions. Any area of the foot or ankle may be involved. In the vast majority of patients the mass is of cosmetic distress or subject to shoe trauma and chronic irritation. Pain is infrequently a subjective finding unless the mass is of sufficient size to impinge on local nerves and blood vessels or is subject to shoe irritation. Carp and Stout, however, in a study of 255 cases of which ten were on the foot, found pain a presenting symptom in 50 percent of the cases.[26] According to Dao (1964), 35 percent of patients give a history of a temporal relationship with previous trauma.[35] Less perceptive patients frequently state simply that they feel that a "bone is out of place."[72] When subadjacent nerves are compressed, the patient may report symptoms comparable to a neuroma—anesthesia, hypoesthesias, paresthesias, pain, burning, aching or weakness of digits. A patient who reports that the lesion at times seems to diminish in size or disappears, only to reappear at a later date, is providing an important diagnostic clue.

Physical examination reveals a fluctuant to tense, unilocular, well defined, soft tissue tumefaction varying in size from 7.0 millimeters to 6.0 centimeters with an average size of 2.0 centimeters in diameter.[26] According to Carp and

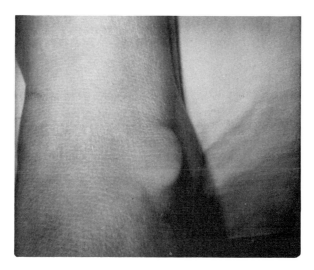

**Figure 3-2A**

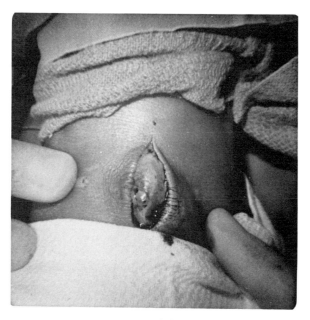

**Figure 3-2B**
Ganglion cyst of the foot and ankle clinically representing a large firm lesion overlying the extensor surface of the foot and ankle. The lesion extended into the ankle joint.

Stout, 30 percent of the lesions palpated elicit tenderness of varying degree.[26] Upon active joint motion, the lesion tends to increase in size, and the patient may simultaneously complain of some vague aching sensation. Lesions on the dorsum of the foot may be very painful with pain and paresthesias radiating to involved, innervated zones. If muscle strength is tested in the digits, a distinct weakness with signs of wasting may be noted.[26] The overlying skin may appear blanched and is freely moveable over the mass while being firmly fixed to deeper soft tissue or underlying hypertrophied bony eminences. When the lesion originates from the tendon sheath rather than the joint, its size becomes accentuated upon digital flexion and extension, is less firm, tends to be multilocular, is more irregular in shape, and is less tender to palpation.[33] Trauma to a cyst may cause hemorrhage into it, producing sudden pain, which makes diagnosis more difficult.[75]

Lesions about the ankle may produce pain or numbness in the heel or may radiate distally into the foot. Plantar lesions are quite infrequent, but, when present, tend to involve the flexor sheath, are quite hard, and are tender to firm pressure. If the lesion acquires sufficient size, one might notice metatarsal separation on x-ray and digital separation in stance, likening it to neuromata. It is not at all uncommon during neuroma surgery to simultaneously excise a ganglion cyst.

Ganglionic cysts produce osseous deformity in two ways. 1) If a lesion attains sufficient size and is of long standing, its expansive nature may produce erosive changes in the cortex or bowing of long bones in accordance with Wolf's law.[51] 2) The masses may also involve metaphyseal bone producing homogenous, well defined, cystic lesions with marginal sclerosis. The lesions may be unilocular or multilocular in nature and usually occur in older individuals more often than its differential counterpart, the unicameral cyst. Franklin reported 17 such lesions involving the lower extremity, 13 in the distal tibia and fibula and four involving the talus.[54] In our experience, it is not uncommon to find these lesions in-

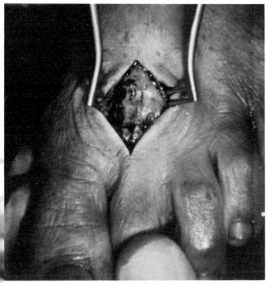

**Figure 3-3A**

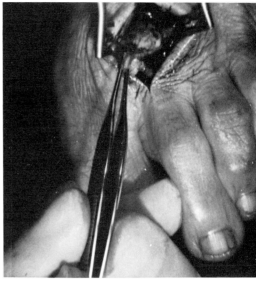

**Figure 3-3B**

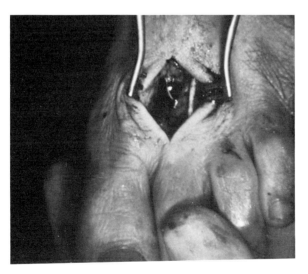

**Figure 3-3C**

Ganglion Cyst. Inter-metatarsal ganglion cysts are frequently seen. The diagnosis is often difficult to make, unless the lesion is somewhat bulging. (A) reveals a surgical view on initial skin incision; a bulging of the lesion. (B) reveals a section of the neoplasm. (C) reveals a surgical cavity that is left after excision. Proper closure of these cavities is necessary to reduce hematoma formation.

volving the first metatarsal head during hallux abducto valgus surgery on patients with osteoarthritis.

*Diagnosis*

The diagnosis of ganglia, in most instances, is based upon clinical symptoms and physical findings. Rarely are such sophisticated techniques as arthrography necessary to establish the diagnosis. On the other hand, arthrography is useful if future surgery is contemplated, for it will not only delineate the cyst, but will also delineate the stalk and its site of origin. To substantiate its value, Pavelka reports a synovial cyst on the knee whose stalk was traced to the achilles tendon via intrasheath injection of Meglutamine Diatrizoate.[103]

In general, those ganglia arising from tendons tend to be less firm, multilocular, and more irregular than their joint counterparts.[33] Those arising from joints tend to increase in size upon joint motion, while those arising from tendon sheath remain relatively constant in size. Ganglia are relatively infrequent in children but, when present, are usually the result of direct insidious trauma. Those of older patients usually are secondary to some intra-articular pathology.[66]

Of significant importance is the realization that ganglia may be present in areas other than the foot though still producing foot symptomatology. Brooks reported several lesions in the popliteal space and around the fibular neck which produced pain or numbness in the foot.[20]

Laboratory studies are non-conclusive and of little value. Should synovialysis be performed on ganglionic contents, the report reveals the fluid to be very similar to normal synovial fluid though more viscous. According to Andren and Elken, its chemical makeup is likened to dialyzed synovial fluid.[3]

*Differential Diagnosis*

Of the differential possibilities, the following have been reported: tubercular tenosynovitis, lipoma, myxoid cyst, sarcomas, fibromas, bursae, osteoma, synovioma, epidermal inclusion cysts, aneurysms, and soft tissue herniations.[26] When

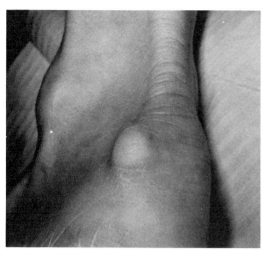

**Figure 3-4A**

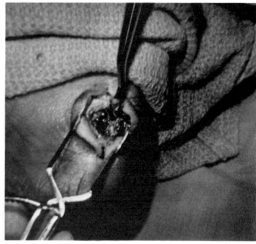

**Figure 3-4B**

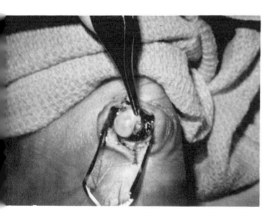

**Figure 3-4C**

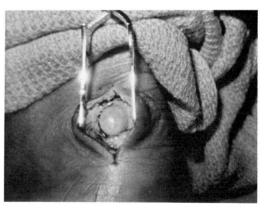

**Figure 3-4D**

Ganglion Cyst (Synovial Cyst). (A) posterior aspect of the foot is perhaps one of the least frequent locations of synovial or ganglion cysts. This lesion closely resembles that of a pump bump, except that it is on the opposite side of the heel. (B) and (C) reveal the surgical exposure and surgical dissection of the lesion. (D) reveals resection of the bony ridge on the posterior aspect of the heel underlying the cyst.

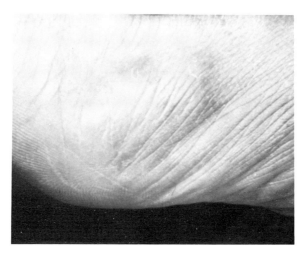

**Figure 3-5A**

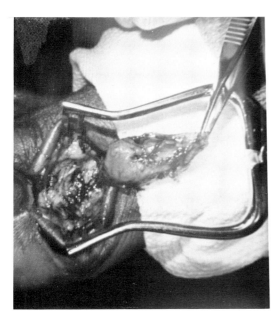

**Figure 3-5B**

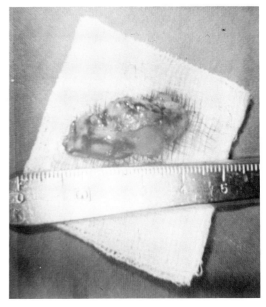

**Figure 3-5C**

Ganglion Cyst. Ganglion cysts are commonly located at the first metatarsophalangeal joint. Clinical diagnosis is relatively easy. (B) and (C) reveal surgical excision of the lesion intact and gross specimen, respectively.

126

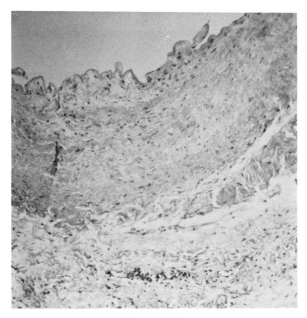

**Figure 3-6**

Ganglion cyst. This lesion shows a cystic cavity lined by a dense connective tissue.

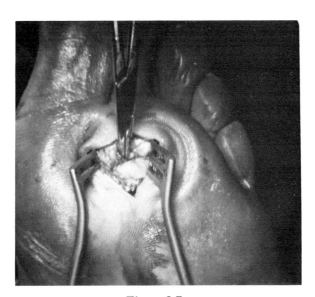

**Figure 3-7**

Synovial Cyst. Synovial cyst on the plantar aspect of the second metatarsal head. This lesion is extremely painful and very infrequently diagnosed. Differential diagnosis in this region may be capsulitis, periostitis or neuritis. Only on indepth examination by palpation of the area will one detect a small, flattened, moveable mass. These lesions on the plantar aspect often become so called "squashed", due to constant weight-bearing pressures.

the lesion involves bone, solitary bone cysts, periarticular pseudocysts of osteoarthritis, and chondroblastomas must also be considered.

## Pathology

Upon gross analysis, a ganglionic cyst appears as a well encapsulated, shiny, cystic swelling, possibly with multiple, adjacent, small cysts. When sectioned, a thick, sticky, clear, amber colored fluid of a soft jelly consistency exudes, and the inner wall is noted to have undergone villous hypertrophy. According to Hansen, a well dissected synovial cyst consists of three parts—an encapsulated main cyst of varying size, ganglionic pseudopods, and microcysts at the site of contact between the ganglion and fibrous capsule or tendon sheath.[68] These structures interconnect but never have an open communication with the joint cavity or tendon sheath although the cyst is invariably bound to these structures by fibrous tissue which may represent reactive fibrosis about the site of perforation.[140]

Microscopically, the cystic swelling contains a mucoid material usually bound by a thin fibrous wall which may be thickened by villous hypertrophy.[66] Stringy collagenous fibers, separated by vacuolated cells of a non-inflammatory nature, are invariably present.

## Treatment

Ganglia may be treated by either conservative or surgical techniques. Of interest, however, is that 58 percent of all ganglia resolve spontaneously with no therapy, and an equivalent number are totally asymptomatic requiring no therapy.[26]

The literature is replete with conservative attempts to eradicate ganglia, each with its own reported degree of success. Some conservative techniques used in the past are immobilization of limb, slow constant compression, rapid abrupt pressure, radiotherapy, baking (massage, and other physical modalities), catgut suture transfixion, and aspiration with subsequent injection and compression. The injections usually consist of the following: 1) sclerosing injections (colloidal gold, 5% sodium morrhuate, iodine, ethanolamine, and phenol), 2) enzyme injections (trypsin and hyaluronidase), and 3) steroid (repository) injections. According to Carp and Stout, regardless of the type of conservative technique employed, recurrences range from 50–78 percent.[26]

Surgical excision of ganglia remains the most effective mode of therapy with a recurrence rate, when the lesion is completely excised properly, ranging between 15–40 percent.[26] Excision is best performed under complete hemostasis so as to facilitate dissection of the cyst with its communicating stalk to the joint or tendon sheath. Those lesions involving the foot almost invariably overlay bony prominences so that simple aspiration with repository steroid injection is usually ineffective on a long term basis. If aspiration indeed fails, surgery is advisable but should be delayed four to six weeks after recurrence to give the ganglion capsular sac sufficient time to regain its strength and thereby decrease the chance of rupturing the capsule during excision. Complete excision requires removal of the main cyst, stalk, subadjacent capsule or tendon sheath, and any underlying bony exostosis if resolution is to be ensured.[75] During excision, care must be taken not to rupture the cyst for two reasons—the contents have a potential to initiate a foreign body reaction, and once ruptured, it becomes extremely difficult to trace the stalk to its point of origin.

Following excision, a void of varying size is left and care must be taken in closure to fill the dead space so as to avoid excessive hematoma formation. Compressive sterile dressings with elastic wrap are of value for a period of two to three weeks postoperative. If significant neurologic symptoms were present, the rate of recovery is related to whether or not the nerve injury was neuropraxic or axonotmesis in nature.[20]

*Prognosis*

Prognosis remains quite favorable in the vast majority of cases.

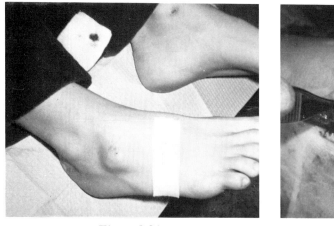

Figure 3-8A

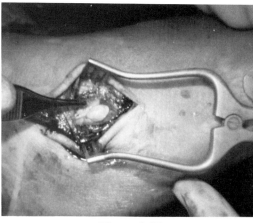

Figure 3-8B

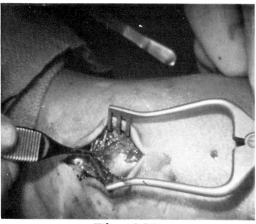

Fibure 3-8C

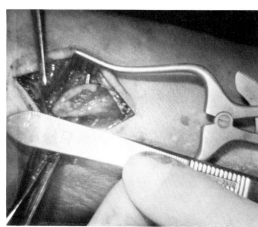

Figure 3-8D

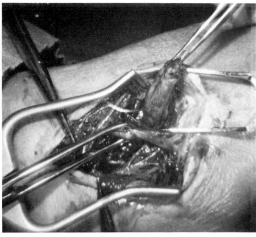

Figure 3-8E

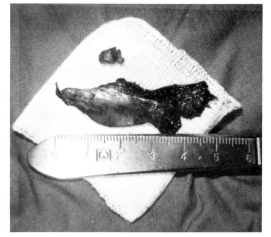

Figure 3-8F

Ganglion Cyst. Ganglion cysts within muscles are not infrequently seen in the foot. This is a relatively large lesion located in the extensor digitorum brevis muscle. The lesion was quite symptomatic, particularly in shoes. Surgical dissection reveals how intricate some of the cystic lesions can be. Surgical exposures reveal various tendinous as well as nerve structures, which this neoplasm courses around. Often ganglion cysts in this area consist of a very thick capsular structure.

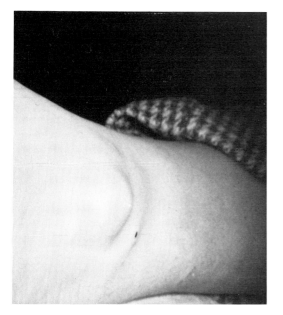

Figure 3-9A

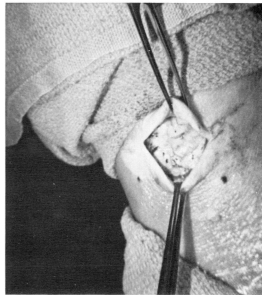

Figure 3-9B

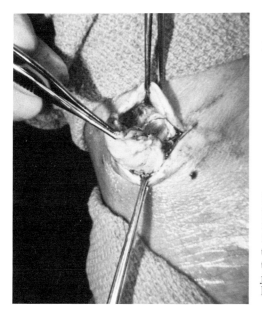

Figure 3-9C

Nodular Tenosynovitis. (A). nodular tenosynovitis of the foot and ankle. Clinical picture reveals a small firm swollen area below the medial malleolus. (B) initial surgical exposure and then (C) surgical dissection of the neoplasm intact. The history is quite interesting from the standpoint that this is a female jockey, and this portion of her foot constantly hits the horse and saddle as she rides.

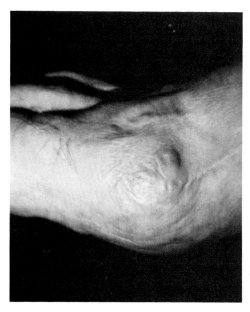

Nodular Tenosynovitis. (A). The clinical picture reveals a small nodular mass on the first metatarsal head. The mass is very firm upon palpation and slightly moveable. (B) surgical exposure reveals a white glistening nodular area. (C) reveals the surgical specimen in gross form. Patient history relates to a ganglion cyst being removed on three previous occasions in this location. After surgical dissection of the lesion, the bony ridge was completely excised and there was no further recurrence.

Figure 3-10A

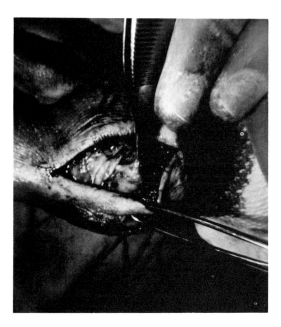

Figure 3-10B

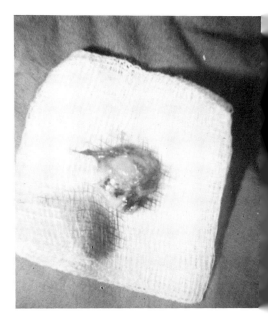

Figure 3-10C

## Giant Cell Tumors of Soft Tissue and Related Villonodular Lesions

### Definition

This category of tumors has been a source of great confusion in regard to nomenclature. Jaffe, Lichtenstein and Sutro (1941) classified these lesions in their classic treatise.[76] They stated that pigmented villonodular synovitis was a giant-cell tumor of synovial membrane; pigmented villonodular tenosynovitis was a giant-cell tumor of tendon sheath; and pigmented villonodular bursitis was a giant-cell tumor of bursal mucosa. Salm and Sissons also regard giant-cell tumors of soft tissue as synonymous with pigmented villonodular synovitis.[121]

### Synonyms

Some of the terminology thought to be synonymous with giant-cell tumors and the pigmented villonodular lesions includes xanthoma, xanthogranuloma, myeloplaxoma, chronic hemorrhagic villous synovitis, giant-cell fibrohemangioma, fibrohemosideric sarcoma, sarcoma, sarcoma fusogiganto cellulare, benign polymorphocellular tumor of the synovial membrane, and malignant polymorphocellular tumor.

### History

The original description of giant-cell tumors is attributed to Broca (1861). The benign nature of the lesion was first recognized by Heurtaux (1891). Extensive reviews of this lesion were published by Tourneux, Bellamy, Garrett, Mason and Woolston, Galloway, Broders, and Ghormley who reviewed 339 cases. This led up to Jaffe, Lichtenstein, and Sutro, who grouped the giant-cell tumors with the pigmented villonodular lesions (1941).

The first report of a lesion thought to be pigmented villonodular synovitis was by Chassaignac (1852). Simon (1865) reported a case involving a large nodule of the knee. Mosin (1909) reported the first case of the diffuse form of this lesion. Many reports followed until the classic review by Jaffe, Lichtenstein, and Sutro.

## Etiology

There is no known etiology. Many authors favor Jaffe, Lichtenstein, and Sutro's theory of a benign inflammatory reaction to some unidentified agent.[76] Because of this, most feel that pigmented villonodular synovitis is not a true neoplasm.

A few reported cases related a history of trauma and the presence of serosanguinous to brownish joint fluid. Reddishbrown or xanthochromic synovium with hemosiderin in the synovium help to support this theory of trauma as a causative agent.[97]

Geschickter and Copeland use giant-cell tumors as a term to describe certain xanthomatous lesions of soft tissue which they regard as originating in sesamoid bones. Many experiments have been attempted to prove that articular hemorrhage initiates growth of the lesion. McCallum, Musser, and Rhangos produced a process resembling villonodular synovitis by repeated injection of autogenous blood into joints of animals and observed identical changes by injection of sterile saline solution.[93] Singh, Grewal, and Chakravarti were able to induce pigmented villonodular synovitis by repeated and prolonged intra-articular injections of colloidal iron as well as autogenous blood.[123] They failed to induce the lesion using injections of plasma and gum acacia and theorized that the iron content of the fluid (usually blood) is important in formation of the lesion. Still other authors feel that these lesions are a tissue manifestation of the disturbance of lipid metabolism. Most feel that these lesions are just benign neoplasms with unknown etiology.[74,97,121]

## Incidence

Pigmented villonodular synovitis and other giant-cell tumors of soft tissue are most commonly found in adults in their third to fifth decades. Authors disagree as to sexual predominance. Most report equal incidence, but others report a more common occurrence among females. There has been no reported racial predominance.

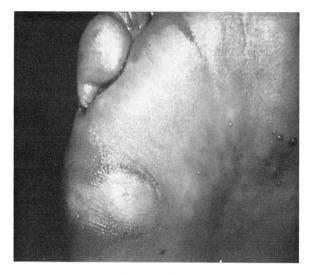

**Figure 3-11**

Giant Cell Tumor. Giant cell tumors are not uncommon to the foot. The relatively large neoplasm involving the plantar surface of the fifth metatarsal head and related area is seen. Clinical picture reveals a very firm and multi-lobulated structure.

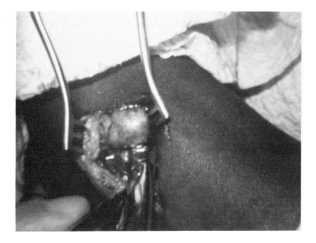

**Figure 3-12**

Giant Cell Tumor. Surgical exposure reveals a giant cell tumor at the lateral aspect of the foot and ankle.

The literature contains very few reported cases of giant cell tumors or pigmented villonodular synovitis involving the foot. This lesion occurs most commonly in the lower extremity, and there are many reported cases involving the ankle joint although the knee is the most common area of the body affected by this lesion, usually in its diffuse form. It is the second most frequent lesion of the hand and is a frequent lesion of the fingers and toes.[53,121]

Salm and Sissons state that true giant-cell tumors of soft tissue are very rare.[121] Most reported cases of pigmented villonodular synovitis do not have bony involvement. Snook reported two cases with bony invasion of the lesion into the shoulder and stated that, until 1963, only 16 cases with bony invasion were reported. One of these cases involved the ankle but none involved the foot.[126]

Gewheiler and Wilson reviewed 300 cases of diffuse pigmented villonodular synovitis in the literature and found that the knee was affected most often, followed by the hip, ankle, tarsus, carpus, elbow, and shoulder in descending order of occurrence.[58]

*Clinical Picture*

The onset is usually insidious and mono-articular. Progression is slow, and years often elapse before treatment is sought. There is sometimes a history of injury. Swelling is usually the first symptom noted; and pain, if present, is usually mild and aching. Acute severe pain denotes pinching or crushing of the villi or nodules and may be accompanied by locking and interruption of joint motion. There may be hemarthrosis if this occurs.

*Diagnosis*

Examination often reveals enlargement of the area with palpable masses, which are generally soft but may be firm. They are irregular, circumscribed, and movable. There is often joint stiffness, with local increase in temperature, but erythema is not usually present.

Most laboratory tests are within normal limits. Aspirated

joint fluid showing serosanguinous or yellow-brown fluid is the most consistent and valuable diagnostic finding.

X-rays show increased soft tissue density and possible cysts in adjacent bones. Arthrograms have been of some success, but arteriograms have not been of value.

## Differential Diagnosis

Differential diagnosis includes tuberculosis of bone, rheumatoid arthritis, osteoarthritis, gouty arthritis, ganglion, and synovial sarcoma. In one series of 29 cases of pigmented villonodular synovitis, ten lesions were originally interpreted as synovial sarcoma.[93]

## Pathology

The histological distinction between giant-cell tumors, pigmented vollonodular synovitis, and xanthomatosis is empirical and not fully understood. There are numerous soft tissue lesions in which numerous giant cells are present, but are not comparable to giant-cell tumors of bone. In pigmented villonodular synovitis the giant cells resemble those in giant-cell tumors.

Pigmented villonodular synovitis is observed in two forms: a) circumscribed with one or more yellow-brown outgrowths, which are either sessile or pedunculated; and b) diffuse, in which the whole synovial membrane is covered with pigmented villonodular outgrowths. This latter is much more common.

Microscopically, there are several lining layers of synovial cells containing pigment; the connective tissue stroma contains hemosiderin-bearing round or polyhedral cells.

Later changes include appearance of foam cells which may contain pigment and, possibly, lipoids in the form of cholesterol esters. Numerous scattered multinucleated giant cells and vascular channels are a feature of the lesion. Eventually, the nodules become fibrotic and collagenize.

Snook reported that by 1963, only 16 cases of pigmented villonodular synovitis had been reported with bony invasion, suggesting that bone involvement is rare with this lesion.[126]

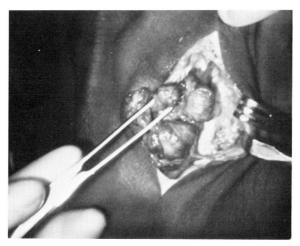

**Figure 3-13A**

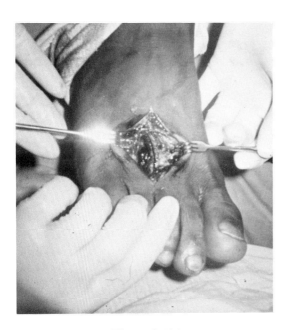

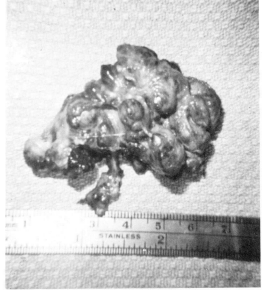

**Figure 3-13B**                    **Figure 3-13C**

Giant Cell Tumor. (A) surgical exposure reveals a
large multilobulated giant cell tumor of the third and
fourth metatarsal interspace. (B) reveals the complete
neoplasm excised, showing the large defect or cavity
created from the excision of the lesion. (C) reveals
the gross specimen showing a multilobulated area.
The lesion was a very dark, yellowish brown color.

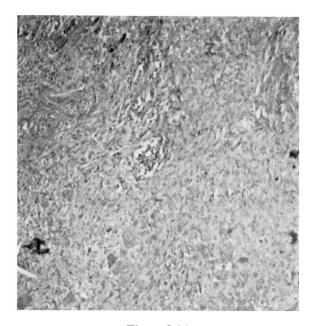

**Figure 3-14**

Giant Cell tumor at tendon sheath origin. The cell population varies from bundles of elongated spindle cells with some collagenous ground substance to mononuclear and multinucleated histocytes.

However, Gewheiler and Wilson disagree and indicate that, although it is rare for the circumscribed form of pigmented villonodular synovitis to produce osseous abnormalities, 50 percent of the total cases of diffuse and circumscribed lesions show positive bony x-ray changes.[58] If there is no invasion of bone, there will be some synovial thickening but no regional decalcification and calcific deposits in the lesion. The cartilage space is usually preserved.[97]

If there is invasion of bone, it appears as one or more discrete intra-osseous cystic lesions, some of which may have slightly sclerotic margins. These are usually located subchondrally and juxta-articular. The surrounding bone is of normal density and the joint space is preserved.[23] The authors have experienced a case in which there was a severe bending of the third metatarsal bone due to the lesions' size, and another case in which the metatarsal head was infiltrated by the lesion. Osteoporosis is rarely seen about an affected joint.[8] Hypertrophic lipping and narrowing of the joint space are uncommon. Feinstein (1974) reported a rare case of this lesion, causing total destruction of a metatarsal head, resembling Freiberg's Infraction.[48]

## Foot Involvement

A true pigmented villonodular bursitis is very rare. Jaffe, Lichenstein, and Sutro reported four cases, one of which was in the ankle joint.[76] Stern reported a case involving cystic degeneration of the first metatarsophalangeal joint and fibular sesamoid and stated that it resembled gouty arthritis on x-ray.[128]

Byers reviewed 126 histologically diagnosed cases, with seven affecting the foot and all the nodular type, and five involving the ankle and of the diffuse type.[23] They also reported a rare case with bilateral involvement of the ankles. De Santo and Wilson reported four cases involving the ankles, with one case in the foot at the navicular and second cuneiform.[39] Galloway, Broders, and Ghormley reported three cases in the ankle joints and three in the tarsal joints.[55]

Jaffe, Lichtenstein, and Suto reported one case in the tibiotarsal joint and one case on the calcaneocuboid joint.

They reported four cases of pigmented villonodular bursitis, one involving the ankle.[76]

Breimer and Freiberger reported a case involving the second toe with cystic degeneration of the middle phalanx.[18] They also reported a case involving the ankle with a history of injury six years previously. Berlin (1970) reported a case of giant cell tumor of the hallux,[14] and Feinstein (1973) reported a case in the foot with extensive bony involvement.[48]

Clark states that the incidence of pigmented villonodular synovitis is one percent of all patients presenting with joint complaints.[30] Most authors agree that the lower extremity is the most common location, with the knee most commonly involved in the diffuse form, and the toes with the circumscribed form.[126]

### Treatment

Most authors agree that surgical excision is the best primary treatment. The use of radiation in any phase of treatment is debated, most feeling that radiation has limited benefit.

Complete surgical synovectomy is the treatment of choice for the diffuse form with local excision for the circumscribed form. If bone is involved, it should be excised or curetted. If the resulting bone defect is sizable, it may be packed with chips or receive a graft.

Radiation is sometimes utilized following surgery to prevent recurrence but should be delayed until there is adequate blood supply to the bone graft.

Byers estimated that with local excision of the circumscribed lesions, there is a recurrence rate of 16–48 percent. Recurrences are treated by further surgery or radiation.[23]

Foster explains the high recurrence rate as being due to an attempt to shell out the lesions, rather than excising them widely, for shelling them out may leave residual parts of the lesion. Thus, because of the diffuse nature of the lesions, they should be widely excised.[53] Johnson emphasizes the importance of removing the tumor en bloc, without penetrating into it, but still estimates a 20 percent recurrence rate.[78]

*Prognosis*

Generally, the prognosis is good providing there has been adequate excision, and there is no bone involvement.

## Synovial Sarcoma

*Definition*

Synovial sarcoma is a primary malignant tumor arising from joint tissues, tendon sheaths, and bursae.

*History*

The clinicopathologic aspects of this disease have been well documented;[6,24,67] and precise histologic criteria have been established for its diagnosis.[67] It is a rare, highly specialized neoplasm, developing predominantly in the extremities and growing, generally, at a slow rate. Approximately eight percent of all malignant neoplasm of the soft somatic tissue are synovial sarcomas. They usually occur as unicentric lesions (with a single growth center) in the middle to older age groups. They may arise not only in joints, but also in tendon sheaths and bursae, all of which contain similarly derived cells. It is of particular interest that the anatomic relationship of synovial sarcoma to synovial structures is often nonexistent. The tumor may be locally invasive, eroding into joint spaces and destroying joint function, as well as metastasizing widely.

It should be remembered that synovial membrane cells, which secrete a lubricating synovial fluid, line the interior of the fibrous capsule and thereby form an imperfect membrane around diarthrodic joints, 25 percent of which are located in the foot. The synovial membrane covers tendons which pass through joints, such as the popliteus tendon in the knee. The membrane is not closely aligned to the inner surface of the fibrous capsule, but is thrown into folds, fringes, or projections composed of connective tissue, fat, and blood vessels. These folds commonly surround the articular cartilage margin.

Equivalent to the synovial membrane in joints are the

synovial tendon sheaths and synovial bursae which have an inner lining of synovial membrane. Synovial tendon sheaths facilitate the gliding of tendons through fibrous and bony tunnels (e.g. the peroneus longus). All tendons crossing the ankle joint are enclosed for part of their length in synovial sheaths (approximately eight centimeters). One investigator believes that the tumor is widely invasive, particularly in the sole of the foot.[87]

## Etiology

The etiological role of trauma is difficult to assess. A history of trauma is probably coincidental to the tumor's development.[24] Of all the cases reviewed by the author, no evidence of synovial sarcoma arising in pre-existing inflammatory joint disease, as reported by the various authors, were found[24] although one author mentions that the tumor may clinically resemble localized arthritis.[81]

## Incidence

The incidence of this tumor is difficult to assess since the histologic diagnosis is often subtle, and extensive sampling of the tumor may be required before its true identity is established. The belief that the tumor arises from synovial joints, tendon, bursae, or adventitious bursae is attractive but unsubstantiated. The lesion may arise "de novo" from undifferentiated mesenchymal cells.[24]

Most reports indicate a slight predilection for males[24,67] although slight female predominance has been reported in some other investigations[6,24] but the sex distinction is not great enough to help in diagnosis.

The tumor is found in all age groups, but there is definitely a peak incidence in early adult life.[6,19,24,67,110,114,141] Why the tumor occurs more commonly between 20-40 years is unknown.[108]

In the study of 78 cases, Codman found the mean duration of the disease from onset of symptoms to death to be 6.5 years, which is relatively long in comparison to other sarcomas. The mean duration of symptoms prior to seeking

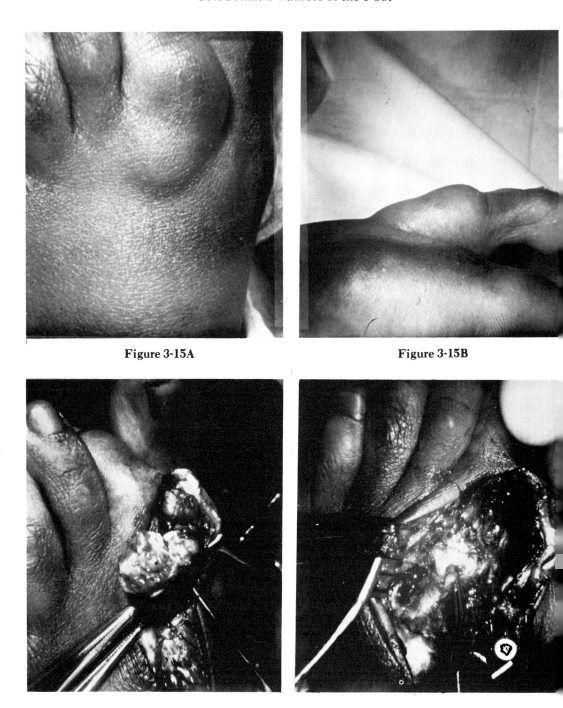

**Figure 3-15A**

**Figure 3-15B**

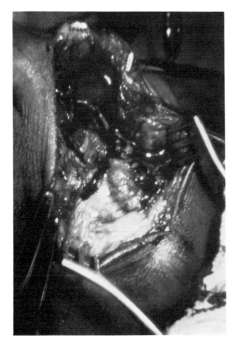

**Figure 3-15E**

**Figure 3-15F**

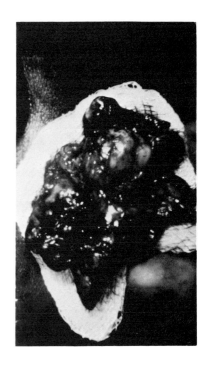

Pigmented Villonodular Synovitis. (A) and (B) clinical pictures reveal a severely swollen second metatarsophalangeal joint and extension of the second toe upon weight-bearing. (C) reveals a large, yellowish, diffused fibro-fatty type of mass being excised from the dorsal aspect of the 2nd MP joint. (D) reveals the invasion into the bony surface of the 2nd metatarsal head. A portion of the tumor is grasped with the forceps. (E) reveals the dissection of the second metatarsal head due to bone involvement. (F) reveals the large gross specimen and closure of the wound.

medical attention was 2.3 years in a group of patients who had subsequently died from the tumor.[24] Thirty-six percent of 13 patients had pain or palpable tenderness for periods ranging from one month to 18 years prior to the appearance of a palpable mass at that same site.

Ariel and Pack found that about one year elapsed from onset of symptoms until the patient sought medical attention. They attribute this to the relatively mild nature of the symptoms.[6]

## Clinical Picture

Since synovial sarcoma is a rare malignant neoplasm, developing at a slow rate, its early recognition is difficult.[67,108] Although pain is present in many patients, it is not severe, and pain may or may not be preceded by a history of trauma.[67] The onset is best characterized as insidious.

The most common presenting complaint in one series was the presence of a tumor, with tenderness and disability as less frequent findings.[108] In another series, of 134 patients, over 97 percent had a palpable mass or swelling; approximately 60 percent had pain and/or tenderness; ten patients had noted sensory or motor disturbance distal to the lesion; six patients had lost six to twenty pounds; and three had sufficient evidence of inflammation to consider an acute inflammatory process.[24] Ariel and Pack reported a mass or tumor only 50 percent painful as the presenting clinical feature.[6]

It is evident that swelling which causes little discomfort and grows slowly is the most common presenting clinical feature. However, rapid growth may occur occasionally.[141]

According to Giannestras, the presenting complaint in the foot usually is an enlarging, painless mass, with physical examination revealing a fixed or non-fixed, non-tender tumor.[60]

## Diagnosis

Accurate diagnosis of synovial sarcoma is usually impossible prior to surgical examination, and most authors conclude that histologic examination is the only reliable means

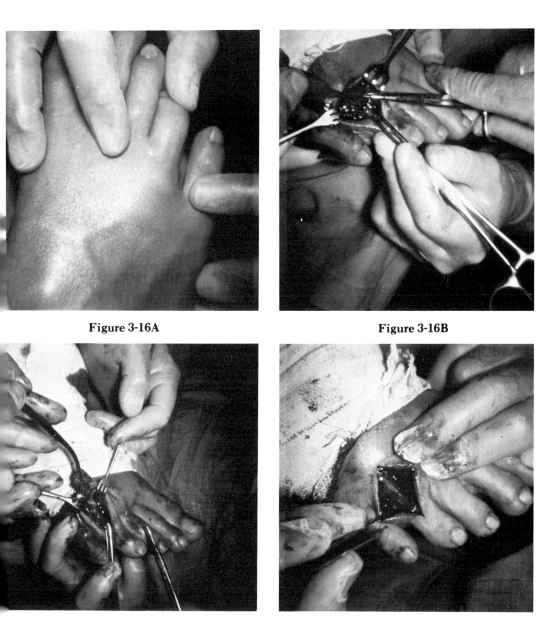

**Figure 3-16A**

**Figure 3-16B**

**Figure 3-16C**

**Figure 3-16D**

Nodular Tenosynovitis. (A) reveals a small swollen area above the fourth metatarsal head. The area happens to be extremely painful and developed after acute physical activity over a period of approximately two months. (B) reveals the isolation of the lesion and its close adherence to the long extensor tendon of the fourth toe. (C) reveals the complete dissection of the lesion off of the tendon and surrounding subcutaneous tissue. (D) reveals a cavity from which it was excised.

of diagnosis.[67] An incisional biopsy of the tumor causes the least surgical trauma. Once the diagnosis is established, definitive surgery can then be employed.

King believes a clinical diagnosis is possible by the discovery of a nodule attached to a tendon or occupying a position next to a tendon sheath, which has rapidly increased in size,[80] but in none of the nine cases reported by Briggs was a correct preoperative diagnosis made, the clinical impression in five cases being benign bursal cyst.[19]

The possibility of a diagnosis by x-ray is variable, especially when the tumor is not close to a joint and has no evidence of calcification,[108] for the tumor may present truly as an ovoid, soft-tissue mass of increased, uniform density, with smooth outlines.[56] Occasionally, calcific deposits may be present, but adjacent bone and soft tissue reaction is uncommon. In one series of 134 tumors, 57 had positive radiographic findings.[24] Of these, 31.6 percent had tumor calcification and 10.6 percent had evidence of adjacent bone invasion and erosion.

## Differential Diagnosis

Synovial sarcoma can easily be mistaken, in the foot and elsewhere, for an innocuous ganglion[67] or a tendon sheath tumor.[19,60] However, when a palpable tumor exists, consideration must be given to the possibility of a malignant soft tissue tumor such as fibrosarcoma, myxosarcoma, neurogenic sarcoma, liposarcoma, or xanthosarcoma, as well as synovial sarcoma.

While synovial sarcoma is composed almost entirely of mesothelial cells, it is questionable whether they are derived from the normal synovial cells of joints, tendon sheaths, or bursae. The tumor seldom projects into those synovial structures, even though it is in close proximity to them.[67] Therefore, it is rare that an actual joint lining or tendon sheath is affected. In contrast, synovial hyperplasia, giant cell tumors, hemangiomas, and other non-malignant lesions almost always involve the synovial tissue themselves.

## Pathology

Synovial sarcomas are composed of two elements, both of which are neoplastic and are as inseparable as the lining of joint, tendon sheath, or bursae and the supportive tissue upon which these cells rest.[108] These two types of cells are designated as fibrosarcomatous and synovoid elements and are invariably intermingled.[67]

The lesions vary in their gross appearance from solitary, well-defined nodules to irregular masses, that may be several centimeters in diameter.[114] There are no gross features that are pathognomic for synovial sarcoma.[108] Extension along fascial planes is common and obvious infiltration into surrounding muscle and fascia is universal.[24] Hence, the tumor starts as a focal area and grows into the surrounding structures. The gross tumor can be nodular and molded by the density and resistance of the tissues into which it grows. The tissue is basically a pale, creamy pink, "fleshy" mass as are the majority of sarcomas. Red and yellow mottled areas from hemorrhage and degeneration may be seen.[67] Some tumors are quite hard when fibrosis and calcification occurs.

A feature that leads an inexperienced surgeon into the tactical error of enucleation of the tumor is the characteristic of the mass to grow and push the connective tissue around it into a pseudocapsule. Enucleation results in recurrence in almost all cases.[108]

## Foot Involvement

Most authors have found this tumor to be more frequent in the lower extremity. The sites at or below the knee in order of frequency are: knee area, foot, ankle, lower leg, and great toe. Pack revealed eight cases in his study. Lichtenstein found eight synovial sarcomas, three of which were in the foot, two in the ankle area, one on the plantar area, and one in the thigh.[87]

Raben studied 38 cases with the following general distribution: foot—11, hand and fingers—18, knee—seven, hip—four, forearm—three, buttock—two, and elbow—three.[110]

Briggs reported one out of nine cases on the foot.[19] King

presented seven cases of synovial sarcoma of tendon sheaths, one in the toe, and two in the ankle.[80] Ariel and Pack reviewed 25 cases treated during the period between 1953–1963; 72 percent of these were found in the lower extremity. They found the following distribution in the lower extremity: knees—five, thigh—five, groin—two, buttocks—two, foot—one, and ankle—one.[6] Bennet made a study of 32 specimens registered at the Armed Forces Institute of Pathology during 1941–1945 and found the following locations in the lower extremity: knee—eight, thigh—five, upper leg—four, ankle—three, foot—three, and tendo-achilles sheath—one.[12] Allen found the knee, foot, thigh, ankle, hand and elbow as the most frequent sites.[1] Tillotson in a study of soft-tissue tumors on the sole of the foot, found seven cases of synovial sarcoma. Their behavior did not differ in regard to prognosis or metastasis from those found elsewhere in the body.[138] He found six in the sole and one in the medial arch. Coley and Pierson cite one case out of 15 as present in the sole of the foot.[32]

Cases at Henry Ford Hospital (1958–1968) showed only four cases of synovial sarcomas—three of the knee, and one of the great toe.[138] Cadman, in a series of 134 cases at the Mayo Clinic (1905–1960), found 95 (70%) in the lower extremity, with a distribution as follows: thigh—35, knee—21, foot—19, leg—10, ankle—six, groin—three, and hip—one. They also found three on the toes and one on the finger.[24]

Some cases which have been reported on the foot will be examined, in order to reinforce in our mind the possible occurrence of synovial sarcoma in this area. Since the diagnosis clinically is difficult, one must include this neoplasm in the differential diagnosis of any pain, tenderness, and/or swelling that has been present for a number of years and has not responded to conservative forms of treatment, especially in a young adult.

King reported a case in a 44 year old who sought treatment for an "infected toe" of one year duration.[80] Examination revealed an enlargement of the left third toe with a fungating mass with elevated edges and an ulcerated base on the plantar aspect of the toe, which was involved distal to the plantar fat pad. Treatment was amputation at the metatarsophalangeal joint. The flexor digitorum longus tendon was apparently involved. Despite this effort at surgical excision, the patient died in 18 months from distant metastases.

Another patient, a 38 year old male, sought attention for a swelling on his right ankle, of two years duration. Examination revealed a slight swelling along the peroneal tendon sheaths and excision revealed a synovial sarcoma. The patient died three months later.

Briggs reported a case of a 30 year old female with a synovial sarcoma on the plantar aspect of the left foot.[19] About ten years previously, she had what was thought to be a simple benign cyst excised. About three years after excision, a swelling developed at the operative site at the base of the great toe which slowly increased in size, causing local pain and ambulatory discomfort. Examination revealed a flattened, lobulated tumor beneath the old scar not attached to the skin. X-rays were negative. Following local excision, the patient received radiation therapy. However, two years later the tumor recurred and grew rapidly; exploration revealed an invasive growth attached to most of the tendons on the plantar surface of the foot. Further x-ray therapy was given but with only temporary relief. Two years later the foot was amputated because of extensive ulceration, with the patient dying a year later due to pulmonary metastasis.

Raben reported seven cases of synovial sarcoma on the foot.[110] Two patients had local excision, and subsequent below-knee amputation, and were still alive five years after diagnosis. One had symptoms eight years before diagnosis and another seven months before diagnosis. A third patient had symptoms two months before diagnosis and died seven years later from distant metastases. A fourth patient, eight years old at the time of diagnosis, had symptoms for seven and one-half years and then died of the malignancy at the age of 16. Another patient, with a synovial sarcoma of the foot, had symptoms for four years before diagnosis, had two local excisions, followed by supra-condylar amputation, but died five years after diagnosis, six months after the amputation.

Their sixth case had a primary foot lesion, but entered the hospital with distant metastasis already present. She was 20 years old and had symptoms for three to four years. Multiple local excisions, followed by radiation therapy and below-knee amputation were tried, but she died within two years. The seventh patient entered the hospital with symptoms for four to five years previous, but, despite local excisions, radiation therapy, and below-knee amputation, he died in one year.

Bennett reported a case of a 22 year old male with a tendo-achilles lesion of seven months duration, who denied any history of trauma.[12] Treatment consisted of local excisions with subsequent recurrence. The patient was still alive four years later.

A 24 year old male, with synovial sarcoma of the heel, who denied any trauma, had been aware of the mass for five months prior to local excision. One month later an above-knee amputation was performed, and the patient was reportedly living with no evidence of metastasis after 40 months.

Thompson reported a case in a 47 year old female with a painful mass, over the plantar surface of the left first metatarsophalangeal joint, for four months. She had had an excision of a spur, ten years previously. Examination revealed a non-tender, small mass enclosed in a bursa on the medio-plantar surface of the joint. Radiographic and laboratory studies were normal. Local excision revealed a low-grade synovial sarcoma. She subsequently had bilateral Keller bunionectomies and is living free of disease ten years later.[135]

### Treatment

The philosophy of Cadman is as follows:[24] "The appropriate therapy for synovial sarcoma must consider soft tissue tumors as a whole. When a surgeon is faced with a soft tissue tumor, it is imperative for him to know the histologic diagnosis before choosing the therapy." Pickren feels that enucleation of soft tissue tumors before determining their histologic characteristic is wrong, for if the tumor is malignant, "the procedure of enucleation has resulted in opening

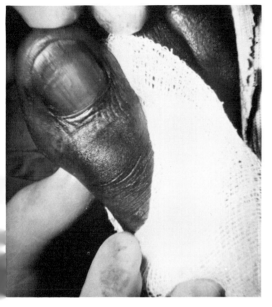

**Figure 3-17A**

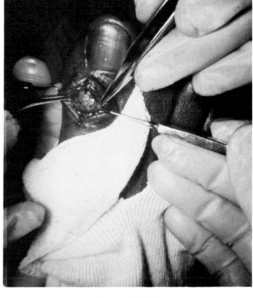

**Figure 3-17B**

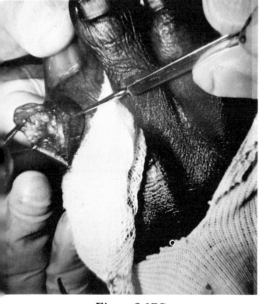

**Figure 3-17C**

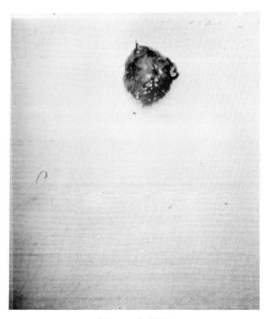

**Figure 3-17D**

Giant Cell Tumor. Giant cell tumors of the digits have infrequently been reported. (A) clinically, the lesion reveals a small swelling of the IP joint of the hallux toe. (B) on the surgical exposure, one sees a small, round, firm, yellowish lesion on the IP joint. (C) reveals a complete surgical dissection. (D) reveals a gross specimen; slight gray streaks are also seen. Clinically it closely resembles that of a small lipoma, except that it is much firmer in nature.

wide planes of tissue so that the tumor may implant centimeters away from its previous border, [and definitive
therapy then becomes more complicated and] may mean that
in order to adequately remove the local tumor, amputation is
required when radical local excision may have sufficed
before the procedure."[108]

When faced with a soft tissue tumor, the procedure of
choice is to remove a small biopsy for diagnostic purposes,
for after a histologic diagnosis is established, the surgeon can
proceed appropriately. "If the lesion is operable, the surgeon
then must design the operation so the area of primary tumor
growth and the immediate lymphatic drainage can be removed. In addition, the procedure must be designed to
minimize and hopefully present the local and distant dissemination which may occur as a result of the operative procedure. Only recently have surgeons become aware of the
dangers of vascular and lymphatic embolization as well as
local implantation which may occur directly as a result of the
operative manipulation and trauma."[95]

Haagensen and Stout are not certain if inadequate surgery renders the tumor more malignant.[67]

When operating upon a patient suspected of having any
malignant neoplasm, the surgeon should intensify efforts to
minimize trauma and handle tissues as gently as possible.
"The skin incision should be well placed and should be of
adequate length so that excessive manipulation of the tumor
will not be necessary."[95] The primary therapy should be
radical surgical extirpation requiring at least the removal of a
one centimeter zone of normal tissue all around the tumor.
"Due to the location of many of these tumors, it is impractical
to do radical local excisions, thus requiring amputation."[108]

Therefore, a carefully limited biopsy and a high immediate amputation (and possible regional node dissection)
provide for the most rational therapy, according to
Haagensen and Stout.[67] The biopsy must be through incision,
not aspiration, because the diagnosis rests on the histologic
architecture of the lesion. The incisional biopsy should be a
limited one, obtaining enough of the neoplasm to make an
adequate histological interpretation. Biopsy of the tissue

should be repaired in layers, with good hemostasis. Extensive exploratory dissections of the tumor or incision of a large portion or of the whole tumor for biopsy are undesirable and may be a serious threat to the patient's life.

Cadman believes local excision to be a poor treatment since seven percent of their patients had recurrence at the primary tumor site.[24] Amputation was the treatment of choice. Cadman also stated that the biologic nature of the lesion is probably the major factor governing the outcome, and early radical surgery achieves only a modest improvement in survival.

Giannestras believes that, in the absence of demonstrable metastasis, the treatment of synovial sarcoma of the foot should be below-knee amputation.[60] Raben believes that for foot, ankle, hand, and wrist tumors, a below-knee or below-elbow amputation is indicated.[110] In Ariel and Packs' series of 25 cases, 12 patients had biopsy and immediate amputation.[6] One with synovial sarcoma of the distal foot had a "conservative" amputation (site of amputation was not specified), and was well 12 years later. Local excision and radical amputation were performed on seven patients, and local excision and radical tridimensional resection were performed on six patients. The best results were in the latter group. a 70 percent recurrence rate with local excision emphasized that conservative therapy seldom, if ever, cures synovial sarcoma. Since the tumor is not encapsulated, the most conservative procedure that should be done is an extensive, tridimensional, local dissection.

Previous treatment with heat, diathermy, and observation were utilized in many of these cases prior to surgery. An extreme example of the lethal nature of this tumor occurred in a one year old girl with synovial sarcoma on the plantar surface of the foot.[6] She died one year later, after a mid-leg amputation. Von Andel emphasized that there is no concurrence of opinion on the best therapy.[141] The principal differences are between extensive local excision or amputation. Regional lymph node dissection and radio-therapy are less frequent treatments. Radiation alone should not be attempted, for it does not destroy a large section of the neoplasm and is futile, even as a palliative measure.[6,24,67,108]

*Prognosis*

Distant metastases usually occur via the blood vessels.[114] Haagensen and Stout reported regional lymph node metastasis in 12 of 104 cases,[67] whereas Ariel and Pack found 19 percent of their patients had metastases to regional nodes and concluded that resection of the nodes was required in the treatment plan.[6] Pickren performed autopsies on five patients and found the pleura to be the most frequent metastasis site, but the lungs, lymph nodes, bone, and pericardium were also sites of involvement.[108] Cadman found the lung involved in 81.4 percent, regional nodes in 23 percent, and bone in 20 percent.[24]

Spread to regional lymph nodes is characteristic and dictates the need for regional node dissection whenever an amputation is performed even in the absence of palpable glands. Even the early well-differentiated lesions that appear histologically innocent carry a grave prognosis and five year survivals are infrequent (approximately 10–25%). Haagensen and Stout's nine new cases and 95 previously reported cases found only three known to be free from evidence of metastasis more than five years after therapy.[67] Lichenstein thinks a ten year survival indicates a permanent cure.[87] Allen believes that even with a limb amputation, prognosis must be guarded.[1] In Ariel and Packs' study of 25 cases, 19 cases showed a 29 percent five year survival rate. In evaluating factors influencing prognosis, the more distant the neoplasm the better the outlook.[6] In one series, the locations of the neoplasms with the best survival were as follows: toe—one, foot—two, lower leg—one, thigh—one, and hand—one. Of those patients with tumors on the buttocks, thigh, knee, and abdominal wall, all had died.

Tillotson believes that the course tends to be longer with repeated local excisions (if this is the primary treatment) for many years.[138] Prognosis is poor, due to a high metastatic rate.

The prognosis varies according to the following

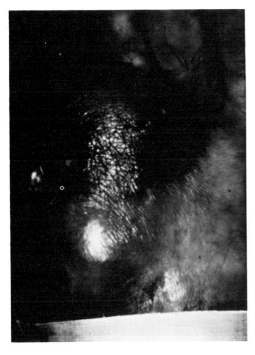

**Figure 3-18**

Benign Synovioma. Benign synoviomas are rare in the foot. In many instances they are somewhat difficult to distinguish between the benign and malignant variety. *(Courtesy Robert Weinstock, D.P.M., Grosse Pt. Farms, Mich.)*

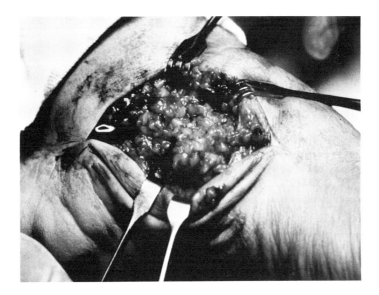

**Figure 3-19**

Synovial Sarcoma. Synovial sarcomas are one of the more frequent malignancies located in the foot. In regard to tumors of muscles, tendons and joints, it is probably the most common of all these malignancies. *(Courtesy of Adolf Galinski, D.P.M., Chicago, Ill.)*

aspects:

1) Age: Recovery is more likely in younger individuals.

2) Rate of Growth: Slower growing tumors remain localized for a longer time and have a better prognosis than the more rapid growing and more diffuse tumors.

3) Treatment: Aggressive therapy is the surgeon's best weapon.

Synovial sarcoma presents a formidable challenge to the clinician, surgeon, radiotherapist, pathologist, and oncologist in spite of its low incidence. Early diagnosis and decision as to the best therapy continue to be the biggest problems.

## Clear Cell Sarcoma

### Definition and History

Clear cell sarcoma is a rare, slowly growing malignant tumor of the extremities found in young adults. It was first described in 1965 by Enzinger as "Clear cell sarcoma of tendons and aponeurosis."[46]

### Incidence

Out of 30 cases reported in the literature, 22 were found to be in the lower extremity, with the foot being the most common site. The distribution in the foot area was as follows: five involving the achilles tendons, seven—the patellar tendon, five—the plantar aspect of the foot, and two—the lesser toes.

### Clinical Picture

The tumor may be described as a usually painless, nonfluctuant, firm, slightly movable swelling or mass. It is sometimes present for many years before treatment, is always attached to tendons and aponeurosis of the upper or lower extremities, is characterized by slow but relentless growth, and has a tendency toward repeated recurrences and eventual metastasis.

*Diagnosis*

Clear cell sarcoma is a slowly growing, painless tumor in the lower extremity of a young adult; x-rays are devoid of any specific feature. Definitive diagnosis can be made only by biopsy.

*Differential Diagnosis*

Clear cell sarcomas must be differentiated from the following tumors:[46]

1. *Synovial sarcoma:* Clear cell sarcomas are painless and slowly growing tumors, located around tendons and apo-neurosis. Histopathologically, they have an "epithelioid" cellular appearance, show mucoid material and hemosiderin, and lack a biphasic cell pattern and pseudo-acinar structures. Histochemically, synovial sarcoma shows moderate amounts of PAS-positive material which resists diastase digestion, while the clear cell sarcomas contain only a few PAS-positive intracellular granules which are removed with diastase.[44]

2. *Fibrosarcoma:* Clear cell sarcoma has no fibroblasts present.

3. *Malignant melanoma:* Clear cell sarcomas contain iron positive granules, have a prolonged clinical course, and are not associated with pigmented skin lesions.

*Pathology*

Grossly, the tumor varies from 2–6 centimeters in diameter and is firm, ovoid, solid, well demarcated, and has a smooth nodular surface. It is surrounded by dense fibrous tissue of varying thickness and is usually gray to white.

Microscopically, the tumor has a homogenous appearance characterized by round or spindle-shaped, pale-staining, epithelioid-like cells, which are arranged in compact nests and fascicles, well defined by septa of fibrous connective tissue. The septa is continuous with dense collagenous structures that cross the tumor and merge with tendinous or aponeurotic tissue. The cells are usually pale-staining and amphophilic with indistinct cytoplasmic borders. The nuclei are round or ovoid and contain a small

amount of dispersed chromatin with centrally located basophilic, deeply-staining nucleolus. Special stains for
characterization[46] include: the periodic-acid-Schiff reaction
(PAS), Rinehart-Abdul-Hai-stain for acid mucopolysac-
charides (AMP), and Gomori's iron stains which show extra-
cellular and intracellular iron.

*Treatment*

The best treatment is adequate surgical excision. If local
excision is not adequate, recurrence is the rule. Metastases
will occur, although months to years later. The most common
sites of metastasis are the regional lymph nodes, lung, heart,
liver, and brain in that order of frequency.

*Prognosis*

Enzinger reports that no significant differences appear
between patients treated early or those treated after several
recurrences.[46] Also, there is no apparent correlation between
the preoperative duration of the symptoms and the length of
survival, as survival periods vary considerably.

**Leiomyoma**

*Definition*

Leiomyomas are tumors which derive from smooth muscle tissue and may be superficial or deep in nature.

*History*

Leiomyomas of the skin are rare and seldom recognized.
According to Fisher[50] and other researchers, there is a belief
that multiple cutaneous leiomyomas arise from the arrector
pilorum muscle, that leiomyoma limited to the genital areas
and nipples arise from the dartoid and mammillary muscles,
and that angiomyomas, or subcutaneous encapsulated
leiomyomas containing thick walled vessels, arise from the
smooth muscles of veins.

*Incidence*

Solitary cutaneous leiomyoma appearing as a firm, red-

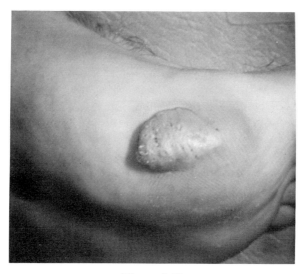

**Figure 3-20**

Superficial Leiomyoma. Leiomyomas of the foot are rare tumors. However, this is a lesion which is believed to have developed in the erector pilorum muscles of the skin. The small pitted hyperkeratotic areas located around the lesion are believed to be due primarily to weight-bearing pressures.

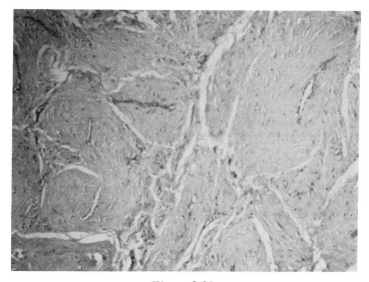

**Figure 3-21**

Vascular Leiomyoma. The tumor is composed of numerous slit-like vascular spaces surrounded by bundles of smooth muscle.

161

dish nodule have been found in seven patients.

Kloepfer[6] believes that the disease is hereditary due to an autosomal dominant gene of incomplete penetrance.[81] A case, reported by Rudner and Schwartz, supports this hypothesis, presenting multiple cutaneous leiomyomas in identical twins.[117]

Duhig and Ayer reviewed 61 cases of vascular leiomyoma and found the greatest number of cases occurring in persons aged 30 to 50 years.[43] The duration of symptoms ranged from two months in one case to 25 years in another. They were twice as common in females than males. By far the greatest number of tumors arose in the lower limbs for, of the 61 cases, 43 arose in or around the foot, the ankle, or the leg below the knee, and of these 23 were on the left and 20 on the right.[43]

### Etiology

Like other muscle tumors, the etiologic agent is unknown. Trauma appears to be one of the more common contributing causes.

### Clinical Picture

The most frequent complaint in leiomyoma is a simple tumor mass or swelling that has grown slowly; however, rapid growth may take place. Most cases were associated with swelling, pain, tenderness, muscle spasm, limited range of motion, or nerve dysfunction (rare). Calcification in the tumor was demonstrated radiographically in several cases. Since many leiomyomas occur on the foot, several patients first noticed discomfort in wearing proper footgear. The most striking clinical feature of the leiomyoma is pain on pressure.

### Pathology

Grossly, leiomyomas vary in size from almost microscopic size to several kilograms. Whereas the larger leiomyomas are usually firm and surrounded by a capsular structure, the smaller tumors are less distinguishable. Leiomyomas are well differentiated tumors composed of in-

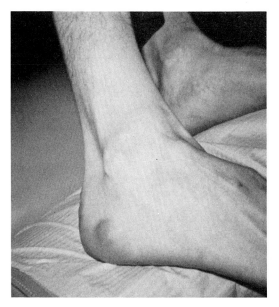

**Figure 3-22A**

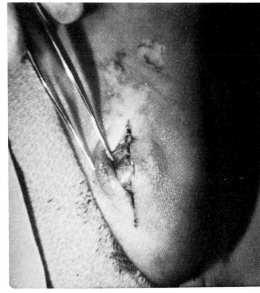

**Figure 3-22B**

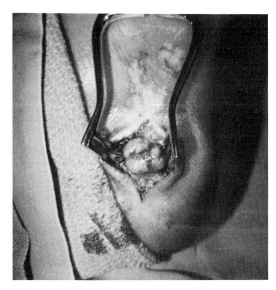

**Figure 3-22C**

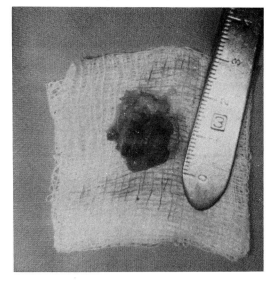

**Figure 3-22D**

Vascular Leiomyoma. (A) clinical picture reveals a very firm, round tumor on the lateral aspect of the heel. The lesion became somewhat painful on pressure. However, it has been present for many years. (B) reveals the lesio lsely underlying the skin. (C) reveals the neoplasm and surrounding tissue being completely excised. (D) reveals the surgical gross specimen.

terlacing bundles of smooth muscle cells with elongated cigar shaped nuclei and intracellular myofibrils. They are usually firm, bluish in color, of rubbery consistency, and nodular on palpation. When surgically opened they have a whitish-grey content with small areas of hemorrhage.

## Differential Diagnosis

Glomus tumor, lipoma, fibroma, and ganglion are the more common benign tumors that can be included. However, we cannot rule out the possibility of a metastatic or primarily malignant tumor by external examination, so that excisional biopsy of the smaller tumors is essential for definitive diagnosis; the larger tumors should either have a biopsy done prior to surgical excision or a frozen section diagnosis during surgery.

## Foot Involvement

Reported cases in the foot are rare; however a number have been reported. Gate reported a malignant leiomyoma (leiomyosarcoma) of the ankle, the lesion later metastasizing to the inguinal nodes.[57] Rakow described an angioleiomyoma on the lateral surface of the right foot in a 71 year old man.[112] It was relatively painless, but bled several times as a result of trauma. It was a well defined, circumscribed mass attached to the skin by a pedicle.

Bulmer described four cases of leiomyoma in the foot, two on the dorsum and two on the sole.[21] One of his cases involved a 26 year old female who had suffered a crushing injury in her right foot. She had developed pain and loss of dorsiflexion in the first metatarsophalangeal joint. Seven years later she was surgically treated for hallux rigidus. Incision of the skin at that time revealed a subcutaneous tumor overlying the capsule of the first metatarsophalangeal joint. The joint was found to be normal. Fourteen months later the joint was once again stiff and painful and a second exploration revealed recurrence of the leiomyoma. Another case by Bulmer involved a 61 year old female with a painful left great toe, due to traumatic injury. Nine months later, an area of swelling was noted on the plantar aspect of the second metatarsal neck. A preoperative diagnosis of glomus tumor was made, but surgical exploration revealed a leiomyoma. The tumor was removed but recurred three years later, and was again surgically excised.

Haug and associates reviewed the literature and found three cases involving the foot.[71] As early as 1868, Aufecht described a leiomyoma over the right medial malleolus originating from the saphenous vein, in a nine year old child. Another case reported by Borchard (1906) occurred, in a 44 year old male, over the left malleolus also originating from the saphenous vein and present for two years.[21,43,62]

A third case reported by Schnyder (1914) involved a leiomyoma over the lateral malleolus of a 27 year old female. The lesion was described as an asymptomatic, firm, nodular swelling, originating from the dorsal metatarsal vein.

Perles and Roth (1968) reported on a 50 year old caucasian woman who presented a palpable subcutaneous mass on the medial side of the left heel area, near the Achilles tendon insertion. The mass hindered normal ambulation with certain footgear and was surgically excised. The leiomyoma was well encapsulated and could be easily removed. Since the tumor occurred in a region in which no hair was evident, the authors felt that this leiomyoma arose from the tunica media layer of a regional blood vessel.[106]

McCain and Galinski (1969) reported a palpable subcutaneous leiomyoma, 0.5 centimeter in diameter, on the lateral aspect of the right heel area in a 59 year old female. The mass was very painful when foot gear was worn. It was found to be well encapsulated and apparently arose from a blood vessel since the tumor was composed of blood vessels encircled by smooth muscle cells. The authors felt that tumors of this nature were usually found on the dorsal surface of the extremities although cases have been reported on the plantar surface. The author's personal experience has shown equal involvement on the dorsal or plantar surface with one case on the lateral border of the heel in our three cases. They also felt very strongly that leiomyomas of the extremities may not be as rare as the literature reports them to be.[92]

**165**

A vascular leiomyoma was reported by Lobbato (1963) in a 45 year old female who complained of a painful mass on the plantar aspect of the left foot, present for two months. Examination revealed a freely movable mass between the second and third metatarsals. Excisional biopsy revealed a well delineated tumor composed of regular, interlacing, smooth muscle fibers with scattered vascular channels.[89]

## Treatment

Surgical excision of the entire tumor mass, with meticulous dissection, is the only form of treatment.

## Prognosis

If completely excised, surgery is curative. However, if surgical excision is incomplete, recurrence is the rule.

## Leiomyosarcoma

### Definition

Leiomyosarcomas are rare malignant tumors of smooth muscle origin, the malignant counterpart of the more common leiomyoma. The majority of smooth muscle tumors develop in the uterus (myometrium). Less commonly, they may be found in the gastrointestinal tract and other tissue including the retroperitoneum, vascular, and osseous tissues.

### History

Historically, Perl (1871) is credited with the first report of a leiomyosarcoma arising from a major vein, a leiomyosarcoma of the inferior vena cava. The first case of leiomyosarcoma of the femoral vein was described by Haug (1954) in which a painless swelling was noticed below the right knee of an adult male, subsiding when the leg was raised. Sixteen months later, the swelling had spread up the thigh and surgical excision showed a mass overlying the right femoral vein, diagnosed as a leiomyosarcoma.[71]

Dorfman and Fishel (1963) reported a leiomyosarcoma of the greater saphenous vein of a 56 year old male, over the medial aspect of the right thigh, just above the popliteal area. Histologically, the tumor involved the adventitia of the vein, and merged with the outer muscle layers of the media.[40]

Botting and Soule (1964) described 18 cases of smooth muscle tumors in children, eight were leiomyomas and ten leiomyosarcomas. They concluded that these tumors had no predilection for specific location when compared to those found in adults.[15]

In a review of the literature of skin and bone origin by Evans and Sanerkin, a primary leiomyosarcoma of bone was described in a 73 year old male. Radiographically, there was an extensive osteolytic lesion of the upper end of the left tibia, with extension into the joint. Histologically, the tumor was a typical leiomyosarcoma, differentiating it from an osteogenic sarcoma.[47]

In a French paper, Leturque described a profuse cutaneous nodular leiomyosarcoma with associated polyglobulinemia found over the leg and thigh.[86]

Cheek and Nickey (1965) reported several cases of leiomyosarcoma of venous origin.[27] Allison (1965) reported a leiomyosarcoma of the femoral vein in a 45 month old girl who had a swelling in the groin. A firm mass resembling a lymph node and attached to the saphenous vein was removed at the sapheno-femoral junction.[2]

Crosby and associates (1965) discussed a case of leiomyosarcoma of the right iliac vein in a 59 year old female complaining of swelling of the right leg during the preceding four months. The severe unilateral edema and painful leg were treated with anticoagulants (for venous obstruction) and a Jobst support stocking. The patient returned two years later with the same symptoms and at that time the mass was surgically excised.[34]

Johnson reported a leiomyosarcoma of the superficial femoral vein. The tumor occurred in a 67 year old white female and was apparently asymptomatic, except for the presence of a firm nodular mass measuring 6 x 7 centimeters located in the right inguinal area.[79]

White (1971) reported a case in an 86 year old female, who presented with pain of the left foot and ankle and edema extending from below the medial malleolus to the forefoot. The primary diagnosis of osteoarthritis was made, and she responded well to conservative treatment. However, two years later a palpable subcutaneous mass appeared just below the medial malleolus which was painful on ambulation or at rest. A leiomyosarcoma was diagnosed by biopsy and a below-the-knee amputation performed. No evidence of metastasis was found.[143]

### Incidence

Hare and Cerny, in a review of 200 soft tissue sarcomas, found that leiomyosarcomas comprised 6.5 percent of the cases.[69] In Stout's review they were the third most frequent sarcoma, the majority being found in the uterus (77%), while the gastrointestinal tract was the second most common location.[132]

Leiomyosarcomas of the lower extremity arise primarily from veins. Thorjnarson found that 11 percent of soft tissue sarcomas were of smooth muscle origin.[137] In a study by Stout, of 105 cases of primary soft tissue malignancy, only two cases of leiomyosarcoma of vascular origin were noted. Until 1963, only twenty cases of leiomyosarcoma of vascular origin had been reported in the world literature.

Patients with leiomyosarcoma of veins ranged in age from 27–83 years although these lesions have been found in children as young as four years. There seems to be a greater predominance in females with no apparent reason to account for this fact.

### Etiology

No etiologic factors have ever been proven although origin from previous leiomyomas is well known.

### Foot Involvement

Foot involvement has been reported, but with extreme rarity.[143]

### Clinical Picture

Clinically these tumors are often confused with their

benign counterpart, leiomyoma, with signs and symptoms being very similar. Accurate biopsy is needed to confirm one's suspicion. According to Cheek and Nickey, the symptomatology and clinical findings vary according to the venous channels involved. Those involving superficial veins or peripheral deep veins produce a palpable mass in nearly every case. Whereas, when the superficial veins are the site of origin, edema or thrombophlebitis does not occur due to the collateral circulation that develops. The masses show slow, continuous growth without symptoms, although the rate varies from one to another.

When the deep peripheral veins are the site of origin, such as the femoral vein, intermittent or persistent edema, sometimes with thrombophlebitis, may be observed. Most of these tumors are associated with a long history of symptoms, especially when of inferior vena cava etiology due to their slow growth. In the cases review by Cheek, eight demonstrated edema of the lower extremity.[27]

### Differential Diagnosis

The occurrence of leiomyosarcoma has been so rare that any small sarcoma could be a differential diagnosis clinically. Histologically it could possibly be confused with a leiomyoma.

### Pathology

The pathology of leiomyosarcomas is the same whether of vascular or some other origin. Stout, reviewing leiomyosarcoma of subcutaneous tissues, believed that the frequency of mitosis was the most significant histological criterion of malignancy.[133] He indicated that a smooth muscle neoplasm, showing an average of one mitosis in every five high power fields, should be considered malignant, that is, a leiomyosarcoma with the degree of malignancy proportional to the number of mitotic figures.

### Treatment

The only possible hope for cure rests upon complete surgical excision. Radiation therapy and chemical therapy are of little value. Recurrence, therefore, is frequent due to the difficulty in complete extirpation of the tumor without radical surgery. Often amputation is the treatment of choice.

### Prognosis

As noted above, prognosis is poor because of the difficulty in total removal of the tumor and therefore its high rate of local recurrence and metastasis.

## Rhabdomyoma

### Definition

A rhabdomyoma is a rare, benign, true neoplasm originating from skeletal muscle. It has been confused in the literature with myoblastoma and rhabdomyosarcoma.[42,49,52,99,103]

### History

Dowling reported that until 1966 only 14 true examples of rhabdomyoma could be found in the literature.[42] Because of the rarity of this benign skeletal muscle tumor, knowledge of it is extremely limited. In the early literature, there was confusion with regard to the distinguishing features between benign and malignant tumors of skeletal muscle origin (i.e. rhabdomyomas and rhabdomyosarcomas). Many early articles still were not certain that a distinction could be made between malignant or benign varients. Parson (1965) stated that no true case of rhabdomyoma had ever been reported in the literature other than that of the fetal variety, which is located predominantly and almost exclusively in cardiac muscle tissue.[102]

### Incidence

No bonafide case of rhabdomyoma has yet been reported in the foot or even in the lower extremity. Cases which were originally reported as rhabdomyoma in the lower extremity were later shown to be granular cell myoblastomas.

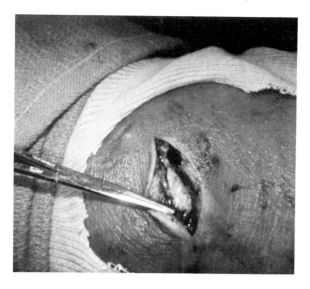

**Figure 3-23A**

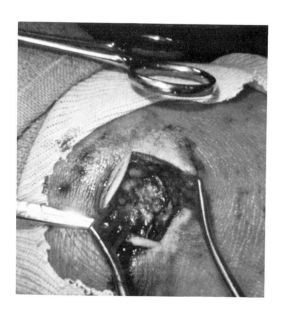

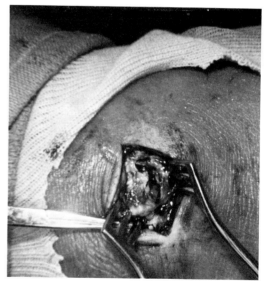

Dowling reported that of all rhabdomyomas he found in the literature, 75 percent were in males between the ages of three and 35 years.[42] Cardiac muscle was the primary tissue involved. Foot emphasized that rhabdomyomas could occur in the lower extremity, but reported no cases.[52]

*Clinical Picture*

Because rhabdomyomas have never been reported in the lower extremity, characteristic signs and symptoms cannot be discussed. (Rhabdomyosarcomas are rare, but do occur in the lower extremity.) Non-specific signs and symptoms of any soft tissue tumor, however, would probably include pain, and an enlarging mass.

(The only radiologic evidence of rhabdomyoma that can be demonstrated is an apparent increase in the soft tissue density. However, this radiographic finding is common in many soft tissue tumors and cannot be considered a true differentiating diagnosis.)

*Diagnosis*

According to some authors, there are several criteria for the diagnosis of a benign rhabdomyoma, in contrast to a rhabdomyosarcoma. These symptoms include: soft tissue swelling of very long duration; a tumor arising strictly from skeletal muscle in the adult type since the fetal type is associated with cardiac muscle containing cells with cross-striations; the presence of an intact capsule without evidence of invasion which is histologically benign and shows no evidence of anaplasia or metaplasia; and the absence of giant cells and mitotic features.

*Differential Diagnosis*

Differential diagnosis of rhabdomyoma must be made with synovioma since both these two originate near joints. Rhabdomyoma, however, has the masses of fibers and synovium coagulum.

*Foot Involvement*

Rhabdomyomas are extremely rare tumors and its

presence on the foot may be nonexistent. Our review of the literature has not provided us with any reported cases on the foot.

*Pathology*

Rhabdomyomas can only be identified by histopathological and histochemical means. The presence of cross-striations in the tumor cells is the crucial point for identifying this skeletal muscle tumor and differentiating it from a granular cell myoblastoma. Some of the differential features between rhabdomyomas and granular cell myoblastomas are as follows: vacuolization is present in rhabdomyomas but absent in granular cell myoblastoma (GCM); cytoplasmic myosin crystals are demonstrable in rhabdomyomas, but not in GCM; cells of rhabdomyomas are much larger, with much more variation in shape from those of the GCM; rhabdomyoma cells have a true cytoplasmic membrane; rhabdomyomas do not have an affinity for the PAS stain, while the granular particles of granular myoblastoma do.[9,10,25,36] (This may be the most important differential feature and the easiest to document.)

Grossly, the tumor is bulky, has a light brown or tan color, is elongated, and usually occurs in the belly of the muscle involved.[36] Types of rhabdomyomas are nodular, cellular, mixed, and cystic. Those distinguished as being nodular are soft and grayish, with markings produced by muscle bundles alternating with connective tissue stroma. The cellular are more opaque, yellowish or reddish, soft, and more diffuse. The mixed are varied in appearance, similar to a teratoma, while the cystic have bundles of intertwining strands of muscle fibers supported by embryonic connective tissue which may encircle blood vessels. The cells of all four gross types seldom exhibit similar adult characteristics.

*Treatment*

Successful treatment of rhabdomyoma can only be accomplished by complete excision of the tumor.

## Prognosis

If the pathologist reports no tumor on the resection margins, the prognosis is generally favorable. With incomplete excision, recurrence is likely.

## Rhabdomyosarcoma

### Definition

A rhabdomyosarcoma is a combined sarcoma and rhabdomyoma containing striated muscle fibers.[41]

### History

Considering the large amount of voluntary muscle in the human body, rhabdomyosarcomas seem to occur very infrequently. Weber (1854) first described a "localized enlargement of the tongue" in a 21 year old male.[142] His treatment was by excision, but the mass later reappeared. It was examined and found to be of striated muscle cells in all stages of development from embryonic to adult forms.[130] Many reports on striated muscle tumors appear in the literature. Rhabdomyosarcomas are of very variable gross characteristics, appearance, and rate of growth. They affect both sexes at all ages and have been found in many cases, systems and regions of the body.

### Etiology

The etiology is unknown, but Perk and Maloney reported the isolation of a virus which induces rhabdomyosarcoma in mice and revealed an alarming predilection for muscular tissue.[104] However, the only etiological factor that has been recorded in man has been chronic irritation due to an ununited fracture of the femur, followed by a tumor of the thigh. Two such cases have been reported.[101] In Stout's study of 121 cases, 14 had a history of some trauma in the location of the neoplasm.[130]

**174**

*Incidence*

As previously mentioned, rhabdomyosarcomas can affect various regions and organ systems of the body. Findings by Stout indicate that "the more common areas affected are the genito-urinary system, kidney, bladder, prostate, testes, spermatic cord, uterus, vagina, round ligament, ovary, upper respiratory and alimentary tracts, and orbit; and sporadic examples have been found in the lungs, breast, esophagus, and brain. In addition, there have been reports of cases which have developed in striated muscles and other soft parts of the body."[130] In almost every case the tumor developed with or was attached to a striated muscle.

The literature indicates a slight preponderance in males with the greatest number of cases involving patients in the fifth and sixth decades; however, the tumor has been found in infancy and old age. Stout states that of the 121 cases, the most common area involved was the lower extremity.[130,136,144]

Saavedra and Martin in a study of 35 cases of rhabdomyosarcoma reported a higher incidence of pleomorphic rhabdomyosarcoma in the extremities of older patients. The pleomorphic rhabdomyosarcoma, because of its location in the extremities and because it may remain localized for a long time, offers a more favorable prospect of surgical cure than other variants of rhabdomyosarcoma. Of the seven alveolar rhabdomyosarcoma studied, four were situated on the extremities.[118]

*Clinical Picture*

Muscle tumors are usually asymptomatic except for some local manifestations, such as swelling, pain, limitation of motion, or interference with function. Commonly the only symptom is a localized swelling.[130] The mass usually appears de novo, is often painless, and seldom interferes with function or causes limitation of motion. Perhaps this is the reason why patients seek advice in later stages. Increase in size may be rapid or very slow. "The deep situation and muscular involvement produces a moderately firm, deep seated mass which is of very limited mobility."[180] Occasionally, the growth of the rhabdomyosarcoma compromises the overlying skin and the tumor fungates. Pleomorphic rhabdomyo-sarcomas are more commonly found in the lower extremities of older patients, while the alveolar rhabdomyosarcomas are usually found on the extremities and the head and neck of young adults. The embryonal tumor arises chiefly on the head and neck of children, while the botyroid form is usually found in hollow viscera and body cavities of infants.

Metastases takes place through the blood and lymphatic systems as well as direct local invasion. In Stout's series of 121 cases, 38 patients had metastases with the lungs being the most common site. The median age for this neoplasm in Stout's study was 42.1 years, with ages ranging from birth to 84.[130]

## Diagnosis

If the astute clinician finds a fairly well-defined tumor of soft to firm consistency within a muscle that is growing rapidly and is painless, with or without skin involvement, he should consider the possibility of a rhabdomyosarcoma arising from a voluntary muscle. However, to make a positive diagnosis, a biopsy of the lesion must be taken.

Rosenberg describes the value of arteriography in the diagnosis of soft tissue tumors of the extremities.[115] Three rhabdomyosarcomas showed small, tortuous vessels, with arteriovenous communications and puddling of contrast material in vascular spaces. Arteriographic studies were also helpful in differentiating benign from malignant lesions, delineating the extent of neoplastic involvement, detecting metastases, and planning surgical therapy.

## Differential Diagnosis

The rhabdomyosarcoma may be confused with any soft tissue tumor, especially the liposarcomas and fibrosarcomas. Liposarcomas form bizarre giant cells but the nuclei are very apt to be pyknotic, and intracellular fat globules are always present in some part of the tumor. Fibrosarcomas can be confused with rhabdomyosarcoma because the cells are often elongated, and connective tissue fibers are usually present between them.

*Pathology*

The gross characteristics of the tumor vary greatly, especially with regard to its texture and consistency, due to the amount of collagen within it. Generally, it is somewhat soft and reddish brown and may be mottled with various shades of red and gray from hemorrhage and necrosis. It can be (and often is) circumscribed.

The cell of the rhabdomyoblastic tumor is variable in size and assumes one of three different shapes—rounded, strap-shaped with two or more nuclei arranged in tandem; or racquet shaped with a single nucleus; or one expanded rounded end and a tapering body extending outward. The cytoplasm is often granular and generally acidophilic. With special staining, either cross striations, longitudinal myofibrils, or some suggestion of their formation should be seen. However, the formation of cross-striations and longitudinal myofibrils may vary in embryonic and adult myoblasts. Marchland (1885) found that the tumor cells are sometimes vacuolated with glycogen.[130] "These vacuoles in cells of giant size, peripherally arranged with cytoplasmic strands separating them and radiating outward from the nucleus have been called spider cells."[130] It must be noted that Thompson reported that in 39 of his cases, not one contained spider cells.[136]

Rakov stated that essential features for a diagnosis of a rhabdomyosarcoma include: polymorphism of the tumor cells, presence of spindle cells, presence of giant cells, peculiar arrangement of the stroma, and the existence of fibrils in the cytoplasm which may be striated.[111]

*Foot Involvement*

Of Stout's 121 cases, only one rhabdomyosarcoma was found on the foot.[130] The case involved a 66 year old female with a small purple nodule on the medial aspect of her right foot in the area of the longitudinal arch, which was occasionally painful. She stated that it had grown slowly beneath the intact skin in the early stages, but after growing two years and eight months, by the time of surgery, the tumor was a large, fungating, ulcerated mass. The foot was then amputated and no other follow up was mentioned.

Horn and Enterline reported one case involving the sole of the left foot in a 44 year old white male. After treatment by amputation, the tumor had metastasized and the patient died nine months later.[74]

The largest study of embryonal rhabdomyosarcoma was by Soule and Associates (1969) which involved 235 cases. Of the patients in the study, the average age was 25.5. There were eight lesions involving the foot and one on the ankle.[127]

Linscheid and Associates (1965) reported a study of 87 cases at the Mayo Clinic between 1905 and 1961. The median patient age was 55; 46 percent involved the lower extremities with only one case involving the dorsum of the right foot.[88] Foot involvement is rare.

*Treatment*

Many types of therapy have been attempted on these tumors, but mainly radiotherapy, excision and/or amputation, or a combination of these methods.

The results were poor in the cases of 12 patients treated with roentgenography as the sole method of therapy; the tumor was resistant to the treatment in the ten patients who died. Preoperative radiation was used in 14 cases and postoperative radiation in 35 patients. Since surgery was performed, it is difficult to assess the effect of the radiation. In one case, postoperative radiation failed to prevent a local recurrence of the tumor.[130] We may assume that radiotherapy is generally of little value in the treatment of rhabdomyosarcomas in ordinary doses. It is possible that roentgen therapy in larger doses, pushed to the limits of tolerance would be beneficial, but this remains to be determined. The danger, of course, is concomitant destruction of normal tissue.

Local excision in 80 cases was found to have some merit in a few instances, but a majority of 63 patients all had recurrences or metastases; and of these, 36 had subsequent operations.[130] The most common complication of surgery was inadequate excision. Primary amputation or amputation after biopsy was carried out in 16 cases. Of these, seven patients were not followed, two died following surgery, and six had recurrences or metastases. Only one had a good result. In a large number of cases the best results can be obtained upon early diagnosis followed by radical excision or amputation.

*Prognosis*

The clinician should be careful in predicting the probable duration in any case of rhabdomyosarcoma. Stout studied 48 cases which were followed from onset until death.[130] Of these, the mean duration was 30 months, with the extremes being two months and 162 months. The average was 24.9 months. There is also a reported case in the literature lasting for 50 years. The duration of the tumor before treatment was 23.2 months in 84 cases studied; however, five cases had a long duration of from nine to 50 years before treatment was undertaken. If these were omitted, the mean duration for 79 cases would be 10.7 months.[130]

It has been shown that lesions of the upper extremity have a better prognosis than those of the lower extremity, and the more distal the lesion, the better the prognosis. However, the prognosis is still poor.

The postoperative course is most favorable when the diagnosis has been made early and the surgery radical; but this is an unpredictable malignant tumor, with a generally poor outcome.

## Bibliography

1. Allen, R.A., Woolner, L.B., and Ghormley, F.F.: Soft tissue tumors of the sole. *JBJS*, **37A**: 14, 1955.
2. Allison, M.F.: Leiomyosarcoma of the femoral vein: report of a case in a child. *Clin. Pediat.*, 4: 28–31, Jan., 1965.
3. Andren, L. and Elken, O: Arthrographic studies of wrist ganglia. *JBJS*, **53A**: 299–302, 1971.
4. Angervall, L., and Stener, B.: Clear cell sarcoma of tendons: a study of four cases. *Acta Pathologica et Microbiologica Scandinavica*, **77**: 589–597, 1969.
5. Arean, V.M. and Marcial-Rojas, R.A.: Rhabdomyosarcoma in children. *Amer. Jour. Surg.*, 93: 143–146, 1957.
6. Ariel, M.I. and Pack, G.T.: Synovial sarcoma: a review of 25 cases. *NEJM*, **268**: 1972, 1963.
7. Armed Forces Institute of Pathology Files, 1961–1965.
8. Arthaud, J.B.: Pigmented villonodular synovitis report of 11 lesions

in non-articular location. *Amer. Jour. of Clin. Path.*, **58**: 511–517, 1972.

9. Assor, D. and Thomas, J.R.: Multifocal rhabdomyoma: report of a case. *Eng. Arch. Otolaryng. (Chicago)*, **90**: 489–491, 1969.
10. Battifora, H.A., Eisenstein, R., and Shild, J.A.: Rhabdomyoma of larynx: ultrastructural study and comparison with granular cell tumors (myoblastomas). *Eng. Cancer*, **23**: 183–190, 1969.
11. Becker, W.F.: Hydrocortisone therapy in ganglia. *Industrial Med. and Surg.*, **22**: 555–557, 1953.
12. Bennett, G.A.: Malignant neoplasms originating in synovial tissue (synovioinota). *JBJS*, **29**: 259, 1947.
13. Berg, J. and McNeer, G.: Leiomyosarcoma of the stomach: a clinical and pathological study. *Cancer*, **13**: 96–101, 1960.
14. Berlin, S.J.: Giant cell tumor of the foot. *JAPA*, **60**: 389–392, 1970.
15. Botting, A.J. and Soule, E.H.: Smooth muscle tumors in children. *Cancer*, No. 6, **18**: 711–720, 1965.
16. Bowerman, J.W. and Muhletaler, C.: Arthrography of rheumatoid synovial cysts of the knee and wrist. *Jour. Canad. Assoc. of Radiol.*, **24**, 1973.
17. Bowman, J.T.: Rhabdomyosarcoma of striated muscle origin in pre-adolescent children. *Jour. Pediat.*, **55**: 620–634, 1959.
18. Breimer, C.W. and Freiberger, R.H.: Bone lesions associated with villonodular synovitis. *Amer. Jour. Roent.*, **79**: 618–629, 1958.
19. Briggs, C.D.: Malignant tumors of synovial origin. *Ann. Surg.*, **115**: 413, 1942.
20. Brooks, D.N.: Nerve compression by simple ganglia: a review of 13 collected cases. *JBJS*, **34B**: 391–400, 1952.
21. Bulmer, J.H.: Smooth muscle tumors of the limbs. *JBJS*, **49B**: no. 1, 1967.
22. Bunnell, S.: *Surgery of the Hand*, 1st ed. J.B. Lippincott, Co., Phila., 1944, p. 682.
23. Byers, P.D.: The diagnosis and treatment of pigmented villonodular-synovitis. *JBJS*, **50B**: 290–305, 1968.
24. Cadman, N.L., Soule, E.H., and Kelly, P.J.: Synovial sarcoma on analysis of 134 tumors. *Cancer*, **18**: 613, 1965.
25. Cantin, J., Moneer, G.P., Chu, F.C., and Booher, R.J.: The problem of local recurrence after treatment of soft tissue sarcome. *Eng. Ann. Surg.*, **168**: 47–53, 1968.
26. Carp, L. and Stout, A.P.: A study of ganglia with special reference to treatment. *Surg. Gyn. & Obst.*, **47**: 460–468, 1928.
27. Cheek, J.H. and Nickey, W.M.: Leiomyosarcoma of venous origin. *Arch. Surg.*, **90**: 396–400, 1965.
28. Childs, P.: Rhabdomyosarcoma of skeletal muscle. *Brit. Jour. Surg.*, **37**: 230–234, 1949.
29. Chung, S.M.K. and Jones, J.M.: Diffuse pigmented villonodular synovitis of the hip joint. *JBJS*, **47A**: 293–303, 1965.

30. Clark, W.S.: Pigmented villonodular synovitis. *Bull. Rheum. Dis.*, **8**: 161–162, 1958.

31. Coe, G.C.: Primary rhabdomyosarcoma of the heart. *Ann. Int. Med.*, **52**: 1124–1138, 1960.

32. Coley, B.L. and Pierson, J.G.: Synovioma: report of 15 cases with review of literature. *Surgery*, **1**: 113, 1937.

33. Crenshaw, A.H.: *Campbell's Operative Orthopedics.* Vol. I, II, 5th ed., C.V. Mosby Co., St. Louis, 1971, pp. 383–385, 1377–1378, 1441.

34. Crosby, V.G., Lawrence, M.S., et al: Leiomyosarcoma of the right iliac vein: a case report. *Ann. Surg.*, **164**: 924–926, 1966.

35. Dao, L.: A new method of treatment of ganglia and synovial cysts. *Jour. Occup. Med.*, **6**: 217–220, 1964.

36. Das Gupta, T.K. and Brasfield, R.D.: Tumors of muscles and synovial tissues. *Eng. Cancer.*, **21**: 379–385, 1971.

37. De, M.N. and Tribedi, B.P.: Skeletal muscle tissue tumor. *Brit. Jour. Surg.*, **28**: 17–28, 1940.

38. Derbyphire, R.L.: Observations of the treatment of ganglia. *Amer. Jour. Surg.*, **112**: 636, 1966.

39. DeSanto, D.A. and Wilson, P.D.: Pigmented villonodular synovitis. *JBJS*, **21**: 531, 1939.

40. Dorfman, H.D. and Fishel, E.R.: Leiomyosarcoma of the greater saphenous vein. *Amer. Jour. Clin. Path.*, **39**: 73–78, 1963.

41. *Dorland's Illustrated Medical Dictionary*, 24th ed., Saunders Co., Phila., 1957.

42. Dowling, E.A.: Rhabdomyoma, a rare, benign neoplasm of skeletal muscle. *Eng. Alabama Jour. Med. Sci.*, **3**: 133–136, 1966.

43. Duhig, J.T. and Ayer, J.P.: Vascular leiomyoma: a study of 61 cases. *Amer. Arch. Path.*, **65**: 424–430, 1959.

44. Dutra, F.R.: Clear cell sarcoma of tendons and aponeurosis: three additional cases. *Cancer*, **25**: 942–946, 1970.

45. Enterline, H.T. and Horn, R.C., Jr.: Alveolar rhabdomyosarcoma. *Amer. Jour. Clin. Path.*, **29**: 356–366, 1958.

46. Enzinger, F.M.: Clear cell sarcoma of tendons and aponeurosis: an analysis of 21 cases. *Cancer*, **18**: 1163–1174, 1965.

47. Evans, D.M. and Sanerkin, N.G.: Primary leiomyosarcoma of bone. *Jour. Path. and Bact.*, **90**: 348–350, 1965.

48. Feinstein, M. and Rubin, L.: Pigmented villonodular synovitis. *ACFS Jour.*, **Vol. 12**, no. 3: 77–83, 1973.

49. Fisher, E.R. and Wechsler, H.: Granular cell myoblastoma—a misnomer. *Cancer*, **15**: 936–954, 1962.

50. Fisher, W.C.: *Leiomyoma of the Skin.* Armed Forces Institute of Path., 1963.

51. Fisk, G.R.: Bone concavity caused by a ganglia. *JBJS*, **37B**: 663–675, 1955.

52. Foot, H.C.: *Identification of Tumors.* Lippincott Co., Phila., 1948.

53. Foster, L.N.: The benign giant cell tumors of tendon sheaths. *Amer. Jour. Path.*, **23**: 567–576, 1947.

54. Franklin, H.S. and Dahlin, D.C.: Ganglion cyst of bone. *Mayo Clin. Pro.*, **46**: 485–488, 1971.

55. Galloway, J.D.B., Broders, A.C., and Ghormley, R.: Pigmented villo-nodular synovitis. *Arch. Surg.*, **40**: 485, 1940.

56. Gamble, F.O. and Yale, I.: *Clinical Foot Roentgenology.* Williams and Wilkins Co., Baltimore, 1966, p. 113.

57. Gate et al: Leiomyoma *Bsoefranc D. Reum.* Straab, 1939.

58. Gewheiler, J.A. and Wilson, V.W.: Diffuse biarticular pigmented villonosular synovitis. *Radiology*, **93**: 137–142, 1969.

59. Ghooi, A., Hazir, M., et al.: Rhabdomyosarcoma. *Jour. Indian M.A.*, **45**: 10, 1965.

60. Giannestras, N.J.: *Foot Disorders—Medical and Surgical Management.* Lea and Febiger, Phila., 1973, p. 617.

61. Goldman, R.L.: Multicentric benign rhabdomyoma of skeletal muscle. *Cancer*, **16**: 1609–1613, 1963.

62. Goodman, A.H. and Briggs, R.C.: Deep leiomyoma of an extremity. *JBJS*, **47A**, no. 3, 1965.

63. Grahame, R., Ramsey, N.W., and Scott, J.T.: Radioactive colloidal gold. *Ann. Rheum. Dis.*, **29**: 159–163, 1970.

64. Gray, H.: *Anatomy of the Human Body*, 28th ed., G.M. Gross (ed.), Lea and Febiger, Phila., 1966, pp. 295, 299, 515.

65. Greenfeld, M.M. and Wallace, K.M.: Pigmented villonodular synovitis. *Radiology*, **54**: 350–356, 1950.

66. Gristma, A.G. and Wilson, P.D.: Popliteal cysts in adults and children. *Archives of Surg.*, **88**: 357–363, 1964.

67. Haagenson, C.H. and Stout, A.P.: Synovial sarcoma. *Amer. Surg.*, **120**: 826, 1944.

68. Hansen, O.H.: On the treatment of ganglia. *Acta. Chir. Scand.*, **136**: 471–476, 1970.

69. Hare, H.F. and Cerny, M.J.: Soft tissue sarcoma: a review of 200 cases. *Cancer*, **16**: 1332–1337, 1963.

70. Harland, W.A. and Clamen, M.: Leiomyosarcoma of the inferior vena cava with clinical features of Chiari syndrome. *Can. Med. Assoc. Jour.*, **83**: 1064–1066, 1960.

71. Haug, W.A. et al.: Primary leiomyosarcoma of femoral veins. *Surgery*, **38**: 410, 1955.

72. Hicks, J.D.: Synovial cysts in bone. *The Australian and New Zealand Jour. of Surg.*, **26**: 138–143, 1956.

73. Hoffman, G.J. and Carter, D.: Clear cell sarcoma of tendons and apo-neurosis with melanin. *Archives of Path.*, **95**: 22–25, 1973.

74. Horn, R.C. and Enterline, H.T.: Rhabdomyosarcoma: a clinicopatho-logical study and classification of 39 cases. *Cancer*, **11**: 181–199, 1955.

75. Inman, V.T.: *DuVries Surgery of the Foot,* 3rd ed. C.V. Mosby Co., St. Louis, 1973, p. 389.
76. Jaffe, H.L., Lichtenstein, L., and Sutro, C.J.: Pigmented villonodular synovitis, bursitis, and tenosynovitis. *Arch. Path.,* **31**: 731–765, 1941.
77. Jayson, M.I.V. and Dixon, A. St. J.: Valvular mechanism in juxta articular cysts. *Ann. Rheum. Dis.,* **29**: 415–419, 1970.
78. Johnson, E.W., Jr.: Adjacent and distant spread of giant cell tumors. *Amer. Jour. Surg.,* **109**: 163–166, 1965.
79. Johnson, L.H. and Shands, W.C.: Primary leiomyosarcoma of femoral veins. *Surgery,* **38**: 410, 1955.
80. King, E.S.J.: Malignant tumors of tendon sheaths. *Aust. and New Zealand Jour. Surg.,* **10**: 338, 1941.
81. Kloepfer, H.W. and Krafchuk, J.: Hereditary multiple leiomyoma of the skin. *Amer. Jour. Human Genetics,* **10**: 48–52, 1958.
82. Kogstal, O.: Malignant sarcoma. *Acta. Rheum. Scand.,* **16**: 81, 1970.
83. *Lancet:* Rhabdomyosarcoma. Feb., 1965.
84. Larmon, W.A.: Pigmented villonodular synovitis. *Med. Clin. North Amer.,* **49**: 141–150, 1965.
85. Leiomyosarcoma of the skin. *British Jour. of Derm.,* Editorial, **79**: 305–306, 1967.
86. Leturque, M.P.: Leiomyomatose cutanée nodulaire profuse avec polyglobulie. *Soc. de Derm et de Syph.,* 1966.
87. Lichtenstein, L.: Tumors of synovial joints, bursae and tendon sheaths. *Cancer,* **8**: 816, 1955.
88. Linscheid, R.L., Soule, E.H., et al: Pleomorphic rhabdomyosarcomata of the extremities and limb girdles. *JBJS,* **47A**: 4, 1965.
89. Lobbato, V.J.: Vascular leiomyoma. *JAPA,* **53**: 355, 1963.
90. Mahour, G.H., Shoule, H.E., et al: Rhabdomyosarcoma in infants and children: a clinical pathological study of 75 cases. *Jour. of Pediat. Surg.,* **2**: 5, 1967.
91. Masson, P.: *Human Tumors.* Translated by S. Kobernick. Wayne State Univ. Press, 1970.
92. McCain, L.R. and Galinski, A.W.: Pedal leiomyoma: a case report. *JAPA,* **59**: 399–400, 1969.
93. McCallum. D.E., Musser, A.W., and Rhangos, W.C.: Experimental villonodular synovitis. *S. Med. Jour.,* **59**: 966–970, 1966.
94. McClatchie, S.: An example of a clear cell sarcoma of tendon. *E. African Med. Jour.,* **46**: 524–526, 1969.
95. McDonald, G.O.: Preventive measures against metastasis and local recurrence in cancer surgery. *Proc. Nat. Cancer Conf.,* **6**: 19, J.B. Lippincott Co., Phila., 1970.
96. McEvedy, B.V.: Simple ganglia. *Brit. Jour. Surg.,* **49**: 585–594, 1962.
97. McMaster, P.E.: Pigmented villonodular synovitis with invasion of bone. *JBJS,* **41A**: 1170–1183, 1960.
98. Messe, A.A. and Sasson, L.: Leiomyosarcoma: a diagnostic challenge. *JAMA,* **174**: 1706–1711, 1960.

99. Murphy, G.H., Dockerty, M.B., and Boders, A.C.: Myoblastoma. *Amer. Jour. Path.*, **25**: 1157–1181, 1949.

100. Pack, G.T. and Eberhart, W.F.: Rhabdomyosarcoma of skeletal muscle: report of 100 cases. *Surgery*, **32**: 1023–1064, 1952.

101. Palumbo, L.T., Leisbitz, M., and Corcoran, T.E.: Rhabdomyosarcoma of the thigh: report of a case. *Arch. Surg.*, **60**: 806–816, 1950.

102. Parson, H.G. and Puro, H.E.: Rhabdomyoma of skeletal muscle. *Amer. Jour. Surg.*, **89**: 1187–1190, 1965.

103. Pavelka, K., Susta, A., and Streda, A.: Giant cyst of the calf in patient with rheumatoid arthritis. *Scand. Jour. Rheumatology*, **1**: 145–150, 1972.

104. Perk, K., Maloney, J.B., et al: Further studies of the relationship of rhabdomyosarcoma virus to muscle tissue. *Amer. Jour. of Cancer*, **2**: 43–51, 1967.

105. Perl, L.: Ein Fall von Sarkom der Vena Cava Inferior. *Arch. Path. Anat.*, **53**: 378, 1871.

106. Perles, D.B. and Roth, S.B.: Leiomyoma of the foot. *JAPA*, **58**: 394, 1968.

107. Petenza, A.D. and Winslow, D.J.: Rhabdomyosarcoma of the hand. *JBJS*, **43A**: 700–708, 1961.

108. Pickren, J.W., Valenzula, L., and Elias, E.G.: Synovial sarcoma. *Proc. Nat. Cancer Conf.*, **6**: 795, 1970.

109. Pinkel, D. and Pickren, J.: Rhabdomyosarcoma in children. *JAMA*, **175**: 293–298, 1961.

110. Raben, M., Calabrses, A., Higinbotham, N.L., and Phillips, R.: Malignant synovioma. *Amer. Jour. Roent. and Rad. Therapy*, **93**: 145, 1965.

111. Rakov, A.J.: Malignant rhabdomyoblastomas of the skeletal musculature. *Amer. Jour. of Cancer*, **30**: 455, 1937.

112. Rakow, R.B.: Leiomyoma of the foot: a case report. *JAPA*, **56**: no. 1, 1966.

113. Rigby, C.: Rhabdomyosarcoma, the pathology in children. *Proc. Royal Soc. Med.*, **59**: 411–412, 1966.

114. Robbins, S.: *Textbook of Pathology.* Saunders, Philadelphia, 1967.

115. Rosenberg, J.C.: The value of arteriography in the treatment of soft tissue tumors of the extremities. *Jour. Int. Coll. Surg.*, 1964.

116. Rothenberg, A.J. et al: Unusual manifestations of rhabdomyosarcoma. *Arch. Intern. Med.*, **118**: 446–448, 1966.

117. Rudner, E.J. et al: Multiple cutaneous leiomyoma in identical twins. *Arch. Derm.*, **90**: 81–82, 1964.

118. Saavedra, J.A., Martin, R.G., and Smith, J.L.: Rhabdomyosarcoma, a study of 35 cases. *Annuals of Surg.*, **157**, No. 2: 186–197, 1963.

119. Sakurai, O. and Toda, A.: Primary leiomyosarcoma within the femoral vein. *Clin. Orth.*, **44**: 197–202, 1966.

120. Salaguarda, F.: Leiomyoma of the inferior vena cava. *Path.*, **105**: 405, 1964.

121. Salm, R. and Sissons, H.A.: Giant cell tumors of soft tissues. *Jour. Path.*, **107**: 27–39, 1972.

122. Scott, P.M.: Bone lesions in pigmented villonodular synovitis. *JBJS*, **50B**: 306–311, 1968.

123. Singh, R., Grewal, D.S., and Chakrovarti, R.N.: Experimental production of pigmented villonodular synovitis in the knee and ankle joints of rhesus monkeys. *Jour. Path.*, **98**: 137–142, 1969.

124. Smith, J.H. and Pugh, D.G.: Roentgenographic aspects of articular pigmented villonodular synovitis. *Amer. Jour. Roentgen.*, **87**: 1146–1156, 1962.

125. Smout, M.S. and Fisher, J.H.: Leiomyosarcoma of the saphenous vein. *Can. Med. Assoc. Jour.*, **83**: 1066–1067, 1960.

126. Snook, G.A.: Pigmented villonodular synovitis with bony invasion: report of two cases. *JAMA*, **189**: 424–425, 1963.

127. Soule, E.H. et al: Embryonal rhabdomyosarcoma of the limbs and limb girdles. *Cancer*, **23**: 1336–1346, 1969.

128. Stern, A.L.: Pigmented villonodular synovitis: a case report. *JAPA*, **56**: 26–27, 1966.

129. Stobbe, G.D. et al: Embryonal rhabdomyosarcoma of head and neck of children. *Cancer*, **3**: 826, 1950.

130. Stout, A.P.: Rhabdomyosarcoma of skeletal muscles. *Ann. of Surg.*, **123**: 447, 1946.

131. Stout, A.P.: Sarcoma of soft tissue. *Cancer*, **11**: 210, 1950.

132. Stout, A.P.: Leiomyosarcomas of superficial soft tissues. *Cancer*, **11**: 844, 1958.

133. Tandler, B., Rossi, E.P., Stein, M., and Matt, M.M.: Rhabdomyoma of the lip: light and electron microscopical observations. *Eng. Arch. Path. (Chicago)*, **89**: 118–127, 1970.

134. Taylor, A.R. and Rana, N.A.: A valve, an explanation of the formation of popliteal cysts. *Ann. Rheum. Dis.*, **32**: 419–421, 1973.

135. Thompson, D.E., Frost, H.M., Hendrick, J.W., and Horn, R.C.: Soft tissue sarcoma involving the extremities and limb girdle: a review. *Surg. Med. Jour.*, **64**: 33, 1971.

136. Thompson, G.C.V.: Rhabdomyosarcoma of skeletal muscles. *Med. Jour. Aust.*, **2**: 359–361, 1951.

137. Thorjnarson: 1961, per Allison, M.F., *Clin. Ped.*, 1965.

138. Tillotson, J.F., McDonald, J.R., and Jones, J.M.: Synovial sarcoma sarcomota. *JBJS*, **33A**: 459, 1951.

139. Toyama, W.M.: Familial popliteal cysts in children. *Amer. Jour. Dis. Child.*, **124**: 586–587, 1972.

140. Turek, S.L.: *Orthopaedics: Principles and Their Application*, 2nd ed. J.B. Lippincott Co., Phila., 1967, pp. 639–640.

141. von Andel, J.G.: Synovial sarcoma—a review and analysis of treated cases. *Radiologiq Clinica et Biologica*, **41**: 145, 1972.

142. Weber, J.: by Pack and Eberhart. *Surgery*, 1952.

143. White, A.G.: Leiomyosarcoma of the foot. *Proc. Roy. Soc. Med.*, **64**: 56–57, 1971.
144. Willis, R.A.: *Pathology of Tumor.* Butterworth, London, 1953, pp. 740–758.
145. Wolfe, R.D. and Giuliano, V.J.: Double contrast arthrography in the diagnosis of pigmented villonodular synovitis of the knee. *Amer. Jour. Roent., Radium Therapy and Nuclear Med.*, **110**: 793–799, 1970.
146. Wyatt, R.B., Schochet, S.S., Jr., and McCormick, W.F.: Rhabdomyoma: light and electron microscopic study of a case with intranuclear inclusions. *Eng. Arch. Otolartyn, Chicago*, **92**: 2–39, 1970.

# Section IV

# Nerve Tumors

## Neuroma: Morton's and Traumatic

### Definition

In the practice of Podiatric Medicine, the neuroma accounts for a significant amount of patient concern. The overwhelming majority of neuromas found in the foot are of the Morton's or intermetatarsal type. However, one must be cognizant of the possibility of an amputation-type neuroma. The amputation neuroma appears as a small, solid, white mass or as a semi-firm, spotted yellow cystic mass; whereas the intermetatarsal neuroma usually appears as hypertrophy of a section of nerve having a white appearance.[121]

Neuromas of the intermetatarsal type, or Morton's neuromas, are not true neoplasms, however, they may be confused with true neoplasms such as neurilemmomas, schwannomas, and neurofibromas.

### Synonyms

Neuromas are often referred to by one of a number of synonyms, such as perineural fibroma, metatarsal neuroma, plantar interdigital neurofibroma, and Morton's toe.

### History

The phenomenon of the intermetatarsal neuroma was first alluded to by Durleuber (1845), who described a neuralgic affection of the plantar nerve between the third and fourth metatarsal bones.[52]

Dr. T.G. Morton (1876) described 12 cases of neuralgia, relative to the metatarsal parabola: "The metatarsophalangeal joints of the first, second and third toes are often found on a line with each other; the head of the fourth metatarsal is found to be from one-eighth to one-fourth of an inch behind the head of the third; while the head of the fifth is from three-eighths to a half an inch behind the head of the fourth. Thus, while the joint of the third is slightly above, the joint of the fifth is considerably below the metatarsophalangeal joint of the fourth, the base of the proximal phalanx of the fifth toe is brought on a line with the neck of the fifth opposite the neck of the fourth."[80]

Dr. Morton explained that the fourth and fifth metatarsals have greater lateral mobility than the others and that the fifth metatarsal has considerably more motion than the fourth. He observed that the lateral pressure brings the head of the fifth metatarsal and the fifth toe into direct contact with the base of the proximal phalanx and the head and neck of the fourth metatarsal and, to some extent, the extremity of the fifth metatarsal rolls above and under this bone. Because of this relationship and the mobility of the fourth and fifth metatarsals, Dr. Morton said "Under certain circumstances a bruising or pinching of the digital branches of the lateral plantar nerve between the fourth and fifth metatarsals, may account for the neuralgia over the fourth metatarsophalangeal joint and fourth digit."[80] He attributed the greater incidence in women to fashionable shoes which were tight and narrow, thus causing the fifth metatarsal to be pressed against the head and neck of the fourth metatarsal, with the phalanx of the fifth toe being especially forced down upon the head of the fourth.

Thus, Dr. T.G. Morton gives us an early account of a metatarsalgia involving the fourth metatarsal and digit. Since that time it has been found that the condition he described was indeed due to a neuroma in the third intermetatarsal space.

Dr. Erskine Mason (1877) reported a case with pain at the second metatarsophalangeal joint, in which he suspected involvement of the digital branch of the medial plantar nerve.[68]

Dr. Woodruff (1890) proposed that the symptoms we now ascribe to a neuroma, were due to a subluxation of the metatarsophalangeal joint. His cases were unique in that his patients were people not accustomed to much standing or walking, not having relaxed ligaments, not having flatened metatarsal arches, and with no history of injury. Furthermore, his patients derived no benefit, and were actually made worse by exercises such as standing on the tiptoes.[125]

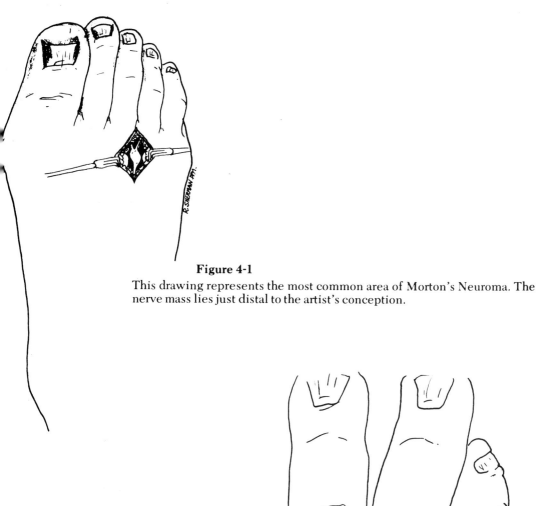

**Figure 4-1**

This drawing represents the most common area of Morton's Neuroma. The nerve mass lies just distal to the artist's conception.

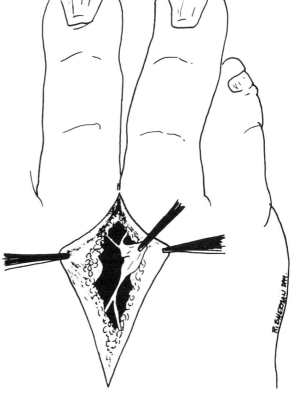

**Figure 4-2**

epresentative drawing of Morton's Neuroma during surgical excision.
'erve should be severed just distal to the bifurcation of the medial and
.iteral branches of the plantar nerve proximally and distally.

Dr. E.H. Bradford (1891) agreed with T.G. Morton and desribed how pain may radiate up the leg in severe cases.[10]

Dr. A.E. Hoadley (1893) was the first to identify and resect a neuroma as a cure for metatarsalgia. Dr. Hoadley disagreed with Dr. T.G. Morton's original description, in that he felt that in the ordinary foot the third, fourth, and fifth metatarsal bones do not fall sufficiently short to allow the head of the bone to fall against the neck of the next medial metatarsal. Dr. Hoadley agreed that the fourth and fifth metatarsals are more mobile but did not accept the possibility that they might slide above or underneath each other. He also felt the idea of the involved nerve being pressed between two adjacent metatarsal heads was invalid, since the nerve lies below the transverse metatarsal ligament and not between the metatarsal heads. He did feel that lateral compression, regardless of metatarsal length, would cause the foot to fold upon itself so as to bring the plantar surfaces of the metatarsal heads into proximity and thus involve the digital nerve. In this regard, it is the internal branch of the external plantar nerve which is usually injured since it lies just where the foot makes the sharpest fold.

Thus, Dr. Hoadley was the first to propose involvement of the inter-digital nerve as a cause for the metatarsalgia. He was also the first to do an operation for this condition, other than the resection of the metatarsophalangeal joint. The following is his account of the first neuroma excision, done on a young lady, whose symptoms are quite typical. "I cut down on the bottom of the foot and without any difficulty found the digital branches of the external plantar nerve. They are comparatively superficial. I found a small neuroma, and I regarded it, on this nerve; it might have been nothing more than an inflammatory thickening of the nerve, it was about seven-eights of an inch long and nearly one-eighth inch in diameter and red. The resection was prompt and perfect cure. It has been four or five years since the operation and there has been no return of the neuralgia and no trouble whatever. The wound healed by first intention and in ten days all signs of there having been a cut in the bottom of the foot was gone save the fine line of a scar."[40]

192

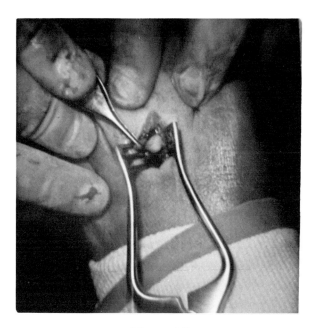

**Figure 4-3**

Ganglion Cyst. Ganglion cyst is not frequently encountered in conjunction with the Morton's Neuroma. Other lesions we have encountered in this area are those of rheumatoid nodules.

Dr. A. Polloson (1899) proposed the theory that metatarsalgia was caused by a certain laxity of the transverse metatarsal ligament, thus permitting a partial collapse of the arch formed by the five metatarsal heads. He thought that probably the third metatarsal head became dislocated downwards to compress the nerves running along each side of it against the heads of the neighboring bones.[91] He was the first to use the term anterior metatarsalgia, instead of neuralgia.

Dr. Tubby (1912) gave a clue as to the true cause of the paroxysmal pain when he described the plantar digital nerves as being thickened and red.[52]

Betts (1940)[6] and McElvenny (1943)[73] described the presence of a neuroma located on the lateral branch of the medial plantar nerve.

Bickel and Dockerty (1947) gave more insight as to the location and nature of the neuroma. In their series, they found that neuromas occur in two different sites along the plantar nerves. The neuroma may be found at the bifurcation. The second site is proximal to the bifurcation, in the medial branch of the plantar nerve.[7]

*Etiology*

The current explanation of the etiology of neuromas can best be understood by appreciating the neuroanatomy of the area. The following explanation is based on 18 cadaver dissections performed by Baker and Kuhn. The fourth digital nerve is formed by the union of the lateral most branch of the medial plantar nerve and a communicating branch from the lateral plantar nerve. Before union these two branches lie below the belly of the flexor digitorum brevis muscle and the plantar aponeurosis, just proximal to the heads of the metatarsals. At this point, it penetrates the aponeurosis and passes beneath the transverse metatarsal ligament. Just distal to the ligament it turns upward into the web space between the third and fourth toes and divides into the medial and lateral branches which supply the adjacent sides of the third and fourth toes.[1]

The Morton's neuroma may be found in any web space of the foot; however, it is most commonly found at the base of

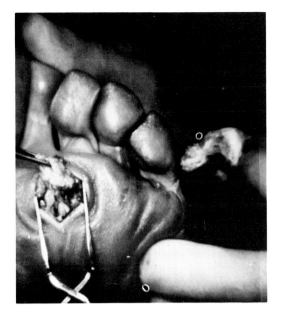

**Figure 4-4A**

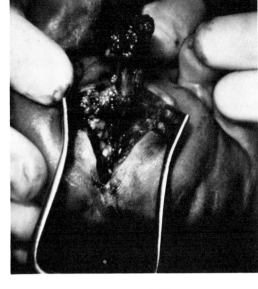

**Figure 4-4B**

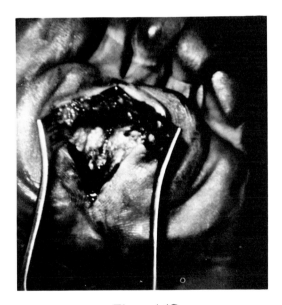

**Figure 4-4C**

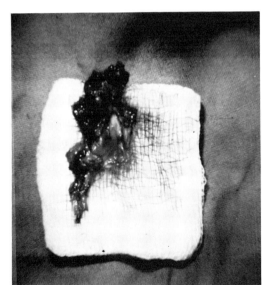

**Figure 4-4D**

Traumatic Neuroma. The most common location for
traumatic neuromas are in the metatarsal region and
usually underlies the second metatarsal head. These
are extremely tender lesions and are frequently associated with Morton's syndrome. (B) reveals a surgical dissection of the lesion.

(C) and (D) reveal the defect after the lesion has been
excised and the gross specimen, respectively.

the web between the third and fourth toes. Because of the anastomoses of the medial branch of the lateral plantar nerve and the lateral branch of the medial plantar nerve, increased immobility may result.[25] Kravette stated that hyperextension of the metatarsophalangeal joint could cause impingement of the plantar nerve against the intermetatarsal ligament. He included biomechanical causes of hyperextension of the metatarsophalangeal joint, hammer toe deformities, and high heel shoes as causes of nerve impingement. Furthermore, a plantar-grade force from above, fracture in the area, and a sudden hyperextension could cause impingement or a stretch on the nerve.[58] Exact locations of the neuromas along the nerves have been discussed previously.

The amputation neuroma is produced by what some authors refer to as the "drive" of a nerve cell and its axon in the spinal cord, in an effort to reattach itself to the now amputated portion. The axons of the cut end of the nerve growing into the soft tissue end of the stump turn back on themselves, thus producing a small ball of nerve tissue. When these neuromas occur in normal soft tissue, one or two inches above the stump end, they will not be sufficiently troublesome to require treatment. Only those neuromas which may have become attached to scar tissue on the stump end or are buried in the bone produce symptoms requiring surgical excision.[116]

## Incidence

Pincus found an increased frequency of interdigital neuropathies in females.[89] Duncan found intermetatarsal neuromas to be four times more frequent in females than males.[25] The type of shoe worn by females is generally accepted as the reason for this disparity. No other predisposing factors are evident. Neuromas, both the intermetatarsal or amputation types, can be found at any age. The reader is referred to the chart in the section on Foot Involvement, which illustrates studies involving the location and frequency of intermetatarsal neuromas and indicates the preponderance of females to develop neuropathies with the third interspace being the most favored site.

Traumatic Neuroma. Traumatic neuroma with vascular malformations. (A) clinical view of the plantar surface of the foot reveals a soft tissue bulge between the second and third metatarsals. The bulging of the soft tissue tumor creates a spreading of the second and third toes. (B) and (C) reveal the surgical dissection of the lesion and complete surgical exposure as it is being excised.

This patient has an equinus foot, which has been subjected to constant trauma.

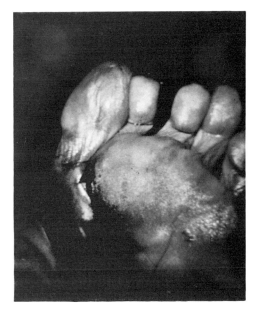

Figure 4-5A

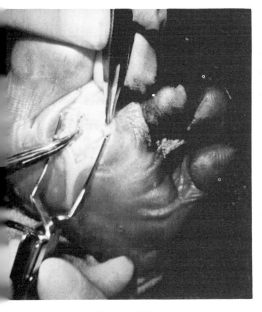

Figure 4-5B

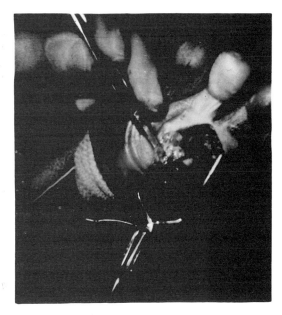

Figure 4-5C

*Clinical Picture*

The signs and symptoms of the intermetatarsal neuromas have been described and documented long before their etiology was discovered. Neuroma pain is typically described as being localized near the fourth metatarsal head. The intensity is classically described by many authors as being so intense that the patient has to stop walking, take off his shoe, and massage the painful area. In severe cases, the pain may radiate up the leg, into the adjacent toes, or medially toward the other metatarsal heads.

The pain may be dull or throbbing with severe tenderness. Most often the pain is spasmodic, but it may be constant. Nocturnal pain, if present, is usually not severe. Massaging the foot may relieve the pain momentarily, however recurrences are inevitable. The recurrences are variable and become more frequent as time goes on. Between attacks there may be no pain. Paresthesias, with numbness and tingling, may or may not be present in the adjacent sides of the toes.

Upon inspection of the foot, its shape is normal in most cases; in some cases a mild depression of the transverse arch has been noted. The skin of the involved area appears normal. No external signs of circulatory changes have been noted. Radiologically, no abnormality is apparent.

Occasionally, a nodule can be palpated in the involved web space. If large and interdigitally located, there may be spreading of the toes when standing. Sharp pain may be elicited upon lateral compression in the involved web space.

Mulder described a diagnostic clinical test wherein the patient's foot is clasped around the metatarsal heads with the fingers of the left hand while the thumb of the right hand exerts a firm pressure on the sole of the foot at the site of the suspected neuroma. Presence of a neuroma produces a palpable click caused by the tumor escaping into the sole of the foot from between the metatarsal heads.[82]

Injection of the site with local anesthetics provides relief for the duration of the anesthesia; but injection of corticosteroids provides little benefit.

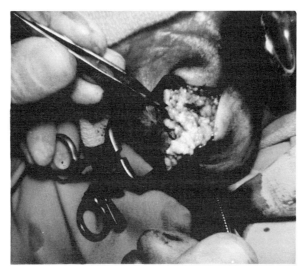

**Figure 4-6A**

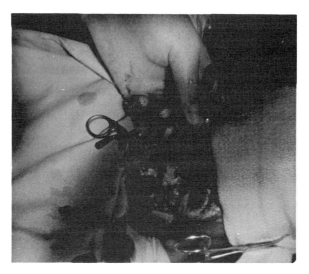

**Figure 4-6B**

Traumatic Neuroma. Traumatic neuromas of the heel are not frequent lesions and are often misdiagnosed. These are often associated with heel spur deformities of the foot and should be carefully evaluated. These lesions are often moveable in the transverse plane and are quite sensitive upon palpation. Differential diagnosis is that of nerve entrapment, sciatica, metabolic disease, calcaneal spurs.

Pain caused by an amputation neuroma is of a shooting type. The remainder of its clinical picture, with the exclusion of the palpable click, closely resembles that of the intermetatarsal neuroma.

## Differential Diagnosis

In considering the presence of a neuroma, differential diagnoses should include Buerger's disease, polyarteritis, sciatica, arthroses or bursitis of the metatarsophalangeal joints and ganglion cysts. Neuromas must also be differentiated from true nerve tumors, neurileommomas, or Schwannomas. These true nerve tumors are encapsulated, well defined, and, without invading adjacent tissue to compress them. The tumors are composed of Schwann cells that encase the axons of the peripheral nerve foot.[100] Schwannommas and neurilemmomas may occur at any age and show no sex predominance. The tumors often occur on the flexor surfaces of the extremities and usually spare the feet.[102]

## Pathology

In recent years, a number of pathological studies have been completed in order to determine the true nature of the neuroma. Gross examination reveals that a marked yellowish-white, fusiform thickening of the plantar nerve is usually present. Upon careful dissection, a white fibrous connective tissue encasing the digital nerve is found.[83] A definite line of cleavage between the tumorous swelling of the nerve and the surrounding tissue has not been detected.[124] Cases have been reported where a round, bulb-like appearance similar to an amputation neuroma has been seen. Frequently, a digital vessel is found in the fusiform swelling.[83]

The average size of a neuroma is approximately 15 centimeters in length and half the diameter of a lead pencil. Neuromas have been reported as large as 2.5 centimeters in length and 1.0 centimeter in diameter. The consistency of a neuroma is firm; however, in early lesions, the tissue may be edematous.

Upon histological examination, Bickel and Dockerty made the observation that early lesions present spotty inter-

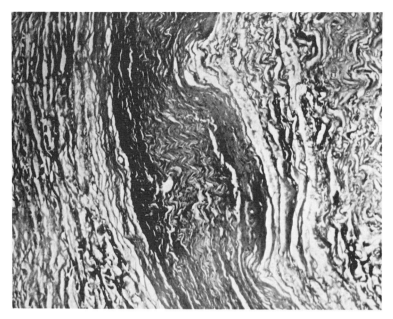

**Figure 4-7**
Traumatic Neuroma. This tumor shows a triangle of
nerve fibers in a dense fibrous matrix. Adipose tissue
surrounds the neuroma.

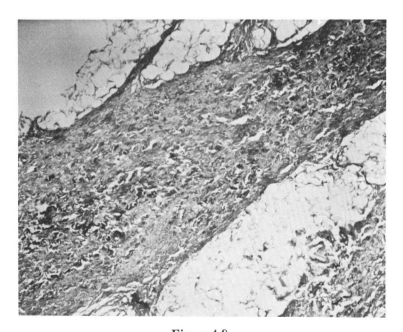

**Figure 4-8**
Morton's Neuroma. The general pattern is that of a
peripheral nerve which is irregular and distorted.
Many axons are missing and Schwann cell sheaths
are thin and elongated.

stitial edema, with swelling and demyelinization of the entire trunk. This may progress to show marked proliferation of the neurilemma nuclei, thus giving a picture of pronounced cellularity. In certain instances, the formation of tissue clefts or small cysts within the substances of the nerve was found to be due to a combination of edema and proliferation. Lesions of long-standing presented moderate to severe fibrosis and hyalinization affecting the nerve bundles. This, however, appeared to represent invasion from without, rather than primary nerve change.[7]

Ringertz divided the histological changes into four major categories, which included fibrosis, endoneural edema, demyelination of the nerve, and vascular changes. The fibrosis was found to be perineural. Milder cases presented only slight thickening and condensation of the perineural capsule, with only slight separation of the nerve bundles. Loose interstitial tissue or adipose tissue was present, which separated the nerve from adjacent arteries, synovial sheaths, and joint capsules. With more marked fibrosis there was a separation of the nerve bundles by a compact mass of connective tissue, which also bound the nerve to the surrounding structures and embedded the larger trunks of the interdigital arteries. Small bursal cavities have also been found embedded in the connective tissue mass. Endoneural fibrosis is present in some cases although it is not marked. No proliferation of Schwann cells has been reported by any of the investigators nor has infiltration with inflammatory cells been reported. This would indicate that the tumor is not a true neoplasm.

Varying amounts of endoneural edema were found, within the nerve bundles, separating the nerve fibers. No edema has been seen in the perineural connective tissue. The amount of demyelination was quite variable. There is a certain correlation between intraneural edema and demyelination, but this is not constant. The amount of demyelination and fibrosis showed no correlation.

Arterial changes consisted of proliferation of the subintimal layer and the elastic structures. These changes occurred mainly in the larger arteries, the interdigital trunks, and their larger branches (down to a diameter of about 75

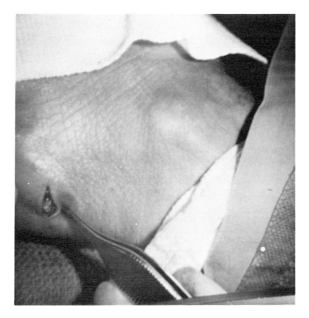

**Figure 4-9A**

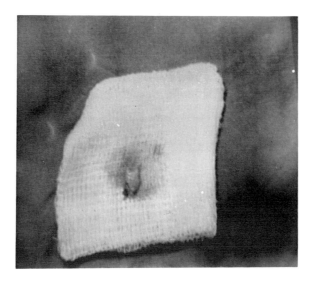

**Figure 4-9B**

Traumatic Neuroma. Traumatic neuromas located in the arch of the foot. (B) reveals the surgical gross specimen.

microns). Slight changes consisted of a hyperplasia of the tunica elastica with multiplication of its lamellae. More advanced changes involved formation of connective tissue cushions, very rich in elastic tissue, rendering the lumen irregularly constricted and slit-shaped. In certain instances, a fibrous mass, less rich in elastic tissue, filled the remaining lumen. This mass contained endothelium-lined spaces, resembling the recanalized vessels in organizing thromboses; however, no recent thromboses were evident.

The smaller arteries, especially the intraneural, were usually unchanged. Intimal changes of an atheromatous type and other calcifications were not found. No changes were found in the media. Due to marked perineural fibrosis, arteries embedded in connective tissue showed condensing of the tunica adventitia. Inflammatory infiltration of the artery was not encountered.

Veins often showed mild changes, consisting of superficial intimal cushions rich in elastic fibers.[95]

In his series of pathological examinations, Hauser found that, in patients with a prolonged convalescence from neuroma surgery, there was a localized endarteritis obliterans. The endarteritis occurs concurrently because of trauma or inflammation of the vessels; it is believed that convalescence may be retarded due to an inadequate blood supply to the area.[39]

To determine whether the observed nerve changes were characteristic of patients with a clinical picture of Morton's neuroma or whether they were common findings in non-symptomatic patients, both Ringertz and Nora did examinations of post-mortem cases of similar age and with no history of foot problems resembling Morton's neuroma or cardiovascular disease; they found a high incidence of both fibrosis and endarteritis in the control cases. As a matter of fact, in many instances, these changes were more severe than in the patients who had the clinical symptoms. In the controls, Ringertz found that the endarteritis was more constant in cases over forty years of age. The endoneural edema and demyelination were found much less frequently in control cases.[83,85]

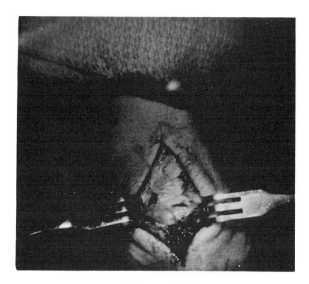

**Figure 4-10A**

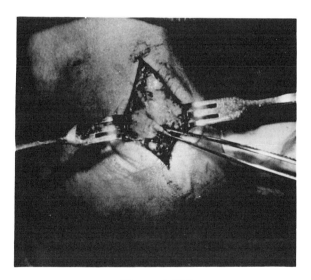

**Figure 4-10B**

Traumatic Neuroma. Surgical exposures (A) and (B) reveal a traumatic neuroma in the posterior aspect of the heel and Achilles tendon, respectively. The area appears as a white glistening mass.

205

Kline observed that, because of partial injury to the nerve, a swollen firm nerve may be present. Furthermore, a small neuroma with endoneural connective tissue proliferation may have poor axonal penetration through the proliferated area. However, a large neuroma with epineural and perineural scarring may have an intact internal architecture.[55]

Mathews found that in two to three days the proximal end of an amputated nerve begins vigorous regrowth. In three weeks, the nerve appears as a neuroma, histologically. The Wallerian degeneration is restricted to a distance of one or two nodes of Ranvier in the proximal segment as it "empties" the distal nerve sheath. To prevent a collapse of the epineurium, Schwann cells rapidly fill in. The proximal end acquires a cap of fibroblasts and proceeds to cicatrization. Only a few regenerating axons penetrate this barrier. Fibers that do penetrade the barrier may wander long distances in fascial planes and with blood vessels. The myelination keeps pace with growing neuraxons both inside and outside the neuroma. Once formed, little change occurs in the neuroma. Avascularity is prominent and is responsible for the whitish fibrous appearance of the neuroma.[69]

Mathews further observed that the outer cap of connective tissue is continuous with the perineurium of the intact nerve trunk. Within the neuroma, there is a mixture of Schwann cells and proliferating neurofibrils. Orderliness is lost in the neuroma, with resulting chaotic tangles of neurofibrils. In older neuromas, calcification and connective tissue are increased at the expense of the nerve fibers.

Mathews asserted that a fusiform swelling appeared on the intermetatarsal neuroma and that compression of the axon within the swelling caused pain. Repeated concussion of the nerve altered the vascularity, thereby precipitating proliferation of the connective tissue, so that hyalinization followed.[69]

## Foot Involvement

Neuromas have been the most commonly reported lesion in the foot and to describe individual cases would be some-

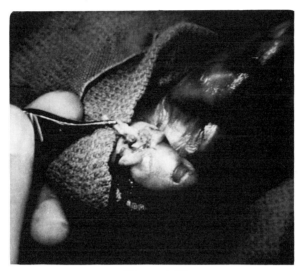

**Figure 4-11**

Traumatic Neuroma. Digital traumatic neuromas are very frequently encountered. They are often associated with painful corns.

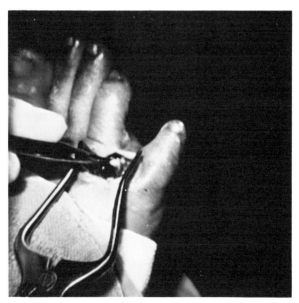

**Figure 4-12**

Traumatic Neuroma. Traumatic neuroma underlying a painful soft corn between the fourth and fifth toes.

what redundant. The reader can evaluate the following chart with regard to number of cases, sex, and location of neuromas. (See page 210.)

*Treatment*

The treatment of the intermetatarsal neuroma historically has followed three main schools of thought. According to the first school, Morton's approach to chronic cases was excision of the irritable metatarsophalangeal joint and the surrounding soft tissue.[80]

The second school is represented by Dr. Polloson, who believed that therapy must be directed at the laxity of the transverse metatarsal ligament. He recommended padding the sole of the foot to help prevent the descent of the offending metatarsal head.[91] (Others believed the convexity of the transverse arch could best be helped by gymnastic exercises to strengthen the muscles of the sole of the foot).

In the third school, Dr. V.P. Gibney, who believed that flatfoot was a contributing factor, constructed a shoe which would help support a flatfoot and spread the metatarsal heads. He chose a Spanish last, which raises the arch of the foot. In conjunction with this, the boot was laced snugly across the ball of the foot. The heel a modified French type, which is elongated and throws the body weight well upon this part of the foot.[33]

Current concepts in the treatment of intermetatarsal neuromas divide themselves into conservative and surgical. The conservative approach includes injection therapy and metatarsal pads and bars in order to redistribute weight-bearing. The injection of Vitamin B (1,000 mcg) has been reported to be of some benefit for small lesions.[39] The effects are probably reserved for very early symptoms where the involved nerve has just begun to be irritated and demyelination has just begun. Injection therapy with local anesthetics produces anesthesia in the involved area, but only for the duration of the anesthetic. The injection of corticosteroids into the involved area may be of some benefit if mild inflammation has occurred. However, corticosteroid injections will be of little or no benefit with an advanced neuroma. It is helpful

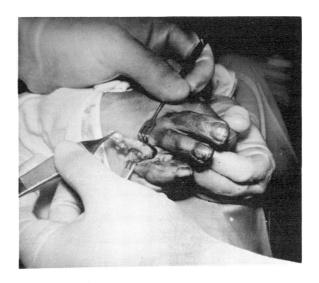

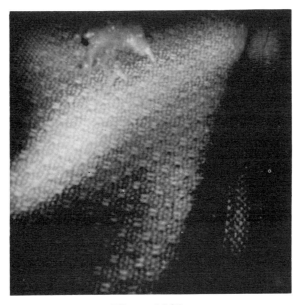

**Figure 4-13B**

Morton's Neuroma. Surgical dissection of Morton's neuroma. (B) reveals surgical specimen as a fleshy ill defined mass.

## MORTON'S NEUROMA — CASE REPORTS

| Reporter | Year | Nr. of Cases | Nr. of Lesions | Females | Males | Age | 1st/2nd | 2nd/3rd | 3rd/4th | 4th/5th |
|---|---|---|---|---|---|---|---|---|---|---|
| Morton, T.G.[80] | 1876 | 15 | 15 | 13 | 2 | 25-40 | | | 15 | |
| Mason, E.[68] | 1877 | 1 | 1 | | 1 | 21 | 1 | | | |
| Bradford, E.H.[10] | 1891 | 16 | 16 | 13 | 3 | 25-40 | | 1 | 15 | |
| Guthrie, M.B.[40] | 1892 | 2 | 2 | | 2 | Young | | | 6 | |
| Hoadley, A.E.[40] | 1893 | 6 | 6 | 5 | 1 | | | | 6 | |
| Morton, T.S.K.[81] | 1893 | 6 | 6 | 6 | | 22-45 | | | 6 | |
| Gibney, V.P.[33] | 1894 | 6 | 6 | 4 | 2 | 22-48 | | | | |
| Baker & Kuhn[1] | 1944 | 11 | 14 | 10 | 1 | 24-57 | | | 14 | |
| Swart, H.[113] | 1944 | 1 | 1 | 1 | | 24 | | | 1 | |
| Bickel & Dockerty[7] | 1947 | 18 | 25 | 16 | 2 | 25-67 | | | | |
| Winkler, H.[124] | 1948 | 20 | | | | | | | | |
| Ringertz, N.[95] | 1950 | 17 | 18 | 13 | 4 | 30-58 | | 2 | 14 | 2 |
| May, V.R.[70] | 1956 | 15 | 15 | 12 | 3 | 13-52 | | 1 | 14 | |
| McKeever, D.[74] | 1956 | | 74 | | | | | | | |
| Litchman, H.N.[64] | 1964 | 21 | 21 | 19 | 2 | 40-65 | | | | |
| Nora, P.F.[83] | 1965 | 43 | | 32 | 11 | 40-65 | | 2 | 39 | 1 |
| Kite, J.H.[53] | 1966 | 105 | 115 | 101 | 4 | 19-77 | | 13 | 102 | |
| Hauser, E.[39] | 1971 | 100 | 116 | 96 | 4 | 40-60 | | 52 | 44 | 4 |

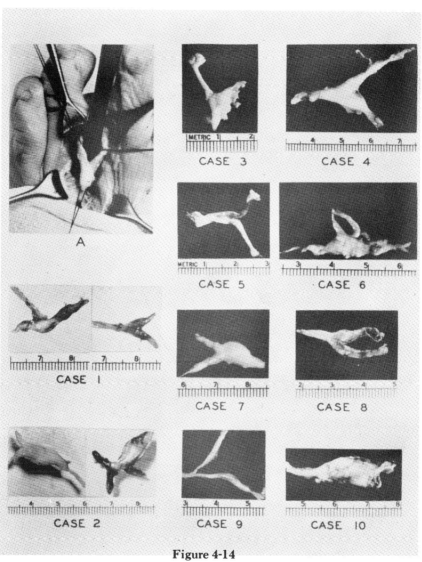

**Figure 4-14**

Illustrations reveal the different sizes and shapes of a Morton's neuroma between the third and fourth metatarsal interspace.

(Courtesy of The Journal of the National Association of Chiropodists, 39:3, March, 1949.)

in differentiating whether the symptoms are due to bursitis or truly those of a neuroma, as the corticosteroid may provide marked relief in the case of bursitis.

Surgical approaches to the intermetarsal neuroma divide themselves into dorsal and plantar approaches. The most accepted technique today is the one described by R.T. McElvenny and is found in most texts dealing with surgery of the foot.[73]

Amputation neuromas are best dealt with by prevention during surgery. Current concepts of amputation surgery, agreed upon by most surgeons, dictate that nerves are best handled by isolation, gentle retraction distally into the wound, and clean division with a sharp knife allowing the cut ends to retract proximally to the level of the bone section.[117] Ligation of the nerve is not indicated; if there is an accompanying blood vessel, the vessel should be ligated separately, with no sutures around the nerve itself.[61]

Pataky found that, when the ligated digital nerves of monkeys were injected, at the time of ligation, with triamcinilone acetonide, less scar tissue formed around the stump and less cellular disorganization occurred to the stump.[86] Smith and Gomez found that with the injection of triamcinilone acetonide into the wrists of 34 patients with neuromas, 19 received relief of paresthesias and tenderness.[109] Huber and Lewis injected alcohol three-quarters to one inch above the plane of section and prevented neuroma formation.[42]

Russel and Spalding found that repeated percussion of amputation neuromas was helpful in relieving pain.[103] Furthermore, Rubin and Kuitert demonstrated that by the use of ultrasound vibrator therapy there was a decrease or disappearance of amputation neuroma pain.[99]

The severed proximal end of the nerve has been implanted both into bone and into the proximal section of the nerve itself in efforts to prevent neuroma formation.[9,88] The severed proximal end has been encased in tight-fitting caps composed of silicone,[26] silver, cellophane, vitallium, or glass,[92] thereby preventing the formation of amputation neuromas. The injection of the severed nerve with tannic acid, gentian violet,[93] or 20% formaldehyde[36] likewise inhibited neuroma formation. However, Lambert found that phenol may encourage the formation of a severely painful neuroma.[61]

## Prognosis

With an intermetatarsal neuroma, the best chance of a cure rests with the surgical excision of the neuroma, but the best treatment of an amputation neuroma is careful surgical dissection and prevention.

## Neurofibroma and von Recklinghausen's Disease

### Definition

Neurofibromas are true neoplasms of nerve. When multiple, the condition of neurofibromatosis or von Recklinghausen's disease is present. Individually, the tumors are the same, whether single or multiple. Again, this lesion may occur singly i.e. without neurofibromatosis or a neurocutaneous syndrome, but this is the exception and not the rule.

Neurofibromatosis is a congenital, ectodermal defect characterized by cutaneous hyperpigmentation and multiple nerve tumors originating from elements of both the central and peripheral nervous systems. It is classified among the phakomatoses or neurocutaneous syndromes, along with Sturge-Weber syndrome, von Hippel-Lindau syndrome, tuberous sclerosis complex, and ataxia telangiectasia.

### Synonyms

Molluscum fibrosum, von Recklinghausen's disease, molluscum pendulum, elephantiasis neuromatosa, molluscum simplex, multiple neuroma, neurinomatosis, neuromatosis, and plexiform neuroma.

### History

Terlesius (1793) was the first investigator to describe multiple fibrous tumors of the skin. Wishart (1822), Hesselbach (1824), and Royer (1835) reported numerous cases of similar fibrous tumors associated with mental illness. Smith (1849) is credited with being the first to fully describe the multiple cutaneous and subcutaneous tumors associated with the disease. Von Recklinghausen (1882) described in detail a disease he called multiple neurofibromatosis and correlated the specific etiologic, clinical and pathologic aspects of the neoplastic disorder, as well as its pathogenesis. Marie and Bernard Chauffard (1896) described the pigmentary changes associated with the disease. Alex Thomson (1906) wrote the first text on the disease and found it to be hereditary. Since these early years, scores of researchers have written about the disorder and the literature is filled with clinical cases and studies.[57]

## Etiology

The cause of neurofibromatosis is unknown. It is inherited as a Mendelian dominant trait in 50% of the cases. Sporadic or isolated cases probably are due to the result of mutation of the dominant gene. The mutation rate is estimated at $1 \times 10^{-4}$ per gamete per generation.[17]

## Incidence

Von Recklinghausen's disease can affect any age, sex, race, color, or nationality. According to Brasfield (1972), in a study of 110 patients, the age range in which the disease was most common was 30 to 40 years; there was a greater incidence in females.[11] (See Table I.) In a smaller study by Feinstein (1972), the average age was 31, and 80% of the patients were female.[28] However, most reports agree with the stated age distribution, but generally acknowledge equal sex distribution. The disease is scattered world-wide, but has a somewhat higher incidence in the Caucasian race.

The disease is estimated to occur in approximately 1:2,500 births, with a greater incidence among the mentally retarded.[56,108,114]

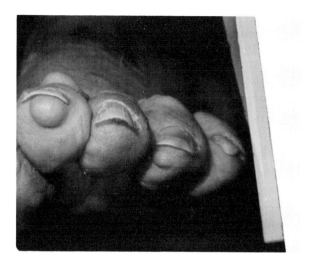

**Figure 4-15A**

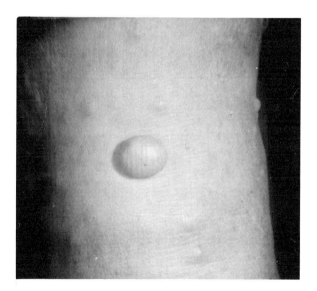

**Figure 4-15B**

Neurofibroma. Multiple neurofibromas of the foot
and ankle. History of von Recklinghausen's disease.

215

## TABLE I

| Age (Years) | Males | Females | Total |
|:-----------:|:-----:|:-------:|:-----:|
| 0– 9 | 14 | 7 | 21 |
| 10–19 | 11 | 10 | 21 |
| 20–29 | 12 | 7 | 19 |
| 30–39 | 8 | 18 | 26 |
| 40–49 | 6 | 6 | 12 |
| 50–59 | 3 | 4 | 7 |
| 60–69 | 2 | 2 | 4 |
| Total | 56 | 54 | 110 |

### Clinical Picture

A patient with neurofibromatosis rarely enters the podiatrist's office because the majority of cases of neurofibromatosis are so mild as to be unrecognized, or so severe as to require the patient to be confined to a mental institution. The patient who does recognize the appearance of an unexplained soft tissue mass usually experiences no significant discomfort, the soft mass posing only a cosmetic problem. Occasionally, however, the mass may be tender, produce a neuralgic type discomfort, or merely paresthesias. The tender nodule is usually accompanied by some degree of muscle weakness; and atrophy may be apparent.[7] Frequently, the disease is manifest by only a single lesion, which is detected only incidentialy during a routine podiatric examination. Such patients are said to exhibit a "forme fruste" variety of neurofibromatosis.

Physical examination of patients with von Recklinghausen's disease generally discloses the classical signs of the disease, which may be classified as (a) cutaneous, (b) osseous, (c) nervous, or (d) miscellaneous.

(a) *Cutaneous* The cafe-au-lait spot(s) and neurofibromata represent the hallmarks of the disease. The cafe-au-lait (coffee with milk) spot characteristically appears as an oval, macular, light brown to tan, smooth-bordered lesion, resembling a large freckle. One or several deep brown macules may be seen in the light brown patches. The lesion is usually present at birth, increasing in size and number through the years. The lesions can be located anywhere on the body and may be asymmetrical or bilaterally symmetrical. One or two similar areas of cutaneous pigmentation are commonly found in otherwise normal individuals who show none of the stigmata of neurofibromatosis. These lesions may increase in size and number with age and may precede by many years the appearance of the characteristic cutaneous and sub-cutaneous tumors.

In neurofibromatosis, the areas of pigmentation are usually greater than four in number and, according to Crowe (1956), any patient presenting with more than six spots over 1.5 centimeters in diameter must be presumed to have von Recklinghausen's disease even in the absence of a positive family history.[18] Cafe-au-lait spots are often the first manifestation of the disease in children. ("Axillary freckling," another form of the cafe-au-lait spots, is almost diagnostic.[16]) Patients exhibiting cafe-au-lait spots without associated tumors are referred to as having the forme fruste (i.e., arrested or partial) stage of von Recklinghausen's disease.

The multiple neurofibromata usually make their appearance around puberty, although occasionally earlier or later, and grow to sizes ranging from a few millimeters to several centimeters. The tumors are located either in the dermis or subcutaneous tissue and are usually soft and elastic, but may become firm.[57] The neurofibromata may take two forms, which may occur separately or in combination. The nonplexiform neurofibromata are sessile or pedunculated, discrete tumors, located in the dermis, that may be widely dispersed over the body. A solitary nonplexiform neurofibroma in the absence of the other stigmata cannot be interpreted as von Recklinghausen's disease. A string of "tumor beads" may be palpable along an involved nerve, showing lateral mobility when displaced with a finger. The tumor may be deep-seated and remain quite small, while others may become globoid or pendulous. The overlying epidermis frequently takes on a melanocytic color which tends to fade as the lesions age.

The plexiform neurofibroma is the most distinctive lesion in the syndrome. In contrast to the generally localized character of the nonplexiform neurofibroma, these subcutaneous tumors involve rather large areas, with localized enlargement of several or many nerve trunks.[38] Such hypertrophied nerve trunks form a plexus and are often embedded in a fibrous matrix associated with an overgrowth of surrounding soft tissue. These tortuous and grotesque nerve trunks are said to have a "bag of worms" consistency when palpated. In severe forms, the skin and soft tissue in the area of involvement may hang in thick, loose folds suggesting elephantiasis.[38] Of interest, according to D'Agostino, is that approximately three percent of patients with plexiform neurofibromata undergo malignant transformation to malignant schwannomas or neurofibrosarcomas, while 50 percent of all malignant schwannomas develop in patients with von Recklinghausen's disease.[21]

(b) *Osseous lesions* On the average, approximately 30 percent of patients with von Recklinghausen's disease demonstrate skeletal deformities, with one-third of the involvement affecting joints.[8] Skeletal deformities can occur because of pressure, erosion, or destruction of bone by neurofibromata occurring within the bones or in close proximity to them. All bone changes can be explained by the development of the neurofibromata that involve the nerves supplying the bone, the lymphatics draining the area, or the medullary cavity. In many cases, osseous changes are noted without any tumor in the region, but, rather, at a distant focus affecting the bone indirectly. However, in most cases, the involved bone lies directly beneath the involved subcutaneous tissue. Deforming scoliosis is the most common skeletal lesion occurring in the disease.[126] In some cases, cafe-au-lait spots and scoliosis are the sole manifestations of the disease. However, x-rays may reveal cortical erosions, irregular linear cortical thickening, subperiosteal cysts (brown cysts), and sharply marginated medullary lytic defects with marked soft tissue hypertrophy and hyperplasia.[59,90,104] Osteomalacia and

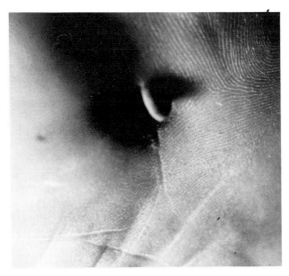

**Figure 4-16**

Neurofibroma. Small pedunculated type of lesion on the plantar surface of the foot. These lesions are usually asymptomatic. *(Courtesy of Richard Gibbs, M.D., New York, New York.)*

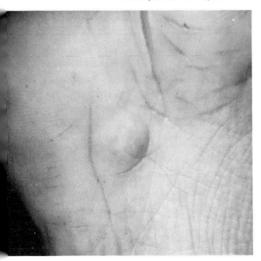
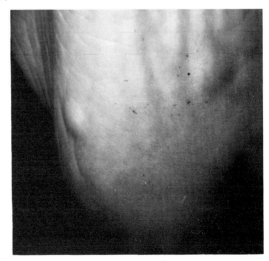

**Figure 4-17A**                    **Figure 4-17B**

Neurofibroma. Neurofibromas on the plantar aspect of the foot are not infrequently seen. They usually underlie the skin and are somewhat soft and fleshy-like in texture. These are most frequently associated with von Recklinghausen's disease.

219

fibrous metaphyseal defects have been noted to occur rather infrequently.[38,76]

(c) *Central nervous system lesions* The disease can involve any part of the central nervious system. Symptoms may range from dramatic, acute, convulsive episodes to subtle delayed speech, impaired hearing, and mental retardation. Crowe noted that the fewer the cafe-au-lait spots the more marked the central nervous system involvement.[17] Nevertheless, rarely does the individual become so severely mentally handicapped as to require commitment to an institution. Meningocele and syringomyelia have also been seen.

(d) *Miscellaneous lesions* In addition to malignant schwannomas and neurofibrosarcomas, other soft tissue malignant neoplasms occur in the disease. Squamous cell carcinomas, fibrosarcomas, pheochromocytomas, malignant melanomas, and basal cell carcinomas have been reported.[56] Periungual fibromas are rarely seen, in contrast to tuberous sclerosis and, when present, are frequently cases of von Recklinghausen's disease combined with abortive forms of tuberous sclerosis. Acromegaly, cretinism, delayed sexual development, hypothyroidism, infertility, Addison's disease, polycystic kidneys, renovascular hypertension, and bladder involvement are rare, but have been reported.[30,76]

## Diagnosis

The presence of multiple cutaneous and subcutaneous neoplasms combined with the cafe-au-lait spots is usually sufficient evidence upon which to make the diagnosis of von Recklinghausen's disease. According to Crowe, if six or more cafe-au-lait spots are present in combination with neurofibromas or axillary freckling, the diagnosis is almost certain.[17] If all three lesions are present they are considered diagnostic. The violaceous color in the more superficial neurofibromas and the tendency of these lesions to buttonhole on digital pressure aid in the differential diagnosis of neurofibromas from other soft tissue tumors. Any patient exhibiting signs of von Recklinghausen's disease must be questioned about familial incidence and must always be examined radiographically for bone pathology.

## Differential Diagnosis

The diagnosis of multiple neurofibromatosis is rarely a problem. Nevertheless, certain disease entities must be considered before a final opinion is rendered. The solitary neurofibroma must be considered in any differential diagnosis of the disease. The solitary neurofibroma is a sporadically occurring neoplasm found in patients who do not have the other stigmata of von Recklinghausen's disease. Its solitary nature is the only differentiating feature of this lesion, for pathologically it is identical to the nonplexiform neurofibroma of von Recklinghausen's disease. The plexiform neurofibroma is rarely, if ever, seen in patients not afflicted with the disease. In addition, the overlying malanotic color of the skin common to the disease is rarely seen in the skin overlying solitary neurofibromas.[38]

The lipoma, either single or multiple, often is the most difficult lesion to rule out. The serrated, lobulated, or irregular border of the lipoma with its long axis lying in a plane horizontal to the subcutaneous fat, as well as its localization to the areas of the body with prominent subcutaneous fat, provide adequate distinguishing features between the two lesions. Lipomas also do not buttonhole upon digital pressure.

The cafe-au-lait spots associated with the disease are classical but, nevertheless, must be distinguished from those that appear in Albright's syndrome. Nevus spilus and Becker's nevus are similar melanocytic lesions but are easily distinguished by the speckled appearance of the former and the hair growth associated with the latter.

## Pathology

The pathological study of lesions associated with the disease centers on the neurofibromas and the cafe-au-lait spots.

Multiple nerve sheath tumors are common to the disease. Solitary and multiple plexiform or nonplexiform neurofibromas are most common, but malignant schwannomas and malignant neurogenic sarcomas are not rare. Apparently, the Schwann cell is the cell of origin for all these lesions. The gross and microscopic appearance of solitary neurofibromas as isolated entities and those associated with the disease are identical, except that in von Recklinghausen's disease the lesions may attain enormous size. Those lesions located in the skin are well circumscribed but not encapsulated, while those located in sites other than the skin and subcutaneous fat are well encapsulated. The mass is rubbery and firm, its cut-surface is grey, homogeneous, and translucent. If a nerve enters the mass, it disappears into the substance of the neoplasm and is not stretched across the surface.[38]

Microscopically, the lesion is located in the dermis or subcutaneous tissue. The tumor cells are usually fusiform and generally arranged in thin, delicate fascicles or small, loosely packed clusters or whorls. Numerous collagen fibrils and a non-organized matrix are noted intercellularly. Axons trapped during the growth of the tumor are frequently seen traversing the lesion. Mast cells, lymphocytes, and melanocytes are found within the lesion, the latter often suggesting that the lesion is a cellular blue nevus. Unlike a schwannoma, in a neurofibroma, axons course through the lesion, while the Schwannoma is a pure nerve sheath tumor, with all neural elements displaced to one side.[38]

The plexiform variety of neurofibroma is a poorly defined type of lesion, and its limits are apt to be impossible to define on gross examination. Numerous tortuous cords and bulbous expansions may protrude from the surface of the specimen. The cut-surfaces show a nonencapsulated, translucent tumor, with a shiny, circumscribed central nodule. The overlying epidermis is often hyperpigmented.[38] Elements of a normal nerve are present, but arranged in a distorted and bizarre fashion. The Schwann cell cords twist, intertwine, and lack an ordinary parallel arrangement. They are associated with a diffuse proliferation of compactly arranged spindle cells, apparently of perineural or epineural origin, into the surrounding tissue.[38] Older lesions exhibit a rather fibrous matrix, whereas younger lesions are more mucinous

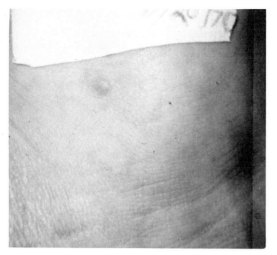
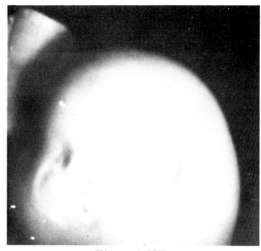

**Figure 4-18A**  **Figure 4-18B**

Neurofibroma. Isolated singular lesion. (A) represents a small neurofibroma of the ankle. (B) represents a neurofibroma in the nail groove. *(Courtesy of Lee E. Friedman, D.P.M., Detroit, Mich.)*

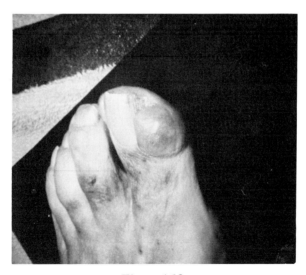

**Figure 4-19**

Plexiform Neurofibroma. Isolated and located in the nail groove area. This lesion has no relationship to von Recklinghausen's disease. *(Courtesy of Gerson Perry, D.P.M., Miami, Florida.)*

in nature. Cross-sections often exhibit numerous hypertrophied nerve bundles coursing through the lesion. The lesion may invade the subcutaneous fat; and, when it does, it will resemble a neurofibrolipoma. Not infrequently, an atypical, hypercellular appearance is noted with an increased number of mitotic figures. This is indicative of a neurofibrosarcoma, but whether or not this is the result of a malignant transformation or is a de novo malignancy is still open to debate.[56] An increased frequency of mitoses is a more reliable index of malignancy than "invasiveness" since benign neurofibromas are not encapsulated, and a certain degree of invasiveness can be seen in almost all the lesions.

The histologic appearance of the cafe-au-lait spots seems to differentiate them from similar pigmentary lesions. Johnson and Charneco reported these lesions to contain more melanocytes and a higher melanocytic activity than similar lesions.[48] Silvers and Greenwood support the belief that giant intracellular pigment granules are characteristic of the disease, but that their absence should not rule out the disease.[107]

## Foot Involvement

The soft tissue and osseous abnormalities that occur commonly, rarely involve the foot. Whether this rarity is absolute or relative to the practitioner's inability to detect the lesions is uncertain. Nevertheless, several researchers have reported both skeletal and soft tissue lesions associated with the disease. The first studies on the leg and feet, done by Halbitz, showed that the nerve lesions were the same in the lower extremity as in the upper.[37] Crowe reported ten patients with dermal and subcutaneous tumors of the soles, which began with a violaceous discoloration and were pathologically diagnosed as neurofibromas.[18] Feinstein, in a review of six cases, reported plexiform neurofibromata about the medial malleoli, subcutaneous nodules on the plantar aspect of both feet, limb shortage, phalangeal cortical thickening, and cafe-au-lait spots on the dorsomedial aspect of a foot.[28] Christenson and Pendborg reported a case of plexiform neurofibroma about the ankle.[14] Hunt and Pugh re-

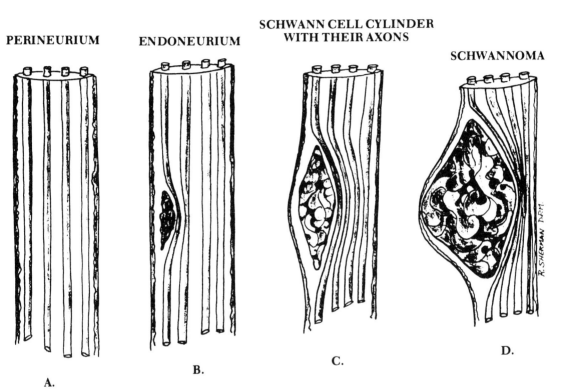

**PERINEURIUM**  **ENDONEURIUM**  **SCHWANN CELL CYLINDER WITH THEIR AXONS**  **SCHWANNOMA**

A.  B.  C.  D.

**Figure 4-20**

(A) represents a normal nerve. (B), (C), and (D) represent a schwannoma developing within a peripheral nerve. Nerve axons do not pass through this tumor but are pushed aside. Surgical treatment is performed by opening the perineurium and excising the nerve lesion without interruption of the nerve axons.[38]

ported two cases of congenital pes cavus associated with the disease.[43] McCarrol wrote of 46 cases of the disease, in which one case showed one short leg and the associated absence of the fifth toe and fifth metatarsal.[72] Moore reported the presence of small misshapen tarsal bones and mottled metatarsals with distorted medullary canals.[78] Friedman stated that cancellous portions of tarsal bones and the first metatarsal showed irregular striations of increased density and some widening of the metatarsal shafts attributed to neurofibromas of the nerve supplying the periosteum.[31] Taylor reported a soft moveable nodule on the plantar aspect of both feet proximal to the second and third toes. The lesions were asymptomatic, but were excised and diagnosed as neurofibromas.[44] Hickey's case is that of a large, soft tissue mass, extending from the first interspace to the third metatarsophalangeal joint on the plantar aspect, which was removed and diagnosed as a neurofibroma. Gamble described a case with multiple, soft, freely moveable neurofibromas on the plantar aspect of both feet.[32]

## Treatment

Palliative therapy remains the only practical treatment for the disease, in general. Although irradiation is of no value, the internist and general surgeon discard ablative surgery as impractical unless signs of malignant transformation are evident. The elective removal of multiple benign lesions indiscriminantly is not justifiable. In addition to treatment of malignant lesions, excision is indicated in cases where the neoplasms are disfiguring, interfere with function, or are subject to trauma and infection.

In podiatry, however, excision of the lesion is more the rule than the exception. The majority of the lesions reported on the foot can be regarded as subject to trauma or infection or may interfere with function. Wide local incision, using a double tourniquet, is recommended. Attempts to curette or shell out the lesion are doomed to failure and recurrence.

## Prognosis

Usually the disease is slowly progressive during the patient's life, but it may remain relatively stationary for long periods. Althugh a benign course is usual, some of the tumors may undergo malignant change to malignant schwannomas or neurofibrosarcomas with their characteristic invasiveness, metastasis, and, usually, death.[56] Sarcomas associated with the disease more commonly arise in deeper nerves, particularly in the extremities. In all cases of plexiform neurofibromas, the prognosis must be guarded. Those lesions appearing in children have a particularly poor prognosis since they grow rather rapidly from the nerve of origin toward the spinal cord. Even wide excision of lesions in children are frequently followed by recurrences at the proximal stump. Death, when it does occur, is usually due to spinal cord compression. Failure to completely excise a lesion frequently results in recurrences with large hypertrophic scars. Metastases, when present, are usually to the lungs and skeletal system, which requires the practitioner to take chest and skeletal x-rays for diagnosis of the extent of involvement of the disease. The cafe-au-lait spots are rarely of any difficulty, but the literature does cite cases of malignant degeneration of these spots into malignant melanomas, requiring careful observation of the lesions during the course of the patient's therapy.[4]

## Solitary Benign Nerve Neoplasms: The Neurilemmoma

### Definition

A neurilemmoma may be defined as a benign nerve neoplasm of neuroectodermal origin comprised of both Schwann cells and collagen fibers.

### Synonyms

A neurilemmoma is also known as a benign schwannoma, neurinoma, encapsulated neurilemmoma, perineural fibroblastoma, and solitary schwannoma.[38]

### Etiology

No specific etiologic agent or cause has been attributed to the neurilemmoma. As with the amputation neuroma and

Morton's neuroma, trauma remains the most likely etiology. Occasionally, the lesions are associated with von Recklinghausen's disease.

*Incidence*

According to Money (1950), neurilemmomas represent .004 percent of all benign soft tissue tumors; in fact, in a study of 361,000 hospital admissions over a 38 year-period, he was able to locate only 13 cases of diagnosed tumors.[77] Fawcett (1967) stated that neurilemmomas are more common in bone but still represent only a fraction of 1 percent of bone neoplasms.[27] Since the lesions are indeed rare, their occurrence within the foot or even the lower extremity is practically non-existent.

These lesions, when present, are, for the most part, solitary, but as many as six have been reported in one patient.[123] Whenever multiple neurilemommas are found, one must investigate whether the patient truly has multiple solitary tumors or is a victim of von Recklinghausen's disease.

There is no age, sex, or race preference, but, according to Marmor (1965), the lesions occur most frequently after the age of 30.[66]

*Clinical Picture*

Schwannomas, in the vast majority of cases, present as asymptomatic soft tissue masses. The lesions are slowly growing and often go unnoticed until found incidentally by the examiner. When symptoms are present, the history usually reveals a duration of approximately five years prior to the patient's visit.[63] The presenting symptoms are, in most cases, dependent upon the location of the tumor. The patient may complain of pain, numbness, paresthesias, hyperesthesias, or weakness of the affected part. When present, the pain may be intractable and not influenced by rest or activity. If the mass acquires considerable size and compresses surrounding vessels, the patient may also complain of swelling, coldness, claudication, or other stages of peripheral vascular disease.

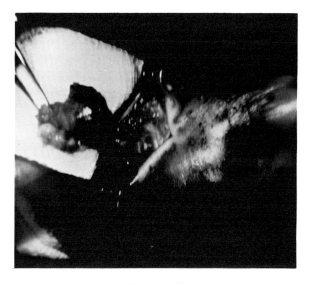

**Figure 4-21**

Neurilemmoma. An extremely rare, benign lesion of the foot. The lesion is located involving the lateral aspect of the fifth metatarsal area. The only symptoms were that of paresthesia and soft tissue swelling could be noticed on palpation.

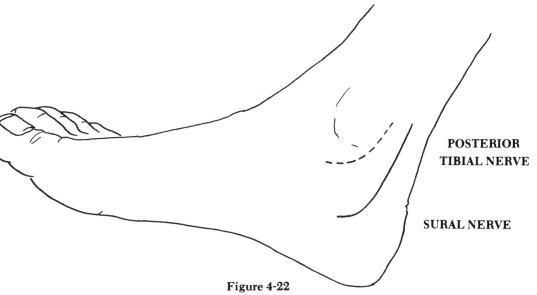

**POSTERIOR TIBIAL NERVE**

**SURAL NERVE**

**Figure 4-22**

This drawing represents surgical approach to various lesions on the medial and lateral aspect of the foot and ankle.

Upon physical examination, an obvious soft tissue swelling may or may not be present. Palpation usually reveals a localized increase in soft tissue mass with variable tenderness. Decreased deep tendon and superficial reflexes may be evident. A positive Tinel sign along the course of the nerve, with sensory loss, is quite common. Lesions that are large enough to palpate usually compress surrounding structures enough to produce diminished peripheral pulses and plethysmographic readings. The lesions may become large enough to produce a cold, cyanotic limb and eventual gangrene.[15] The lesions are usually distributed on flexor surfaces. Nerve conduction studies reveal little if any effect of the tumor, whereas electromyographic studies do reveal some weakness of those muscles innervated by the involved nerve.[123]

## Diagnosis

The diagnosis of a neurilemmoma cannot be made definitively by clinical findings. Symptoms referrable to the neoplasm are common to many soft tissue masses and are consequently of little definitive value. The mass is moveable in its transverse axis and rather fixed in its longitudinal axis. When pigment changes are evident in the overlying skin (cafe-au-lait spots), one must further evaluate the possibility of von Recklinghausen's disease. Biopsy and microscopic examination are the only definitive diagnostic methods.

## Differential Diagnosis

The following differential possibilities must be considered: solitary neurofibroma, multiple neurofibromata (neurofibromatosis), fibroma, neuroma, malignant nerve lesions, giant cell tumor of tendon (sheath origin), osteoid osteoma (when neurilemmoma involves bone), glomus tumor, ganglion, lipoma, and leiomyoma.

## Pathology

According to Stout (1935), neurilemmomas and Schwann cell tumors and are of neuroectodermal origin.[112] The lesions are fusiform, encapsulated masses developing within the perineurium. Unlike a solitary neurofibroma, the nerve fibers are compressed to one side, rather than passing through the tumor itself.[46] Upon gross examination, the lesion has a rubbery consistency and appears more or less homogeneous. Its cut-surface may be homogeneous or slightly nodular and reddish brown, with irregular, yellow, cystic foci. If carefully dissected during removal, the nerve of origin may be recognized. The tumor usually projects from one side and is adherent to the nerve.

Microscopic examination reveals the mass to be contained within a fibrous tissue sheath. The cellular patterns which make up the bulk of the mass are of two types. The first type,, the Antoni type A, is a solid tumor with elongated Schwann cells, straight reticular fibers, and nuclei in vertical or horizontal rows called "palisades". Zones where the palisades are at either end of a bundle of straight reticular fibers may have an organoid appearance (verocay body).[9] The second type, the Antoni type B, is a loose syncytium of anastomosing cells with long slender processes, together with interspersed microcysts probably from degenerating collagen fibers.[45]

Blood vessels are usually prominent, while nerve elements are rarely seen. However, if the neoplasm grows into a nerve (not merely displacing it), axonal elements may be found in the tumor. Rarely does the tumor show evidence of malignant change.

## Foot Involvement

Foot involvement is extremely rare with perhaps less than 20 cases ever reported on the foot. The folowing are unusual cases presenting signs and symptoms involving the foot.

The first cases is that of a patient presenting with pedal edema, a cold, cyanotic left leg, negative pulses, dry gangrene of the left hallux, and weak dorsiflexion of the left foot. Physical examination revealed a palpable mass in the left popliteal space. Exploratory surgery revealed a fusiform mass in continuity with the peronial nerve, which had produced thrombosis of the popliteal artery. Biopsy showed a benign schwannoma of the common peroneal nerve.

The next case involved a patient presenting with numbness in the toes of both feet, decreased knee and ankle reflexes, and hyperesthesias of the lateral aspect of both legs and feet. A biopsy revealed a neurileommoma of the T-11 spinal root.[45]

Another patient complained of a painful mass on the dorsum of the left foot, with irritation and pain on ambulation, which was only partially relieved by non-weight bearing. Physical examination revealed diffuse swelling on the dorsal and plantar aspects of the left foot in the area of the third metatarsal, to the extent that the circumference of the left foot was 3.5 centimeters larger than the right foot. Biopsy revealed a dumbbell-shaped neurilemmoma of the medial and lateral plantar nerves.[51]

In the fourth case, the author's experience revealed a small palpable mass along the mid-shaft of the patients fifth metatarsal. The only symptoms were paresthesia and edema. Biopsy showed a neurilemmoma of a branch of the sural nerve.

The literature occasionally reveals the existence of these lesions in the foot, and the following is a chart representing a 40 year literature review of these cases.

| Number of Cases | Location in Foot | Reference |
|---|---|---|
| 6 | No lesion in foot, only symptoms. | Jacobs[45] |
| 1 | Medial plantar N. | Stout[112] |
| 32 | 4 in foot, with no mention of location. | White[123] |
| 13 | No mention of location. | Jacobs[45] |
| 5 | No mention of location, 4 malignant and 1 benign. | Wardle[119] |
| 1 | Calcaneus. | Cucolo[19] |
| 1 | Jct. medial & lateral, plantar N. | Kaplan[50] |
| 1 | Medial plantar N. | Marmor[66] |

## Treatment

The nerve fibers in a neurilemmoma do not course through the tumor mass; the mass, instead, develops below the perineurium displacing the nerve fibers to one side, or the nerve fibers might surround the neoplasm. This makes it possible to longitudinally incise the perineurium and shell out the mass.[20] The perineurium is resutured, using the nerve sheath as a guide, to retain the proper nerve bundle alignment and avoid sensory-motor transposition.

According to Stout (1935), the vast majority of the lesions are benign, and enucleation of the lesion, after longitudinal dissection of the nerve, produces a cure.[112] Wardle (1957), however, disagrees about possible malignancy, and, therefore, feels that a more aggressive surgical approach should be employed. If bones are involved, the part should be amputated.[119] When difficulty is encountered in enucleating the mass, one must consider the possibility of a malignancy or neurofibroma and proceed in the appropriate manner. If neurolysis is performed, nerve repair should also be attempted.

In the vast majority of patients, any sensory or motor deficiencies quickly return following excision of the lesion although transient aggravation of symptoms postoperatively has been reported.[112]

## Prognosis

Total recovery takes approximately four months and the recurrence rate is low with complete removal of the lesion. If the lesion is inadequately removed, in time the symptoms would most likely return due to further development of the tumor. However, Stout (1935) stated that the prognosis for decrease in symptomatology is good, even if the entire tumor is not removed.[112]

Healing of nerve tissue may take as long as 18 months after the removal of a nerve tumor.

## Malignant Nerve Lesions

*Definition*

The subject of malignant nerve neoplasms appears to be more confusing than it really is because over the years a multitude of different terms has been applied to describe similar peripheral nerve tumors. The controversy basically centers on the cell or cells of origin for these peripheral nerve tumors.

Malignant nerve lesions have been classified into two broad categories: nerve sheath tumors and neuroectodermal tumors.

Nerve sheath tumors arise from either the Schwann cell, perineurium, epineurium, or neurilemma; whereas neuroectodermal tumors are the product of the neural substance, the neuron and ganglia. Of these two broad categories, only those involving the nerve sheath are of real importance to podiatry since, to date, reports of neuroectodermal lesions in the extremities have not appeared in any literature. Nerve sheath neoplasms may be further subdivided into four categories: malignant schwannoma, malignant epithelioid schwannoma, malignant melanocytic schwannoma and nerve sheath fibrosarcoma.

*Synonyms*

1. Malignant schwannoma: malignant neurinoma, malignant neurilemmoma, malignant nerve sheath tumor, perineural fibrosarcoma, neurogenic sarcoma, neurofibrosarcoma, fibromyxosarcoma of nerve, fibrosarcoma myxomatodes, fibrosarcoma of nerve sheath, malignant peripheral glioma, myxosarcoma of nerve sheath, neurilemmosarcoma, sarcoma of peripheral nerve, and secondary malignant neuroma.

2. Malignant epithelioid schwannoma: malignant neurinoma, malignant neurilemmoma, and malignant schwannoma.

3. Malignant melanocytic schwannoma: fusiform cell malignant melanoma, and malignant blue nevus.

4. Nerve sheath fibrosarcoma: fibrosarcoma, neurogenous of nerve, fibrosarcoma myxomatodes, fibrosarcoma of nerve sheath, malignant neurilemmoma, malignant neurinoma, malignant peripheral glioma, myxosarcoma of nerve sheath, neurilemmosacoma, neurofibrosarcoma, neurogenic or neurogenous sarcoma, sarcoma of peripheral nerve, and secondary malignant neuroma.[38]

## History

Data on malignant nerve lesions date back to the late 1800's with reports by French pathologists Delore, Feindel, and Garrè. The most all-inclusive work on the subject, however, is attributed to A.P. Stout, who concluded that the majority of malignant schwannomas was found in patients with von Recklinghausen's disease, either de novo or due to malignant transformation of an existing plexiform neurofibroma.[111] Stewart described malignant nerve neoplasms with histologic pleomorphism, resembling a malignant melanoma but containing no melanin. Stewart and Copeland coined the term malignant epithelioid schwannoma, and suggested that this lesion may bridge the gap between the typical schwannoma or neurogenic sarcoma and melanomas.[110] Michel (1967), in a review of the literature on malignant neurilemmomas with epithelioid elements, concluded that there was no significant difference in the behavior of those tumors with epithelioid elements and those in which they were absent.[75]

## Incidence

Very little statistical information is available on the incidence of the various types of nerve sheath malignancies, although the literature abounds with clinical cases. As stated earlier, the confusion regarding the cell or origin of these tumors has led most investigators to lump all malignant nerve lesions into groups broadly call malignant schwannomas or neurogenic sarcomas. Taking this fact into consideration, the following statistical studies can be more fully appreciated.

Vieta and Pack, in a study of 31 patients with malignant

schwannomas, found that the lesions were more prevalent in females, with a ratio of 3:2. The lesions occurred at practically all ages, with the mean age for females being 35 and males 43.[118] Maseritz, in a study of 192 cases, found an equal sex distribution, and most of the patients (93%) were Caucasians.[67] DasGupta and Brasfield, in the largest study to date (232 cases), found males outnumbered females by 3:2, with an age spread of one through 79 years, but with 42 percent of all lesions occurring between the ages of 30 and 50.[23] In summary, there appears to be more or less equal sex distribution, an average age of 40 years, and a predominant occurrence among Caucasians.

The lesions occur in any part of the body. Maseritz found that 50 percent of his cases had lesions located on the lower extremities, while DasGupta found only 38 percent with involvement of the lower extremity.[67,23] Thompson stated that 24 percent of all malignant schwannomas are associated with von Recklinghausen's disease. White estimated, however, that up to 75 percent are associated with the disease.[115,22] Harkin and Reed compromised and conceded that at least 50 percent of all malignant schwannomas and/or neurogenic sarcomas are associated with this neurocutaneous syndrome.[38] The following table represents a composite of the studies that are available on the incidence of these malignancies:

Compilation of the figures from the table on page 237 indicates the following incidence in the lower extremities:

| | | |
|---|---|---|
| Leg | ......................... | 10.0% |
| Ankle | ....................... | 1.5% |
| Foot ...... 2.7% | Toes ...... | 0.5% |

*Clinical Picture*

There are no characteristic signs or symptoms identifiable with nerve tumors. However, according to Pack and Ariel, the most consistent chief complaint is the presence of a soft tissue mass.[85] In those individuals with von Recklinghausen's disease, in whom these lesions are more common,

**DISTRIBUTION**

| Cases | Age | Sex | Race | Torso | Arms | Thigh | Leg | Ankle | Foot | Toes |
|---|---|---|---|---|---|---|---|---|---|---|
| Pack[85] (32) | * | * | 32-C | * | * | * | 2 | * | 2 | * |
| Vieta[118] (31) | 43-M 35-F | 18-M 13-F | 31-C | * | * | * | * | * | 1 | * |
| Maseritz[67] (192) | * | 96-M 96-F | 179-C 13-B | (99 torso + arms) | | 38 | 33 | 10 | 9 | 3 |
| D'Agostino[21] (24) | * | * | * | * | * | * | 2 | * | * | * |
| Stewart[110] (128) | * | * | * | * | * | * | * | * | 1 | * |
| White[122] (15) | * | * | * | * | * | 1 | 3 | * | * | * |
| Charache[13] (19) | 41 | 8-M 11-F | 17-C 2-B | 8 | | 8 | 3 | * | * | * |
| DasGupta[23] (232) | 30 −50 | 130-M 102-F | 220-C 12-B | (125 torso + arms) | | 53 | 25 | * | 6 | * |
| 673 | * | 252-M | 479-C | (232) | (232) | 100 | 68 | 10 | 19 | 3 |

* No statistics available.
M Male    C Caucasian
F Female    B Black

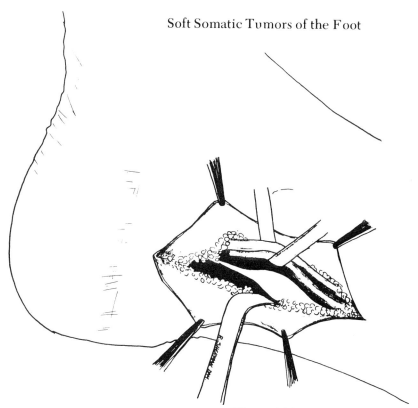

**Figure 4-23**

A representative illustration of an area of the posterior tibial nerve where schwannoma have been reported. Nerve repair at this level should be pursued.

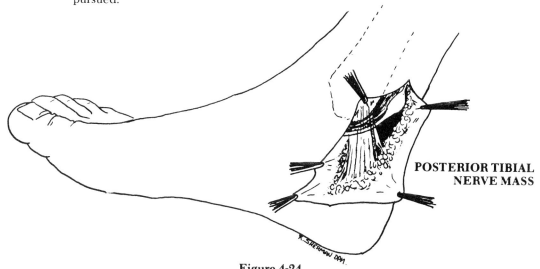

**POSTERIOR TIBIAL
NERVE MASS**

**Figure 4-24**

Nerve tumors at the distal bifurcation of the posterior tibial nerve. Neurinoma as well as neuroma have been reported. Nerve repair at this level should be attempted.

**238**

the recent, more rapid growth of a mass which may have been present without symptoms, causes the patient to seek aid. In other cases, pain, parasthesias, or muscular atrophy may be the presenting symptom long before any definitive soft tissue mass is evident. The tumors are rather slow-growing and, in fact, symptoms, if present, may be present for up to four years before a palpable mass is evident.[85]

All types of nerve sheath tumors are more common on the extremities than the torso. The lesions are basically flexoral in distribution and vary in size from several millimeters to many centimeters. According to DasGupta, in his study of 232 cases, 60 percent of all the lesions are less than 10 centimeters in size.[23] Most lesions are small and rarely increase in size, unless exposed to trauma or incomplete excision, the latter being common with removal of neurofibromas. Following trauma, they may grow rapidly, become necrotic, and metastasize.[13]

The lesions are generally firm and non-tender, skin-colored masses, attached to the overlying skin but freely moveable beneath. According to Holland and Frei, these masses are freely moveable in the transverse axis but not in their longitudinal axis.[41] While the malignant schwannoma is more common in the lower extremity, the malignant epithelioid schwannoma is more common in the upper extremity and tends to take on a fusiform appearance on the flexoral surfaces. The malignant melanocytic schwannoma usually appears as a blue-black flat lesion, but it is extremely rare, and, like its analogue, the malignant melanoma, is usually asymptomatic for years, followed by rapid metastasis and death. The nerve sheath fibrosarcoma is the most common malignant neoplasm of von Recklinghausen's disease and tends to occur in the stump of the nerve after excision of the neurofibroma. These lesions are very malignant but tend to metastasize much later than the malignant epithelioid schwannoma.[13]

It should be noted that the incorporation of a nerve into a tumor mass is insufficient proof that the tumor arose from the nerve. In fact, the majority of malignant lesions that involve nerve are the result of the tumors ability to surround, invade, and destroy adjacent nerves. On the other hand, if a nerve contains or is incorporated into a tumor and the histologic structure is compatible with a nerve sheath neoplasm, this would be conclusive proof of origin in nerve tissue.[57]

*Diagnosis*

The diagnosis of nerve sheath neoplasms, as with any other soft tissue tumor, cannot be made clinically, but rather rests on interpretation of its histopathology.

*Differential Diagnosis*

The most common and important aspect of the differential diagnosis is whether the tumor noticed is malignant. Of the four malignant nerve tumors, the malignant schwannoma most commonly involves the foot and must be differentiated from the benign schwannoma. This differential diagnosis is usually relatively easy when one remembers that the malignant lesion is usually invasive, affects larger nerves, is more common on the lower extremity, and is usually associated with von Recklinghausen's disease.

Fibrosarcomas, desmoid tumors, lipomas, liposarcomas, myxosarcomas, rhabdomyosarcomas, dermatofibroma protuberans, and sclerosing hemangiomas have been reported as differential possibilities.[23,47] The malignant epithelioid schwannoma must especially be differentiated from a pure spindle cell sarcoma and malignant melanoma. The malignant melanocytic schwannoma must be differentiated from the malignant melanoma and spindle cell nevus. The nerve sheath fibrosarcoma must be differentiated from the pure fibrosarcoma.

*Pathology*

Malignant schwannomas are well circumscribed, homogeneous, hypercellular, gray, leathery masses. They may be solitary or arise within or in the vicinity of a plexiform neurofibroma. Those arising within a plexiform neurofibroma show a picture of invasiveness because of the diffuse nature of the tumor of origin. The majority arise along peripheral nerves. They may remain encapsulated or confined within the nerve sheath, expanding it or forming a fusiform mass, whose shape is determined by the density of the surrounding tissue into which the nerve is expanding. Multiple tumors may fuse, and adjacent nerves may become incorporated, producing a false impression of infiltration. The capsule, though it grossly appears as such, is really a pseudocapsule, for the points at which the capsule adheres to bone, fascia, muscle, and vessels frequently contain tumor cells; such points of attachment serve as a nidus for regrowth if the tumor is shelled out rather than being widely resected. The tumor tends to grow along the nerve trunks, rather than into the surrounding tissues, via intraneural, perineural, and perivascular lymph channels. Encapsulated distant satellite nodules may occur. The gross extent of the tumor can often be delimited by observing the thickening and edematous appearance of the perineural tissue.[118] Although the nerve appears to enter and traverse the neoplasm, it is impossible to trace it into the tumor.[23]

The histologic picture is that of a cellular tumor composed of plump spindle cells, with mitoses and hyperchromatic nuclei of variable size. The increased cellularity and nuclear changes are present both within and outside the confines of the perineurium.[38] Russell and Rubenstein described the cells as growing in cords with the nuclei in tandem formation and having a tendency to pallisade.[102] In some areas, these cords form whorls resembling a herringbone pattern. This interlacing pattern of cells and cell bundles often makes it difficult to differentiate this tumor from a fibrosarcoma.

A malignant epithelioid schwannoma resembles a malignant schwannoma, but its cut-surface appears pale gray and flecked with multiple colors. Microscopically, these are similar to malignant melanomas, but contain no melanin. The cells appear round to polyhedral and may be arranged in solid round nests much like a melanoma.[38] The degree of cellular pleomorphism is variable. The lesion is usually confined within the perineurium. A surrounding neurofibroma may be evident if the patient also has von Recklinghausen's disease.

Grossly, the cut-surface of a malignant melanocytic schwannoma is pale gray, with a whorled pattern and irregular areas of pigmentation. Microscopically, spindle cells are arranged in interlacing fascicles with intermingled melanocytes and numerous mitotic figures.[38]

Nerve sheath fibrosarcomas resemble many other sarcomas in having a non-distinctive gross appearance. However, since they are the most frequent malignant neoplasm associated with von Recklinghausen's disease, a direct continuity with the plexiform neurofibroma is seen. Histologically, the tumor cells appear to be fibroblasts, though it is not known whether they are in part or totally of schwann cell origin.[38] The tumors tend to be differentiated from the pure fibrosarcoma by a matrix that is more mucinous than collagenous, but they overlap histologically with malignant schwannomas and assignment of a tumor to either category is often quite arbitrary. The spindle cells are arranged in bundles and whorls. Quick and Cutler graded these tumors based on their histologic degree of malignancy:

Grade I:      Low-grade malignancy. Tumors show mild cellularity, with lage spindle cells, and a firm hyaline matrix.

Grade II:     Moderate-grade malignancy. Tumors show moderate cellularity with large spindle cells in bundles with whorling and little matrix.

Grade III:    High-grade malignancy. Very cellular tumors, with small spindle cells in whorls and large pleomorphic polyhedral cells.[94]

*Foot Involvement*

Foot symptoms associated with these lesions are rare, and the presence of a mass on the foot is practically non-existent. The following cases represent a selective sampling of descriptive cases with foot involvement.

One case is that of a 25 year old female who complained of pain and tingling in her right foot. No inherent foot pathology was noted on examination, and she was treated for "sciatica" for one year with no apparent relief. Following exhaustive studies, a tumor was found in the right gluteal region,[23] a biopsy of which showed a malignant schwannoma of the sciatic nerve.

A case was reported of a 31 year old male, who, while standing on his toes, felt a sudden pain in his foot. He disregarded it until six months later, when pressure against his left second toe produced pain. A slight swelling was then observed, spreading to his calf and the back of his thigh, and worsening in the evening. Two months later he observed a tumor behind his knee. One year later he could not flex his toes. He subsequently lost weight and was admitted to the hospital where a biopsy revealed a malignant schwannoma of the tibial nerve. He died shortly thereafter of metastases.[3]

A 44 year old male complained of a painful, palpable mass proximal to the right lateral malleolus, which became a fungating, ulcerating lesion. A biopsy showed a malignant schwannoma of the peroneal nerve.[118]

Another case is that of a 19 year old female who was seen because of a severely painful hammertoe. Physical examination revealed an associated port-wine nevus and a "congenital peeling" between the toes. Because of the pain, an amputation was performed revealing a previously undiscovered tumor in the region of the metatarsal, diagnosed as a malignant schwannoma. The tumor was excised, but metastasis had already occurred, and the patient died shortly thereafter.[110]

Giannestrous and Bronson (1975) described the most recent case of foot involvement. The malignant schwannoma involved the medial branch of the plantar nerve in a 64 year old male and was unassociated with von Recklinghausen's disease.[31A]

A 33 year old black female presented with a small, firm, painless mass, of seven years duration, on the dorsomedial aspect of her right foot. The lesion was not clinically pigmented. At surgery, the tumor appeared encapsulated and was located within the lower dermis and subcutaneous tissue. Cut-sections of the tumor were gray-pink. The tumor was resected and reported as a malignant blue nevus.[60]

An infant presented with a slowly growing, pea-sized nodule over the lateral and dorsal aspects of the distal phalanx of several toes. The lesions were non-tender and glistening and resembled blisters. They were originally diagnosed as blisters, but, following rupture, they recurred.[47] Excisional biopsy showed them to be neurofibrosarcomas.

Malignant epithelioid schwannomas are extremely rare. They are usually painless, but may present on the foot in the same manner as a malignant schwannoma. To date, no case of this lesion involving the foot or lower extremity has been reported. Their occurrence on the foot and leg, however, is mentioned in passing in several reports.

It is important to note that, as with many other foot problems, though the symptom may be pedal in nature, its origin may be due to a primary lesion located elsewhere. White cites six cases where symptomatology in the foot was due to a lesion in the thigh.[122]

*Treatment*

Because of their relatively infrequent occurrence, little has been published concerning treatment of malignant nerve lesions. Nevertheless, there is no question that extirpative surgery is the only form of treatment.[98] If these lesions are left alone they grow inexorably and eventually metastasize, with death ensuing. According to Stout, they recur in about 20 percent of patients after attempted surgical removal, indicating that it is impossible to know how difficult it is to determine adequacy of local resection.[111] Since cure of these notoriously resistant tumors by any form of radiotherapy is unlikely, early radical surgery is essential.[111]

Again it should be emphasized that although these tumors appear encapsulated, they infiltrate the surrounding muscle, bone, fascia, and blood vessels; attempts to excise or shell out these tumors have invariably failed with resultant local recurrence and probable metastasis.[21] DasGupta recommended en bloc resection of the tumor and tumor bed, with attached muscle, bone and fascia.[23] Lataste suggested that, if, upon gross examination, the lesion merely extends along the course of a nerve, and the nerve of origin can be identified, then the nerve should be resected through a normal segment.[62]

Wardle stated that total radical resection is minimal and if invasiveness is evident, amputation is a necessity.[120] It should be noted that even in what appears to be an innocent fibroma, total excision should be the goal since according to Charche, 12 percent of fibromas of any origin undergo sarcomatous changes due to stimulus of trauma and incomplete excision.[13]

*Prognosis*

In general, malignant schwannomas are locally invasive, with little propensity for metastasis; malignant epithelioid schwannomas and nerve sheath fibrosarcomas are highly malignant; and the malignant melanocytic schwannoma is of undecided behavior.[38] All are resistant to x-ray therapy and frequently recur after local excision. In general, the longer surgical resection is postponed, the greater the likelihood that amputation will be required. Metastases to the lung occur in up to 30 percent of all patients, primarily with malignant epithelioid schwannomas or nerve sheath fibrosarcomas.

Radical resection (or amputation) initially appears to have the best prognosis. In the study by DasGupta, of 103 patients, the following statistics were compiled:[23]

|  | *Patients* | *Recurrences* | *Recurrence Rate* |
|---|---|---|---|
| Local excision | 55 | 40 | 73% |
| Wide resection | 48 | 10 | 20% |

In a similar study by the same author, the five and ten year survival rates were determined, based upon whether wide resection, radiotherapy, or palliative therapy was performed. The following results were obtained:

| | Patients | Recur-rences | Recurrence Rate | | |
|---|---|---|---|---|---|
| | | | 1–2 yrs. | 5 yrs. | 10 yrs. |
| Wide Resection | 132 | 61 | 48% | 50% | 30% |
| Radiation | 54 | 31 | 58% | 40% | 35% |
| Palliation | 31 | 31 | 100% | 2% | 0 |

Malignant nerve neoplasms of the foot, in addition to their intrinsic problems, should alert the practitioner to the possibilities of other tumors elsewhere in the body and the possible need for referral to an oncologist. Up to seven percent of patients with malignant nerve lesions have other primary malignancies, such as in the colon, breast, lymph nodes, lungs, or skin.[23]

## Bibliography

1. Baker, L.D. and Kuhn, H.H.: Morton's metatarsalgia. *South. Med. Jour.*, **37**: 123–127, 1944.
2. Barbalias, G.A.: Neurofibromatosis of the pelvis and bladder. *Del. Med. Jour.*, **45**: 33–37, 1973.
3. Bergstrand, H.: Malignant schwannoma of the tibial nerve. *Amer. Jour. Cancer*, **21**: 588–595, 1934.
4. Berlin, S.J., Donick, I.I., Block, L.D., and Costa, A.J.: Nerve tumors of the foot: diagnosis and treatment. *JAPA*, **65**: 157–166, 1975.
5. Berry, T.A.: Morton's metatarsalgia due to cavernous angioma. *JBJS*, **39B, No. 1**: 124–125, 1957.
6. Betts, L.O.: Morton's metatarsalgia: neuritis of the fourth digital nerve. *Med. Jour. Aust.*, **1**: 514–515, 1940.
7. Bickel, W.H. and Dockerty, M.A.: Plantar neuroma's, Morton's toe. *Surg. Gyn. & Obst.*, **84**: 111–116, 1947.
8. Bingold, A.C.: Joint changes in neurofibromatosis. *JBJS*, **34B**: 76, 1952.
9. Boldrey, E.E.: Amputation neuroma in nerve implanted in bone. *Ann. Surg.*, **118**: 1052, 1948.
10. Bradford, E.H.: Metatarsal neuralgia, or Morton's affection of the foot. *Bost. Med. & Surg. Jour.*, **125, No. 3**: 52–55, 1891.
11. Brasfield, R.D.: von Recklinghausen's disease, a clinical pathological study. *Ann. Surg.*, **175**: 86–104, 1972.
12. Butterworth, T. and Strean, L.P.: *Clinical Genodermatology.* Williams & Wilkins Co., Baltimore, 1962, pp. 103–104.

13. Charache, H.: Neurogenic sarcoma. *Amer. Jour. Surg.*, **41**: 275–280, 1938.
14. Christenson, E. and Pendborg, J.J.: Rare case of neurofibromatosis (plexiform type). *Acta. Odent. Scand.*, **14**: 1–10, 1956.
15. Clifford, J.R. et al: Thrombosis of popliteal artery caused by a neurinoma of the common perineal nerve. *Amer. Surg.*, **40**: 392–394, 1974.
16. Crowe, F.W.: Axillary freckling as a diagnostic aid in neurofibromatosis. *Ann. Int. Med.*, **61**: 1142–1143, 1964.
17. Crowe, F.W., Schull, W.J., and Neil, J.V.: *A clinical, pathological and genetic study of multiple neurofibromatosis.* Charles C. Thomas, Springfield, 1956, pp. 123–245.
18. Crowe, F.W., Schull, W.J., and Neil, J.V.: *A clinical, pathological and genetic study of multiple neurofibromatosis.* Charles C. Thomas, Springfield, 1956, p. 39, 123–245.
19. Cucolo, G.F. et al: Neurilemmoma of peripheral nerves—case report. *Bul. Hosp. Joint Dis.*, **27**: 225–235, 1968.
20. Cutler, E.C. and Gross, R.E.: Surgical treatment of tumors of peripheral nerves. *Ann. Surg.*, **104**: 436–451, 1936.
21. D'Agostino, A.N., Soule, E.H., and Miller, R.H.: Primary malignant neoplasms of nerves in patients with von Recklinghausen's disease. *Cancer*, **16**: 1003–1004, 1963.
22. DasGupta, T.K. et al: Tumors of peripheral nerve origin—benign and malignant solitary schwannomas. *Cancer*, **20**: 228–233, 1970.
23. DasGupta, T.K. and Brasfield, R.D.: Solitary malignant schwannomas. *Ann Surg.*, **171**: 419–428, 1970.
24. Domonkos, A.N.: *Andrew's Diseases of the Skin.* W.B. Saunders Co., Phila., 1971, pp. 803–804.
25. Duncan, T.L. and Wright, J.L.: Plantar interdigital neuroma. *South. Med. Jour.*, **51**: 49, 1958.
26. Evans, L.E. et al: Prevention of painful neuromas in horses. *Jour. Amer. Vet. Med. Assoc,*, **153**: 313, 1968.
27. Fawcett, K.J. et al: Neurilimmoma of bone. *Amer. Jour. Clin. Path.*. **47**: 759–766, 1967.
28. Feinstein, M.H.: Foot pathology associated with tuberous sclerosis and neurofibromatosis. *JAPA*, **62**: 336–350, 1972.
29. Fleming, M.P. and Miller, W.E.: Renovascular hypertension due to neurofibromatosis, report of a case. *Amer. Jour. Roent. Radium Therapy Nucl. Med.*, **113**: 452—454, 1971.
30. Fraument, J.F.: Neurofibromatosis and childhood leukemia. *Brit. Jour. Med.*, **4**: 489–490, 1971.
31. Friedman, M.M.: Neurofibromatosis of bone. *Amer. Jour. Roent.*, **51**: 623, 1944.
31A. Giannestras, N.J. and Bronson, J.L.: Malignant schwannoma of the medial plantar branch of the post tibial nerve. *JBJS*, **57A**: 701, 1975.
32. Gamble, D.E.: Multiple neurofibroma. *JAPA*, **49**: 501–502, 1959.

33. Gibney, V.P.: The non-operation treatment of metatarsalgia. *Jour. Nerv. and Ment. Dis.*, **19**: 589–596, 1894.

34. Gross., S.W. et al: Peripheral nerve tumors. *Neurol.*, **7**: 711, 1957.

35. Guthrie, L.G.: On a form of painful toe. *The Lancet*, **1**: 628, 1892.

36. Guttman, L. and Medawar, P.B.: The chemical inhibition of fiber regeneration and neuroma formation in peripheral nerve. *Jour. Neurol., Neurosurg., and Psych.*, **5**: 130, 1942.

37. Harbitz, F.: Multiple neurofibromatosis. *Arch. of Int. Med.*, **3**: 32, 1909.

38. Harkin, J.C. and Reed, R.J.: Tumors of the peripheral nervous system. Armed Forces Institute of Pathology, *Atlas of Tumor Pathology*, Series 2, Fascicle 3, 1969: 67–95, 107–136.

39. Hauser, E.D.: Interdigital neuroma of the foot. *Surg., Gyn., & Obst.*, **133**: 265–267, 1971.

40. Hoadley, A.E.: Six cases of metatarsalgia. *Chic. Med. Rec.*, **5**: 32–37, 1893.

41. Holland, J.F. and Frei, E., *Cancer Medicine*. Lea and Febiger, Phila., 1973, p. 1859.

42. Huber, C.G. and Lewis, D.: Amputation neuromas. *Arch. Surg.*, **1**: 85, 1920.

43. Hunt, J.C. and Pugh, D.G.: Skeletal lesions and neurofibromatosis. *Radiology*, **76**: 1, 1961.

44. Ivins, J.C., Dockerty, M.B., and Ghormley, R.K.: Fibrosarcomas of soft tissues of the lower extremity. *Surg.*, **28**: 495, 1950.

45. Jacobs, R.L. and Barmada, R.: Neurilemmoma—a review of the literature with six case reports. *Arch. Surg.*, **102**: 181–186, 1971.

46. Jenkins, S.A.: Solitary tumors of peripheral nerve trunks. *JBJS*, **34B**: 401–411, 1952.

47. Jensen, A.R., Martin, L.W., and Longino, L.: Digital neurofibrosarcoma in infancy. *Jour. of Pediatrics*, **51**: 566–570, 1957.

48. Johnson, B.L. and Charneco, D.R.: Cafe-au-lait spot in neurofibromatosis and normal individuals. *Arch. Der.*, **102**: 442–446, 1970.

49. Joplin, R.J.: The proper digital nerve, vitallium stem arthroplast and some thoughts about foot surgery in general. *Clin. Ortho.*, **76**: 199–212, 1971.

50. Kaplan, F.B.: Neurilemmoma of peripheral nerves—case report, *Bul. Hosp. Joint Dis.*, **27**: 225–235, 1968.

51. Kaplan, R.: Neurilemmoma of foot. *JBJS*, **48A**: 949–952, 1966.

52. Kelikian, H.: *Hallux Valgus, Allied Deformities of the Forefoot and Metatarsalgia*. W.B. Saunders, Phila., 1965, pp. 359–368.

53. Kite, H.I.: Morton's toe neuroma. *South. Med. Jour.*, **59**: 20–25, 1966.

54. Kitting, R.W. et al: Removal of an inter-metatarsal neuroma. *JAPA*, **63**: 274–276, 1973.

55. Kline, D.G. et al: The neuroma in continuity. Its pre-operative and operative management. *Surg. Clin. N.A.*, **52**: 1189–1209, 1972.

56. Knight, W.A., Murphy, W.K., and Gottlieb, J.A.: Neurofibromatosis

associated with malignant neurofibromas. *Arch. Derm.,* **107**: 747–750, 1973.

57. Kramer, W.: Tumors of nerves. *Handbook of Clinical Neurology,* North Holland Publ. Co., Amsterdam, 1970, pp. 450–453, 945–950.

58. Kravette, M.A.: Peripheral nerve entrapment syndrome in the foot. *JAPA,* **61**: 457–472, 1971.

59. Kullman, L. and Wouters, H.W.: Neurofibromatosis, gigantism and subperiosteal hematoma. Report of two children with extensive subperiosteal bone formation. *JBJS,* **54B**: 130–138, 1972.

60. Kwitten, J. and Negri, L.: Malignant blue nevus. *Arch. Derm.,* **94**: 66–69, 1966.

61. Lambert, C.N.: Amputation neuroma—prevention in juvenile patients. *Orth. Clin. N.A.,* **Vol. 3, No .2**: 475, 1972.

62. Lataste, J.: Tumors of peripheral nerves. *Presse Med.,* **70**: 213–215, 1962.

63. Lewis, D. and Hart, D.: Tumors of peripheral nerves. *Ann. Surg.,* **92**: 961–983, 1930.

64. Litchman, M.D. et al: Morton's metatarsalgia and its relationship to trauma. *Rhode Is. Med. Jour.,* **47**: 328–331, 1964.

65. Lynch, J.D., Sheps, S.G., Barnatz, P.E., Remine, W.H., and Harrison, E.G.: Neurofibromatosis and hypertension due to pheochromocytoma or renal artery stenosis. *Minn. Med.,* **55**: 25–31, 1972.

66. Marmor, L.: Solitary peripheral nerve tumors. *Clin. Orth.,* **43**: 183–188, 1965.

67. Maseritz, I.H.: Neurogenic sarcoma. *JBJS,* **24**: 586–594, 1946.

68. Mason, E.: A case of neuralgia of the second metatarsophalangeal articulation, cured by resection of the joint. *Amer. Jour. Med. Sciences,* **74**: 445–446, 1877.

69. Mathews, G.J. et al: Painful traumatic neuromas. *Surg. Clin. N.A.,* **52**: 1313–1324, 1956.

70. May, V.R.: Metatarsal neuroma: the etiology and treatment. *South. Med. Jour.,* **49**: 1142–1144, 1956.

71. McCarral, H.R.: Clinical manifestations of congenital neurofibromatosis. *JBJS,* **32A**: 601, 1950.

72. McCaral, H.R.: Soft tissue neoplasms associated with congenital neurofibromatosis. *JBJS,* **38A**: 717–731, 1956.

73. McElvenny, R.T.: The etiology and surgical treatment of intractable pain about the fourth metatarsophalangeal joint. *JBJS,* **34**: 490, 1956.

74. McKeever, D.C.: Surgical approach for neuroma of plantar digital nerve (Morton's metatarsalgia). *JBJS,* **34A**: 490, 1956.

75. Michel, S.L.: Epithelial elements in malignant neurogenic tumors of the tibial nerve. *Amer. Jour. Surg.,* **113**: 404–413, 1967.

76. Mittal, M.M., Gupta, N.C., and Sharma, M.L.: Osteomalaiia in neurofibromatosis. *Jour. Assoc. Physicians India,* **19**: 823-825, 1971.

77. Money, R.A.: Tumors of peripheral nerves. *Aust. New Zeal. Jour. Surg.,* **19**: 239–245, 1950.

78. Moore, B.H.: Some orthopedic relationships of neurofibromatosis. *JBJS*, : 109, 1941.

79. Morton, K.S. and Vassar, P.S.: Neurilemmoma in bone—report of a case. *Canada Jour. Surg.*, **7**: 187–189, 1964.

80. Morton, T.G.: A peculiar and painful affection of the fourth metatarsophalangeal articulation. *Amer. Jour. Med. Sciences*, **71**: 37–45, 1876.

81. Morton, T.S.K.: Metatarsalgia (Morton's painful affection of the foot) with an account of six cases cured by operation. *Ann. Surg.*, **17**: 680-699, 1893.

82. Mulder, J.D.: The causative mechanism in Morton's metatarsalgia. *JBJS*, **33**: 94-95, 1951.

83. Nora, P.F. et al: Morton's metatarsalgia: a misconception. *Ill. Med. Jour.*, **127**: 155–160, 1965.

84. Pack, G.T.: *Tumors of the Nervous System. Treatment of Cancer and Allied Diseases*, Vol. 2, Harper & Row, New York, 1959.

85. Pack, G.T. and Ariel, L.M.: *Tumors of the Soft Somatic tissues.* Hoeber-Harper, New York, 1956, pp. 596–597.

86. Pataky, P.E. et al: Terminal neuroma treated with triamcinolone acetonide. *Jour. Surg. Res.*, **14**: 36–45, 1973.

87. Penfield, W.: The encapsulated tumors of the nervous system. *Surg. Gyn. Ob.*, **45**: 178–188, 1927.

88. Petropoulos, P.C. and Stefanko, S.: Experimental observation on the prevention of neuroma formation. *Jour. Surg. Res.*, **1**: 241, 1961.

89. Pincus, A.: The syndrome of plantar metatarsal neuritis (Morton's toe). *JAPA*, **52**: 746, 1962.

90. Pitt, M.J., Mosher, J.F., and Edeiken, J.: Abnormal periosteum and bone in neurofibromatosis. *Radiology*, **103**: 143–146, 1972.

91. Polloson, A.: *Anterior Metatarsalgia. Lancet*, **1**: 436, 1889.

92. Poth, E.J. and Bravo-Fernandez, E.: Prevention of neuroma formation by encasement of the severed nerve end in rigid tubes. *Proc. Soc. Ex. Biol. Med.*, **56**: 7, 1944.

93. Poth, E.J. et al: Prevention of formation of end bulb neuromata. *Proc. Soc. Ex. Biol. Med.*, **60**: 200, 1945.

94. Quick, D. and Cutler, M.: Neurogenic sarcoma, a clinical and pathologic study. *Ann. Surg.*, **86**: 810–829, 1927.

95. Ringertz, N. and Unander, S.L.: Morton's disease (a clinical and patho-anatomical study). *Acta. Ortho. Scan.*, **19**: 327–348, 1950.

96. Rodin, B.M. et al: Digital traumatic neuroma. A case report. *JAPA*, **63**: 445–456, 1973.

97. Roughton, E.: Anterior metatarsalgia, its nature and treatment. *Lancet*, **1**: 553, 1889.

98. Rowe, S.N.: Surgical treatment of nerve lesions. *Handbook of Clinical Neurology*, Vol. 8, American Elsevier, New York, 1970, pp. 526–527.

99. Rubin, D. and Kuitert, J.: Use of ultrasonic vibrator in the treatment

of pain arising from phantom limbs, scars and neuromas. A preliminary report. *Arch. Phys. Med.,* **36**: 445, 1955.

100. Rubinstein, L.: Tumors of the central nervous system. *Atlas of Tumor Pathology,* Fascicle 6, Armed Forces Institute of Pathology. Washington, D.C., 1972.

101. Russell, D.S. and Rubenstein, L.J.: *Pathology of Tumors of the Nervous System.* Edwards Arnold Publ. Co., London, 1963, pp. 242–257.

102. Russell, D.S. and Rubinstein, L.J.: *Pathology of Tumors of the Nervous System.* 3rd Ed., Williams and Wilkens Co., Baltimore, 1971.

103. Russell, W.R. and Spalding, J.M.K.: Treatment of painful amputation stumps. *Brit. Med. Jour.,* **2**: 68, 1950.

104. Sane, S., Yunis, E., and Greer, R.: Subperiosteal or cortical cyst and intramedullary neurofibromatosis—a case report. *JBJS Amer.,* **53**: 1194–1200, 1971.

105. Seth, H.N. et al: Neurilemmoma of bone—report of a case. *JBJS,* **45B**: 382–383, 1963.

106. Shreve, C.A.: Metatarsalgia neurogenica definitive clinical syndrome. *JAPA,* **64**: 16–24, 1974.

107. Silvers, D.N. and Greenwood, R.: Cafe-au-lait spot without giant pigment granules. *Arch. Derm.,* **110**: 87–88, 1974.

108. Singleton, A.O.: The surgical aspect of neurofibromatosis. *Amer. Jour. Surg.,* **36**: 451, 1970.

109. Smith, J.R. and Gomez, N.H.: Local injection therapy of neuromata of the hand with triamcinolone acetonide. *JBJS,* **52A**: 71, 1970.

110. Stewart, F.W. and Copeland, M.M.: Neurogenic sarcoma. *Amer. Jour. Cancer,* **15**: 1235–1320, 1931.

111. Stout, A.P.: Malignant tumors of peripheral nerves. *Amer. Jour. Cancer,* **25**: 1–36, 1935.

112. Stout, A.P.: Peripheral manifestations of the specific nerve sheath tumor (neurilemmoma). *Amer. Jour. Cancer,* **24**: 751–796, 1935.

113. Swart, H.A.: A new case of metatarsalgia. *West Vir. Med. Jour.,* **40**: 12, 1944.

114. Taylor, P.M.: Case report of neurofibromatosis. *JAPA,* **61**: 272–273, 1971.

115. Thompson, A.: On neuroma and neurofibromatosis. Turnball and Spears, Edinburgh, 1900.

116. Thompson, R.G.: Amputation neuroma. *Ortho. Clin. N.A.,* **Vol. 3, No. 2**: 330–331, 1972.

117. Tooms, E.: Amputation neuroma—prevention in surgery. *Ortho. Clin. N.A.,* **Vol. 3, No. 2**: 385, 1972.

118. Vieta, J.O. and Pack, G.T.: Malignant neurilemmoma of peripheral nerves. *Amer. Jour. Surg.,* **82**: 416–431, 1280–1281, 1951.

119. Wardle, E.N.: Neurilemmoma. *Brit. Jour. Surg.,* **45**: 58–61, 1957.

120. Wardle, E.N.: Nerve sheath tumors. *Brit. Jour. Surg.,* **45**: 58–61, 1957.

121. Weinstein, F.: *Principles and Practice of Podiatry.* Lea and Febiger, Phila., 1968.

122. White, H.R.: Survival in malignant shwannoma, An 18 year study. *Cancer*, **27**: 720–729, 1971.

123. White, N.B.: Neurilemmomas of the extremities. *JBJS*, **49A**: 1605–1610, 1967.

124. Winkler, H. et al: Morton's metatarsalgia. *JBJS*, **30A**: 596–600, 1948.

125. Woodruff, C.E.: Incomplete luxations of the metatarsophalangeal articulations. *Med. Rec.*, **1**: 61–62, 1890.

126. Zorab, P. and Edwards, H.: Spinal deformity in neurofibromatosis, *Lancet*, **2**: 823, 1972.

# Color Plates

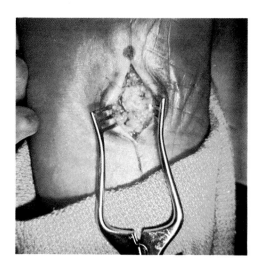 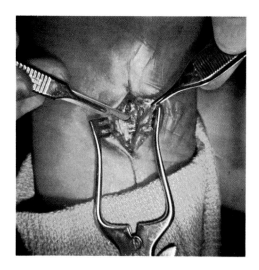

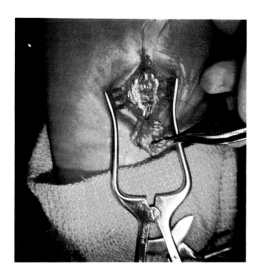 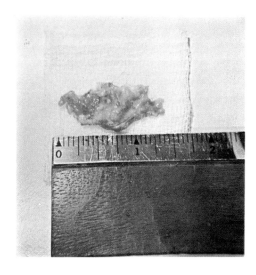

Plantar fibromatosis. This lesion is located in the central portion of the foot and reveals a white glistening very firm mass. The mass is being sharply dissected including the underlying surrounding plantar fascia. The mass measures approximately 4 cm in length. Sutures remain approximately three weeks postoperatively with patient ambulating on crutches as follow-up therapy.

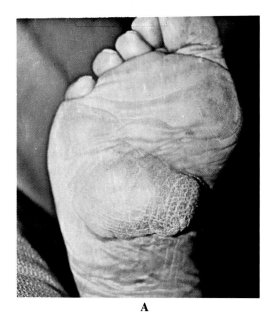

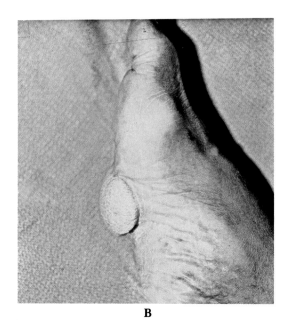

A                                    B

Lipoma. (A). A large multilobulated lipoma of the plantar
aspect of the right foot. Clinically the lesion shows a large
central lesion on the plantar surface and extending to the
fifth toe with another soft tissue mass. (B). Lateral view of
the foot revealing lipoma type lesion showing some
hyperkeratosis due to constant weight bearing on that
area.

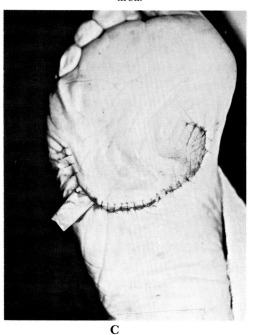

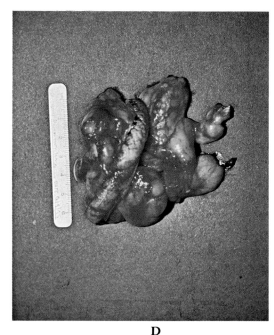

C                                    D

(C) reveals large surgical excision of the plantar lipoma
showing a semi circular type of incision and insertion of a
drain for prevention of hematoma. (D) shows a gross
specimen of the plantar lipoma also showing a small section of the skin that was excised. (Courtesy of Joseph
Orlando, M.D., Towson, Md.)

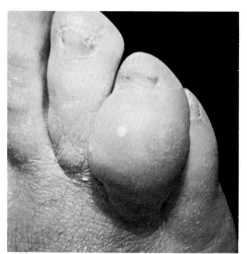

Gouty Tophi. Painful reddened, firm swelling involving the 4th toe on clinical exposure.

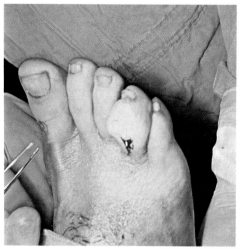

Surgical exposure reveals white, soft to firm material.

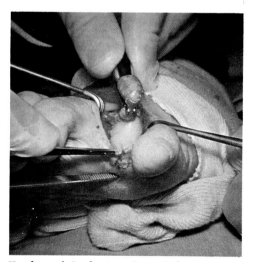

Epidermal Inclusion Cyst. A large cystic lesion located between the 4th and 5th metatarsal shafts. Early symptomatology was that of a plantar callous.

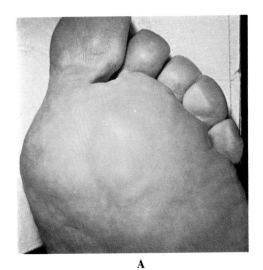

A

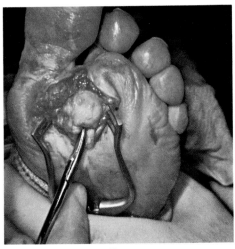

B

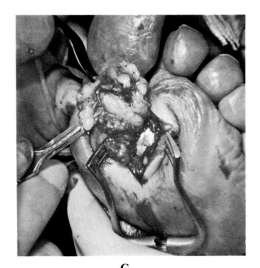

C

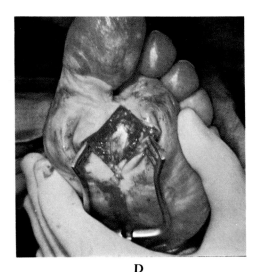

D

Synovial Cyst. (A). These cysts are infrequently found on the plantar aspect of the metatarsal heads, and seldom do they get this large. Clinically, one can see a bulging of the plantar skin. The mass is quite moveable on palpation. (B) reveals the cystic mass bulging out of the incision after the initial skin incision. (C) reveals the excision of the cystic lesion. One can notice how closely adherent it is to the flexor tendon. (D) reveals the lesion completely excised, with the exposure to the flexor tendon.

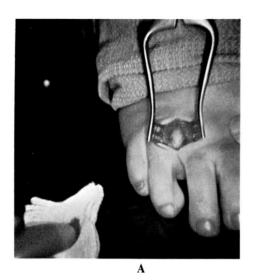

**A**

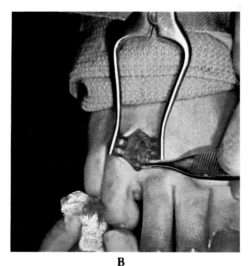

**B**

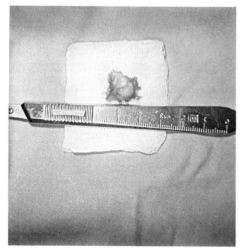

**C**

Morton's Neuroma. Morton's neuromas are the most common nerve lesions located in the foot. The surgical view (A) reveals an extremely large Morton's neuroma between the third and fourth metatarsal. (B) reveals the grasping at the distal aspect of the neoplasm showing surgical dissection toward the proximal bifurcation. (C) reveals complete surgical excision of the neoplasm.

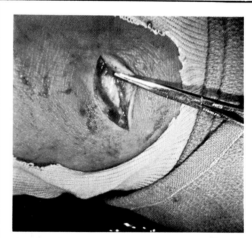

Tendon Cyst. A rare cystic lesion involving tendinous structure on the dorsal-lateral surface of the foot. Unfortunately, very little information is available concerning this entity.

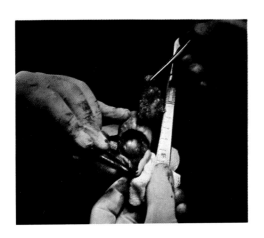

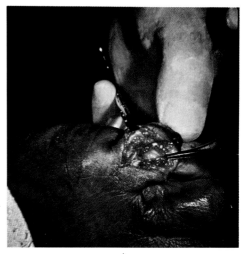

A

Rheumatoid Nodule. Large rheumatoid nodule involving the hallux toe which gave the clinical appearance of that of a ganglion. The patient has no history of rheumatoid arthritis, and it is extremely rare to find nodules without the presence of this disease.

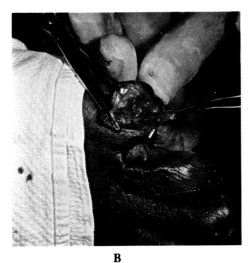

B

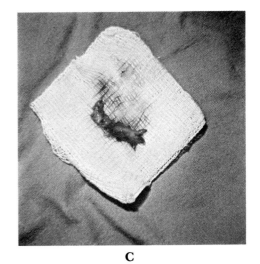

C

Traumatic Neuroma. Extremely large digital traumatic neuroma involving the fifth toe. (A) reveals surgical exposure. (B) reveals the grasping of the neuroma with a hemostat. (C) represents the gross specimen.

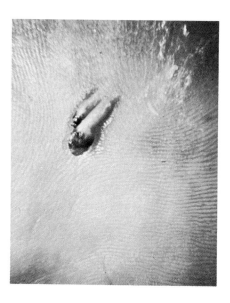

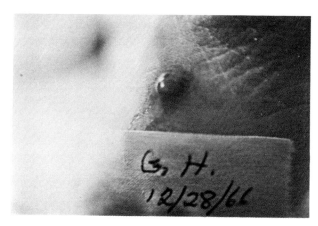

Pyogenic granuloma. Pyogenic granulomas may take most any form and any shape. It is usually reddish in nature; however, some areas may show hyperkeratosis, particularly on the plantar surfaces of the foot. The above two figures are two different appearing lesions of pyogenic granuloma. The "B" lesion may closely resemble that of a melanoma.

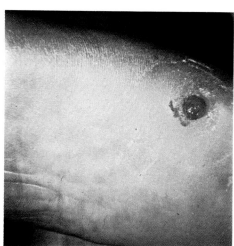

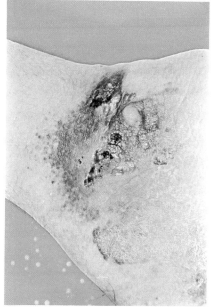

Foreign Body Granuloma. An unusual lesion and vascular in nature on the plantar surface of the foot. This granulomatous type lesion is believed to be due to an insect bite. Differential diagnosis may be that of a melanoma or pyogenic granuloma.

Hemangioendothelioma. This is an extremely rare lesion involving both the foot and the ankle, clinical diagnosis being extremely difficult. (Courtesy of Ronald Goldner, M.D., Baltimore, Md.)

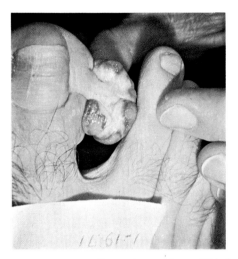
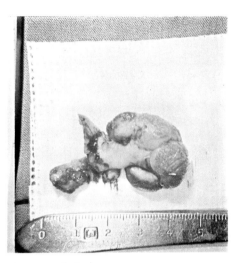

Pyogenic granuloma. This lesion represents a severely large pyogenic granuloma of irregular form. Clinically it may closely resemble a malignancy. The adjacent photograph reveals complete excision and gross specimen.

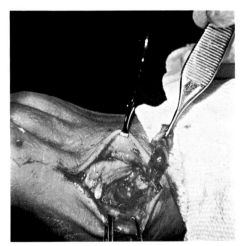
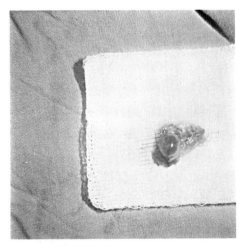

Ganglion Cyst underlying the first metatarsophalangeal joint. The cyst is quite "fluidy" and one can distinguish the central bubble usually seen in early lesions.

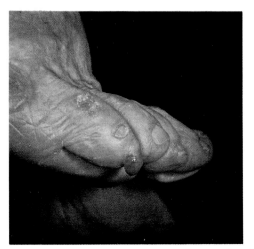

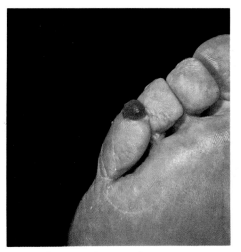

Pyogenic Granuloma. The above two photographs reveal a granulomatous lesion on the distal aspect of the toe. These lesions may reveal chronic drainage and are usually asymptomatic. Surgical excision usually results in a complete cure.

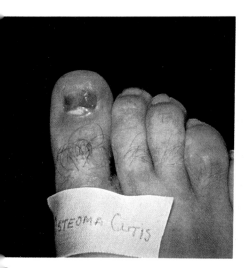

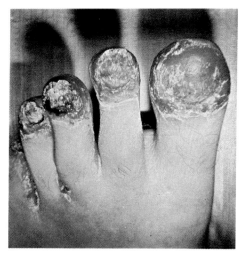

Osteoma cutis. A very uncommon lesion in the foot and usually associated with calcification of soft tissue. It may closely resemble that of a glomus tumor or subungual granuloma. (Courtesy of Stanley Katz, D.P.M., Owings Mills, Md.)

Reiter's Disease. A severe manifestation of draining sinuses, loss of nails, and chronic drainage. Differential diagnosis may be that of squamous cell carcinoma when involving one nail.

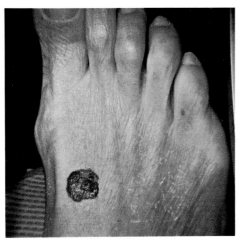

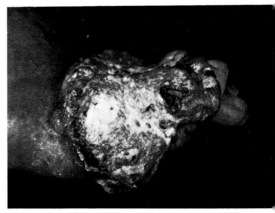

Malignant Melanoma. Large melanoma, dorsal surface of foot undergoing change in size and color. Treatment consisted of radical excision followed by skin graft.

Squamous Cell Carcinoma. A severely discolored lesion largely invading the skin and bony structures of the 4th and 5th metatarsals and digits. Treatment was amputation. (Courtesy Leon Cohen, D.P.M., Carlsbad, New Mexico.)

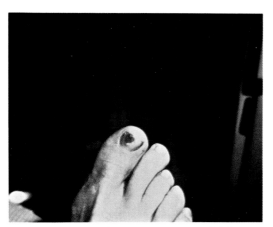

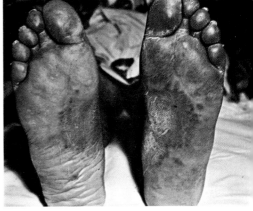

Glomus Tumor. These are very painful lesions usually associated in the nail bed areas of the foot. The most common location is that of the hallux toe. They are usually reddish-blue in nature and exquisitely tender. (Courtesy of James Ganley, D.P.M., Norristown, Pa.)

Kaposi's Sarcoma. The photograph reveals a diffuse and extensive amount of Kaposi's lesion along the plantar surfaces and toes of both feet. The color of the lesions in this individual quite purplish in nature. (Courtesy of William V.R. Shellow, M.D., Beverly Hills, California.)

# Section V
# Vascular Tumors

## Hemangioma

### Definition

Pack and Miller believe that a hemangioma is a neoplasm since there is actual new formation of vessels or proliferation of the vessel wall.[208] Goidonich and Campanicci prefer the designation "hamartoma" instead of "neoplasm".[100]

Hemangiomas, whether neoplasms or hamartomas, are usually benign, only rarely malignant, and are composed of vascular channels and spaces in the skin or the deeper structures of the body.[59]

### History

Bouchet (1856) reported the first case of hemangioma of the synovial membrane. Bajadri (1900), Fulkroger (1903), Keen (1905), Mariotta (1908), Finaly (1914), and Forty (1936) each reported cases of hemangiomas in the muscles of the foot.[59,79]

However, the first report which provided the natural history of vascular nevi was gathered from Lister's studies of 77 cases, comprising 93 lesions (1938).[284]

### Etiology

Reviewing the literature, one cannot find any general agreement as to the etiology and pathogenesis of the hemangioma. Most researchers believe that they are of congenital origin. However, cavernous hemangiomas may also be traumatic although the great majority are congenital.

Fitzwilliams (1911, cited by Waddell) found that, in 645 cases, over 83 percent of hemangiomas were first noticed at birth.[283] Lampe and Latourette, in a study of 600 hemangiomas, found 61 percent were present at birth with 86 percent appearing at birth or within the first month.[149] However, Waisman stated that cavernous hemangiomas occur in less than five percent of the newborn, and that they tend to occur after infancy, with fewer than 33 percent of the lesions occurring in the extremities.[284]

Margelith and Museles,[180,181] and Lampe and

Latourette,[149] stated that a family history of hemangioma was noted in ten percent of their studies of cutaneous hemangiomas in children. We have been unable to find similar findings regarding cavernous hemangioma. Beers and Clark reported one case with a family history of hemangioma going back through three generations.[18] Their case was that of a cavernous hemangioma associated with a short first metatarsal in many persons in the family; however, no direct relationship between cavernous hemangioma and a short first metatarsal could be established.

Jenkins and Delaney, in a study of 256 cases of hemangioma affecting muscles, reported that 47 percent of their cases were of congenital origin and that trauma was the primary factor in 17 percent.[124]

Verrucous hemangiomas develop a progressive hyperkeratotic phase which seems to develop as a response to trauma.[122] Baque believed that a "nervous condition" was a predisposing factor, because the lesion followed the course of nerves with trauma or infection not playing a role.[14]

It has also been reported that carcinogenic hydrocarbons injected into specific strains of white mice are capable of producing hemangiomas.[31]

## Incidence

One of the most common childhood neoplasms is the hemangioma. Some of these lesions disappear early in childhood. White infants have a higher incidence of hemangiomas than do blacks, and they occur twice as often in females as in males. There is a ten to fifteen percent incidence of familial cases.

Lampe and Latourette studied 471 hemangiomas of which 63 percent were cutaneous, 15 percent subcutaneous, and 22 percent mixed.[148] About one-half of these lesions occur on the trunk, one-third on the extremities, and one-sixth on the head and neck.[284]

Berlin, in his literature review of 33 cases of hemangiomas of the foot, reported 30 percent occurring in muscle, 30 percent in connective tissues, 22 percent in bone, 12 percent in nerve, and six percent in tendon.[21]

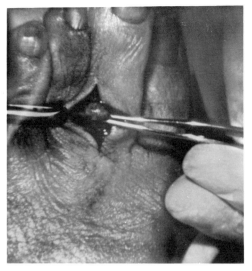

**Figure 5-1**

Capillary Cavernous hemangioma. This illustration reveals a small, vascular tumor at the base of the second toe undergoing surgical excision.

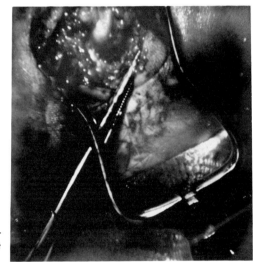

**Figure 5-2**

Cavernous hemangioma involving the metatarsal region of the foot. Clinically, in this particular case the skin gave a somewhat blueish, bulged appearance.

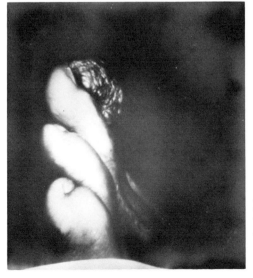

**Figure 5-3**

Verrucous hemangioma. This is an extremely rare variety of hemangioma involving the hallux toe. (Courtesy of Sandford Rosenfeld, D.P.M., Detroit, Michigan.)

Hemangiomas can be classified as follows:[284]

I. Capillary
   A. Port-wine stain
   B. Simplex, Salmon Patch

II. Dermal (Strawberry Mark)
   A. Mature hemangioma
   B. Late Appearing
   C. Hypertrophic

III. Sub-Dermal (Cavernous)
   A. Bone and internal organs
   B. Mature
   C. Hypertrophic

IV. Combined

V. Diffuse, systemic

*Clinical Picture*

A hemangioma usually presents itself at birth or shortly thereafter, and most likely within the first three decades of life. It may start as small as a pea, and enlarge to the size of a grapefruit. It may be deep or superficial.

Clinically, the most common form of hemangioma is the erythema nuchae, characterized by a stain or salmon patch on the skin. This form, seen in one out of three newborn infants, may disappear spontaneously,[149] but the port-wine mark and cavernous lesions do not resolve spontaneously. Venous hemangiomas appear as large, bluish vascular lesions, whereas strawberry hemangiomas (a capillary form) are usually bright red or purplish with well defined margins. Subcutaneous (hypodermal) cavernous types usually have poorly defined borders, but they may be well delineated if dermal. The cavernous hemangioma occurring in muscle has been found most commonly in the lower extremities, frequently involving the quadriceps muscle.[124,243] Benign hemangiomas can be affected in their growth by trauma,[60] infections,[93] or pregnancies.[208]

Pain is the most common symptom and is experienced by compression of a nerve trunk or by direct involvement of a nerve by the tumor. Bonvallet reported that 349 out of 357 cases of hemangioma of skeletal muscle had pain.[31] In cavernous hemangiomas, pain may be present only on movement of the involved part. Pain may be variable and may be associated with paresthesia.

Wiley reported a capillary cavernous hemangioma, "the size of an almond," lying close to the medial plantar nerve, in which pain and paresthesia were present for two years prior to surgical treatment.[290] Of the 33 hemangiomas reported on the foot, pain was the primary symptom in 24. Edema is common and was noted in several cases in which no distinct mass could be palpated.[79,85,128,256] Skin discoloration may be present, when the soft tissue mass is in close proximity to the epidermis, and may be red, brown, blue, or purple.

On palpation, cavernous hemangiomas may vary from soft and spongy to hard and may be either fixed of moveable. Margileth and Museles described their consistency as "worm-like",[181] and Carnevali described it as being "like spaghetti".[43] The tumors range from the size of a pea to that of an orange or larger. Jenkins and Delaney, in their review of hemangiomas of skeletal muscle, stated that the most frequent shape of the tumors was oval in 87 cases, as compared to only 50 which were round.[124] The tumor is usually compressible and pain may be elicited.

Pulsations in the cavernous hemangioma are rare (1.2%), usually being felt distal to the lesion. Forty reported a patient in whom the dorsalis pedis artery revealed "expansive pulsations" in the tumor mass, both proximal and distal to it.[79]

In vascular tumors, the impairment of function and deformities usually occur late. Several cases of deformity have been reported involving the foot and leg,[60,151,186] but only two cases have been reported affecting the foot.[40,216] Shallow, Eger, and Wagner stated, in their review of 335 cases of hemangioma affecting skeletal muscle, that 26 percent had deformities and 25 percent had impairment of function.[243]

*Diagnosis*

Clinical examination may be difficult or inaccurate in delineating the extent of the lesion. There are some reports indicating that the correct diagnosis of skeletal muscle lesions was made as infrequently as 19 percent (before treatment).[243]

Angiography, which may be invaluable in the diagnosis of vascular tumors, has not attracted the attention of clinicians treating hemangiomas. Angiography may outline the vascular anatomy, the extent of the lesion, and its topography.[8,78,152,162] However, Kendrick and his associates expressed the view that angiography was a valuable tool in evaluating a patient with hemangioma.[138] They believed that an angiogram shows the exact boundaries, the localization of the mass, and the number of feeding vessels. On the other hand, Herzberg and Schreiber, after utilizing angiography in three patients with hemangiomas, concluded "their true extent could not be determined."[113] A venogram was performed on one of four cases Berlin studied.[21] However, he indicated "this did not reveal the true depth and vastness as seen at operation."

The result of a study of cases with deep hemangiomas, in which nine angiograms were performed, showed the procedure valuable in five cases, of limited value in three cases, and of no value in one case.[243]

X-ray examination of soft tissue vascular lesions may provide a clue to diagnosis, but the x-ray may be normal or simply show soft tissue swelling. Shallow saw phleboliths in 49 percent of the cases he studied.[243] In some cases, phleboliths may even be palpable on clinical examination.

The oxygen content of the blood in these lesions is normal, whereas, in arteriovenous fistulas, it is usually elevated on the venous side. The skin may be tight over the tumor. The skin temperature is usually normal, except where there is a mild phlebitis. These lesions can be compressed but quickly fill upon release of pressure.

Hemangiomas involving bone are more difficult to diagnose. Radiologically, benign hemangiomas usually cause uniform expansion of involved bones with the formation of cystic cavities. The cortex may be eroded, without expansion of the periosteum, on x-ray. Thomas described it on x-ray as a "soap-bubble effect" in long bones.[277] (This term is commonly used to describe the x-ray appearance of both aneurysmal bone cysts and giant cell tumors.)

## Differential Diagnosis

Since hemangiomas may resemble many other masses of tumors, the differential diagnosis becomes important prior to treatment. The differential diagnosis of soft tissue tumors includes fibromas, lipomas, cysts, ganglions, hematomas, and arteriovenous fistulae.

A hemangioma of bone may produce different bone changes leading to a variety of differential diagnoses, and, for example, may resemble a giant cell tumor, osteitis fibrosis cystica, hyperparathyroidism, Gaucher's disease, or an aneurysmal bone cyst.

## Pathology

There are many theories as to the pathologic development of hemangiomas.[60] Virchow believed that the tumor arose from disease of the vasovasorum and enlargment of pre-existing vessels, due to mechanical influence, during intra- or extra-uterine life.[124]

Ribert believed that the angioma, although congenital in origin, was a true neoplasm which grows independently of its own vascular substance and may invade surrounding structures.[21] Four cases have been described involving the surrounding soft tissue and bones in the foot.[128,142,165,216]

Angiosarcomas are rare and are characterized by the presence of solid masses of endothelial cells infiltrating the stroma. There are four reported cases involving the bones of the foot.[94,277]

The majority of pathological reports indicates that hemangiomas are benign tumors which may suggest a malignant tendency by infiltrating adjacent tissues, rather than by expansion and destruction. As the tumor advances, a responsive endothelial proliferation takes place, increasing the size of the tumor. This creates an associated fibrofatty tissue development around the vessels, as may be seen in fibro- or lipo-cavernous hemangiomas. The response of a fibrofatty mass is due to the response of damaged or destroyed tissue

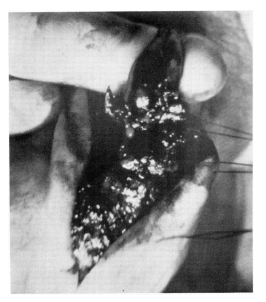

**Figure 5-4A**

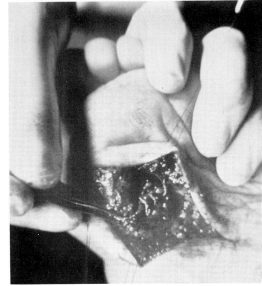

**Figure 5-4B**

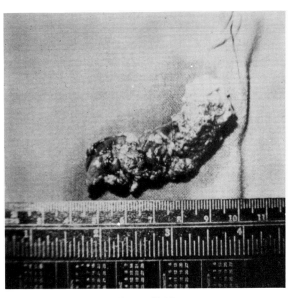

**Figure 5-4C**

Cavernous hemangioma. Surgical view (A) reveals a large vascular cavernous hemangioma on the plantar aspect of the foot. Surgical exposure (B) reveals a large defect after complete excision and (C) reveals a gross description of the neoplasm.

and is a reaction secondary to irritation of surrounding tissues by the tumor.

In muscle, the hemangioma may grow between the muscle fibers causing an expansion of muscle, with fibrosis, or it may involve the perimysium of muscular tissue or the advantitia lining of the vessel causing production of adipose tissue.[122243] The growth of this vascular mass may entrap nerve fibers, which probably accounts for symptoms of pain. Bajardi (cited by Davis) reported a case in which the growth involved the posterior tibial artery and nerve.[59] These tumors may ulcerate, probably due to ischemic necrosis from trauma. Pomerantz and Tunich reported a case in a five year old male, with ulceration developing after x-ray therapy.[216]

Phlebolith formation is a characteristic feature, and may result from calcification of thrombi attached to or within the vessel wall.[85] However, phleboliths involving the vessels of the foot have only been reported in two cases.[42,216]

*Foot Involvement*

Hemangiomas of the foot are somewhat of a rare occurrence. Berlin's review of the literature revealed 33 cases involving all tissue structures of the foot, including bone.[21]

The two most frequent areas of involvement were muscle and connective tissue layers of the foot with tendon and nerve being rarely involved. Since that time the literature has only revealed a few additional cases.

The greatest difficulty encountered in treating this tumor of the foot is due to its infiltrative involvement in other tissue structures creating extreme difficulty for its complete removal.

Hemangiomas may affect any living tissue that has a vascular supply. McNeil and Ray, in their review of 35 cases, state that 28.5 percent show foot involvement.[191] The tumor may be either discrete of diffuse. Johnson and Dogherty reported 93 cases of hemangioma in the lower extremity, 20 being discrete and 73 diffuse.[126] On clinical examination, it appeared that less than 25 percent of the discrete tumors showed infiltration of adjacent normal tissues.

LaSorte (1960) reviewed the reported cases of hemangioma affecting skeletal muscle and reported a total of 399 cases, with 11 cases involving the foot alone.[151]

Harkins reported 24 cases of hemangioma affecting the tendon, with only two cases involving the peroneal and extensor digitorum longus tendons in the foot.[108] Although additional cases of tendon involvement have been reported, no additional cases have been found affecting the foot.[94,108,243]

Hemangiomas of peripheral nerves have been reported infrequently. Losli found a total of seven cases (1952), with two cases affecting the posterior tibial nerve in the heel.[166] Berry[24] (1957) and Giugiaro and Bertola[98] (1958) each reported a case of hemangioma involving the medial plantar nerve, both in the right foot, bringing the total number of cases of nerve involvement in the foot to four.

Bone hemangiomas are also infrequent. Geschickter and Maseritz (1938) reported a total of 14 cases of primary hemangioma of bone, with only one case affecting the foot, and an angiosarcoma of the oscalcis.[94] Since then, other reviews[45,191,277] and cases[142,165] have been presented, bringing the total number of cases of hemangioma or angiosarcoma of bones of the foot to seven.

### Treatment

There are no uniform answers to the questions "Should one treat a hemangioma?" and, if yes, how? In any given case, there may be more than one possible mode of treatment. Surgical excision, cautery, x-ray, or radium therapy and sclerosis are perhaps the most frequent forms of treatment in hemangiomas involving the foot. Cryotherapy has been utilized in cutaneous hemangiomas, but has been described in the treatment of verrucous hemangioma, with complete success in only one case.[14,122]

Sclerosis, a common form of treatment for varicose veins, has been described only once in the foot, with a successful result, following the side-effects of radiation therapy.

X-ray or radium therapy has been described in several cases. Only one case involving soft tissue (muscle) of the foot is reported,[85] whereas it was utilized in five cases of hemangioma of bone.[48,113,138] X-ray or radiation therapy in he-

264

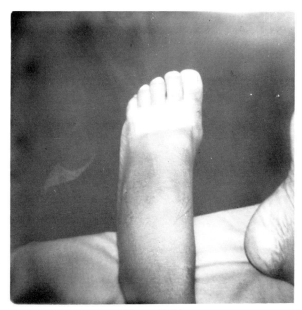

**Figure 5-5A**

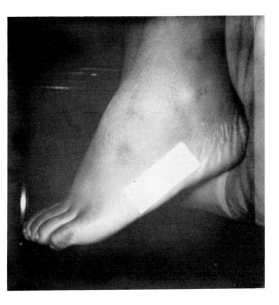

**Figure 5-5B**

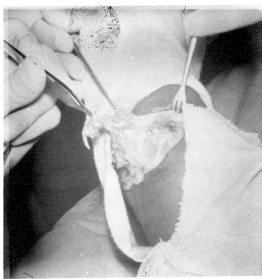

**Figure 5-5C**

Cavernous hemangioma. Cavernous hemangiomas are uncommon in the foot. (A) and (B) reveal an anterior as well as a lateral view respectively, with a great deal of edema. Darkened pigmentation of the skin are areas of extreme tenderness. (C) shows surgical excision of the neoplasm. It gives the appearance, as one of our Italian authors describes it, of spaghetti at some times.

mangioma of bone was used in conjunction with surgical treatment and not as the only form of therapy. Waddell believes cavernous hemangioma to be radiation-resistant.[283] Ackerman and Hart stated that radiation therapy appeared to create osteoblastic predominence with reduction of osteolysis, thus reducing pain and ultimately arresting the growth.[1]

If x-ray or radiation treatment is utilized in the treatment of children, one must be careful to prevent possible damage to the growth centers of the bones. Mau reported a case of hemangioma affecting the lower third of the leg and foot, in which a clubfoot deformity developed after radiation therapy.[186]

Surgical treatment has been used as the total form of treatment in 23 cases involving the foot. Five additional cases involving bone were treated with surgery followed by radiation therapy.[21]

Shallow, Eger and Wagner stated, in their review of hemangiomas of muscle (335 cases), that 79.1 percent (265 patients) were treated surgically, with 90.6 percent cure or improvement rate, and only 1.2 percent (four patients) were treated by amputation.[243]

Surgical treatment is perhaps the treatment of choice in deep hemangiomas involving the foot. However, if complete excision is not possible, the tying-off of as many involved vessels as possible may retard its growth and eliminate symptoms. Of course, one must be extremely careful to prevent hemorrhage and nerve damage.[187,234]

*Prognosis*

The preceding discussion of hemangioma and its treatment indicate a bright prognosis. Most of the affected patients are rid of the problem spontaneously or uneventfully with some kind of treatment.

But, at the same time, one should be aware of some of the complications which may affect the patient, especially the young. One of the complications is thrombocytopenia, affecting mostly infants and some adults.[245] A certain number of tragedies will occur from rapid extension of the inoperable

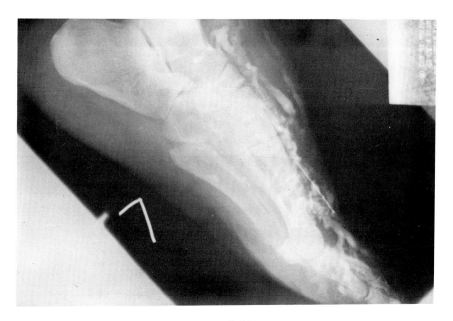

Figure 5-6A

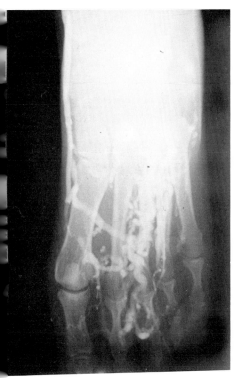

Figure 5-6B

Cavernous hemangioma. Venograms reveal extreme depth and diffuseness of the cavernous hemangioma involving the foot. X-rays of the lateral and anterior view of the foot revealed massive involvement.

lesion, which may ulcerate or even kill the child. Of course, this type of complication is more common in cases where the liver, spleen, lung, or kidney are involved.

Other complications include giant growth, producing huge, grotesque deformity, or ulceration, leading to infection and scarring.[284]

Therefore, hemangiomas, although mostly benign, must be correctly diagnosed and properly treated.

## Pyogenic Granuloma

### Definition

Pyogenic granuloma is a highly vascular benign tumor which arises from connective tissue or mucous membranes and usually results from trauma.

### Synonyms

Kuttner suggested the name "granuloma telangiectales," whereas other authors used the terms "granuloma pediculatum" or "granuloma pediculatum benigrum".[194] There has been a mention of Hartzell's disease and bloody warts.[233] Martens and MacPherson (1956) proposed a descriptive term for granuloma pyogenicum, granuloma gravidarum, juvenile angiofibroma and urethral caruncle, which they called "Fibroangioma", due to similarities between these lesions.[182] Angelopoulos (1971) proposed the term "hemangiomatous granuloma" which he felt accurately expressed the characteristic histopathologic picture (hemangioma-like) and the inflammatory nature (granuloma) of the lesion.[7] Other synonyms for pyogenic granuloma have been mentioned in the literature.[22]

### History

Poncet and Dor (1897) described a lesion in man, which they called "human botryomycosis", because it resembled botryomycosis in castrated horses.[22] Hartzel introduced the term Pyogenic Granuloma due to the lesions' raw appearance and the presence of pus.[111]

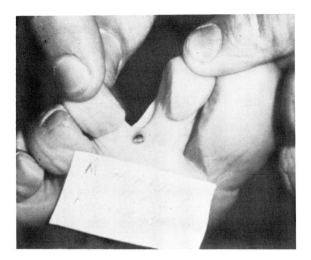

**Figure 5-7A**

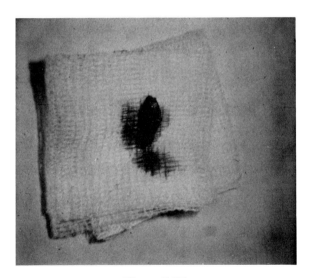

**Figure 5-7B**

Pyogenic granuloma. Pyogenic granuloma occurring in the web space of the second and third toe. A reddish-blue type of macular lesion. (B) reveals surgical excision.

269

*Etiology*

The etiology is still unknown; however, most references indicate that it is due mostly to trauma.[22,23,238,285] Many authors feel that there is a possible relationship to pregnancy.[26,111] Montgomery and Culver found an increase in blood pressure associated with pyogenic granuloma.[196] Zayid reported 19 cases of granuloma pyogenicum, due to smallpox vaccination in Jordan, and suggested that the following factors play a role in the etiology of the lesion: trauma, viral infection, and hormonal influences.[299]

*Clinical Picture*

All age groups are affected with no apparent sex predilection. Most cases involve the Caucasian race. Angelopoulos stated that 60 percent of the reported cases involve individuals between 11 and 40 years of age, although it is fairly commonly seen in children.[7]

Pyogenic granuloma can be found anywhere on the body. The lesion may arise without any history of injury, inflammation, or infection in the area.

The color of an early lesion is usually bright red, with older lesions becoming darker, gray or even black, due to injury and ulceration. Lesions develop quite rapidly at the site of trauma. The shape of the lesions may be papular, nodular or lobulated; the texture may be rough or smooth; the consistency may be firm or soft; they may also be pedunculated with a long stalk, or sessile. On the plantar surface of the foot, they are more likely to be pedunculated, due to pressure; dorsally, the sessile type is more frequently noted.[22] The size usually ranges from 0.5 to one centimeter in diameter.

*Differential Diagnosis*

Pyogenic granuloma must be differentiated from the following:

1. Malignant melanoma: often pigmented, with change in pigmentation and size when originating in a junctional nevus; but up to 75 percent may arise from normal skin.

2. Kaposi's sarcoma: (multiple idiopathic hemorrhagic

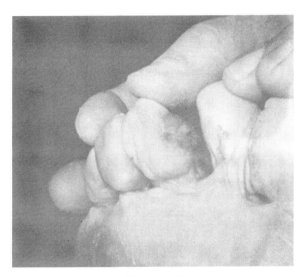

**Figure 5-8**

Pyogenic granuloma. This pyogenic granuloma is quite vascular with moderate amounts of drainage and gives some verrucous type appearance involving the third toe.

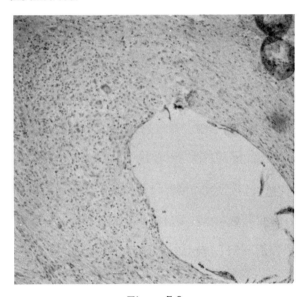

**Figure 5-9**

Foreign body granuloma. The inflammatory reaction consists of many neutrophils, eosinophils, and scattered lymphocytes. Multinucleated foreign body giant cells can be seen surrounding the cystic cavity.

sarcoma); shows slow growth and occurs predominantly in adult males, whereas granuloma pyogenicum is seen in younger adults and has a faster growth rate.

    3.  Cavernous hemangioma: blue, soft, and usually flat.

    4.  Dermatofibroma: slow rate of growth, less vascular than pyogenic granuloma, and usually depressed.

    5.  Blue nevus: dark blue, flat, or elevated.

    6.  Glomus tumor: associated with severe paroxysmal pain in the side of the lesion.

    7.  Verrucae: verruca vulgaris, molluscum contagiosum, hyperkeratotic papilloma.

    8.  Subungual hematoma.

    9.  Paronychia.

   10.  Melanotic whitlow.

   11.  Senile keratosis.

   12.  Eccrine poroma.

*Pathology*

Contrary to some opinion, this lesion is really a capillary hemangioma with secondary ulceration; inflammation is not a primary reaction.[141] As the vascular tissue grows, it stretches the epidermis. This is followed by ulceration, acute inflammation, and necrosis. Neutrophil leukocytes are present early, and, in time, a new inflammatory process develops.

*Foot Involvement*

Pyogenic granuloma of the foot has been a rarely reported entity and has often been confused with that of proud flesh, particularly in the nail bed area.

Berlin's review of the literature (1972) revealed only nine cases reported with four cases being present on the digits and five cases located on the dorsal and plantar surfaces of the foot.[22] Since that time, podiatry literature has only recorded seven other cases, with the digits representing the most frequent location. Even though this entity is infrequently or rarely encountered on the foot it has not been known to cause any difficulty in the eradication.

## Treatment

Even though granuloma pyogenicum is not the usual neoplasm, it must be removed or destroyed completely to prevent secondary infection. Because of the presence of a feeder vessel deep in the dermis, complete excision followed by electrocoagulation of the base is necessary to avoid recurrence. An alternate method, suggested by Pinkus, is removal of the pyogenic granuloma by "slicing and thorough electrodessication."[213] Any excised tissue must be submitted to histopathological diagnosis.

Desforges described a trial of hydrocortisone with occlusive dressings.[61] Kandil and Basile described three successful uses of triamcinolone.[129] Small lesions can be cauterized by application of silver nitrate at weekly intervals.[212] Successful use of penicillin therapy[189] and x-ray therapy[68] as well as liquid nitrogen have also been described.

## Prognosis

The prognosis, after complete excision, is good.

## Glomus Tumors

### Definition

Glomus tumors are painful, bluish to reddish purple nodules consisting of a convoluted arterio-venous communication with an organized anastomosis between a small artery and venule. These peripheral structures are normally located in the stratum reticulare of the skin and, occasionally, in the subcutaneous tissue beneath the subcapillary vessels.

### Synonyms

Synonyms for glomus tumors are glomangioma, angioneuromyoma, Popoff tumor, Barré-Masson tumor, tumeur-du-glomus, and neuromyoarteriole tumor.

### History

Glomus tumors, or subcutaneous nodules which cause excruciating pain, were described more than two centuries ago. William Wood (1812) characterized them as benign growths, associated with acute, spasmodic pain, that are very susceptible to temperature changes.

Muller (1844) described a direct connection between the arteries and cavernous sinuses of the penis. Subsequently, in 1862, he described direct connections between the arteries and the veins in various parts of the body. Similar observations were made by Bourcert (1855) and later by Girard (1895) when the term arteriovenous anastomosis first appeared. Sucquet (1862) described peculiar blood vessels, larger than normal arteries, communicating directly with adjacent veins without the usual interposition of the intermediary capillary network. These were primarily described in the palms and soles.

Hoyer (1877) gave a more detailed description of the glomus body. Kolaczek (1878) reported the first incidence of subungual glomus tumors in the great toe. Mueller (1901) changed the name to perithelioma and Bating-Gaudy in the same year changed the name again to fibromyomatous angioma. Also, Grosser (1901) related the arteriovenous anastomosis and temperature regulation with glomus tumors. In the following year Grosser pointed out that they are not present in the young or aged.[58]

Barre (1922), a French neurologist, was the first to categorize glomus tumors clinically according to the type of pain elicited. Group I consisted of shooting pain localized in the terminal phalanx of the fingers. The patient would beg for relief from pain, even if it meant amputation. Clinical and radiological examinations were essentially negative. In Group II the pain was milder but more prolonged, then becoming very sharp in nature. In this group, radiologic examinations revealed a cystic, circular area in the terminal phalanx surrounded by bony erosion of the terminal phalanx itself.

*Incidence*

Glomus tumors are unusual, but not rare. They are usually solitary, although several cases of multiple tumors have been reported in the literature. There is strong evidence favoring the concept of an autosomal dominant mode of inheritance for the glomus tumors in multiple cases. Horton and Saunders[119] reported that five to ten percent of all their cases were multiple. In the cases with multiple tumors the lesions were usually grouped together in the subcutaneous tissues.[119] Kohout and Stout[263] reviewed 731 cases and noted that multiple lesions in the adult comprised 2.3 percent while in children the incidence rose to 26.3 percent. They felt that the tumor was more common in males than in females. Maley reported the case of a 36 year old white male with bilateral glomus tumors of both hands. He felt that this was the first reported case of a bilateral glomus tumor.[175]

Both sexes appear to be equally affected. However, Law stated that males have a higher incidence of glomus tumors.[154] Horton made conflicting claims and stated that females with glomus tumors have a higher prevalence.[119] And yet Kaplan stated that they occur with equal frequency in both sexes, as stated earlier.[130] Stout[263] was of the opinion that this tumor would be more common in persons of Jewish ancestry; however, there has been no further evidence to substantiate this theory. Other studies also related that these tumors were found more frequently in the Jewish people, but no race was found to be immune to this tumor.[239] One case was reported in a Negro by Lewis and Geschickter and one in a part Inca Indian by Keasbey. All other glomus tumors reported in the literature have apparently been in Caucasians.

Cases of glomus tumors have been reported from the ages of one to 85 years; most seem to occur after puberty with the most common period being between 20 and 40 years of age.

The average age at which treatment is sought is generally during the thirties. The duration of the symptoms has been reported from a few weeks to 37 years. This great variation is apparently dependent upon the severity of the pain and the ease with which diagnosis is established.

The greatest incidence is in areas where there are normal glomuses; however, various other locations have been described as the sites of these tumors, including the thoracic wall, temporal region, scapular region, arms and forearms, thighs, knees, various facial muscles, stomach, omentum, chest, various joints, neck, and penis.

The majority of the sites is almost entirely limited to the extremities. Approximately 67 percent of the cases have been found in the upper extremity and 33 percent in the lower extremity. About one third of the tumors have been subungual, and nearly half have occurred in the digits. Dockerty and Harris reported that the glomus tumor has a higher incidence in the distal aspect of the upper extremity,[63,109] while Saunders stated that he found a higher incidence in the proximal part of the lower extremity.[242] In a series of 144 cases, an attempt was made to determine the relationship between trauma and the formation of these lesions. Even though 20 percent were preceded by definite injury, no true cause and effect relationship was established.

### Clinical Picture

The classical triad of symptoms is pain, tenderness, and temperature sensitivity. Rarely do these tumors not develop pain, but rather are manifested merely as areas of increased sensitivity. The most consistent symptom of the three is pain which is usually excruciating, lancinating, stabbing, or pulsating in character. The pain is generally the first symptom and usually radiates proximally. The pain may also involve a circumscribed area of skin. At first, the pain is intermittent but becomes progressively longer as the paroxysms come more frequently, radiating to greater distances. Between attacks, the patient may be pain free or may experience a continuous dull ache to the affected area.

In some patients, the pain may be so severe and the radiation of pain so extensive that the localizing or "trigger point" may be overlooked or cannot be found. There are many reported cases of intractable pain, having the same characteristics, following trauma to the fingers, in which no tumor could be found, and amputation was the only treatment which yielded relief. Not infrequently, such patients are, unfortunately, classified as neurotic. And this problem deserves careful consideration from the standpoint of compensation.

Elevation of blood pressure frequently produces a striking increase in pain. Relief may be obtained from elevation of the extremity, but, if the blood pressure cuff is raised to a pressure greater than the patient's diastolic pressure, there may be a great increase in throbbing pain. On the other hand, if the veins of the extremities are emptied and the pressure of the cuff is abruptly raised above the systolic level, there may be instantaneous relief of pain. Pressure may also elicit paroxysms of pain that may be fleeting or may persist for several minutes. The pain may also be aggravated by contact, cold, anger, nervousness, or excitement. Heat may also act similarly, although, generally, mild warmth will relieve the symptoms. Pain with a glomus tumor may also be associated with various sympathetic vasomotor disturbances such as increased, local sweating, or Horner's syndrome.

At the onset there is generally no swelling, but, as the tumor enlarges, focal swelling will be noted. Color changes then occur which are directly proportional to the size and depth of the tumor. Changes in temperature also cause striking changes in color of the skin directly over the tumor. The tumor will generally be well circumscribed and moveable in the subcutaneous tissue. When the tumor is subungual, the nail may be curved and thickened with longitudinal striations. The nails are often left uncut because of this severe pain.

The "pin test," first described by Love, may be useful diagnostically if a glomus tumor is suspected, but not visible.[86] The head of a common pin is gently rubbed over the area where the invisible tumor is suspected. When it touches the tumor, the trigger point of the sensitivity is localized. This "trigger point" is so specifically localized that we can press the skin as near as one centimeter to the tumor without producing pain.

A variety of atrophic changes may be demonstrated in the involved extremity, thereby leading to a mistake in the diagnosis of a central nervous system lesion. These atrophic phenomena may be brought about by disuse due to the guarding of the affected part by the patient or vasomotor changes or both. Skeletal postural changes may result from

**277**

carrying the extremity in a certain position in order to obtain relief from pain. A soft, wrinkled skin, associated with extreme hyperhidrosis, may also be present. Noticeable enlargement of the tumor site, or the entire hand or foot, or extremity, is a frequent but not a consistent sign. Alcohol has also been known to aggravate pain corresponding to the vasodilation produced.

Glomus tumors are characteristically located subungually, but they also may be located on the dorsum of the fingers and toes as well as other exposed parts of the body. Digital glomus tumors are often not diagnosed because of lack of familiarity with them. The glomus tumor is not a true neoplasm, but, rather, a hypertrophied normal structure.

Surrounding the vascular channels of the glomus tumors are neuro-reticular formations containing non-medullated nerves and a set of collecting veins. The whole glomus is surrounded by an ill-defined layer of collaginous tissue.

Glomus tumors are generally considered to be benign in nature. However, Symmers also demonstrated that glomus tumors do have the ability to metastasize and cause death. He stated that one year following excision, the patient noted that lymph nodes of the groin, on the same side as the surgery, were enlarging. These lymph nodes were surgically excised and found to be extensively infiltrated by glomus tumor cells, indistinguishable from the glomus cells of the primary tumor originally excised. There was also x-ray evidence of secondary deposits in the lungs. The patient died one year and nine months after excision of the original tumor.[273]

The same author presented another case that occurred in a woman 66 years old. The initial growth was on the skin of her thigh and had been excised five years previously. Apparently, inadequate excision had allowed the tumor to invade deep fascia and underlying muscle. The patient died two years after initial invasion was determined. There were metastases in the abdominal lymph nodes, lungs, brain, liver, and vertebral bodies. In both of these cases the histologic pattern of the metastasizing glomus tumor was identical to the original excised specimen. The only reported case of a single glomus tumor occurring in the foot was reported by

Alberts[3] and Galinski.[86] This glomus tumor was found sub-ungually and again excision was necessary for removal of the mass.

Another author presented a huge atypical glomus tumor which was excised from the thigh of a ten year old white male, and measured 27 x 7 x 3 centimeters. The original diagnosis was cavernous hemangioma, but histologically it was a glomus tumor.

## Diagnosis

If the glomus tumor is extensive and invasive enough, saucer-shaped defects are visualized on the dorsal surface or at the distal tip of the phalanx. If the tumor is bound tightly against the bone and is pulsating and expansive in character, primary radiographic changes will reveal pressure erosion of the adjacent cortical bone. It is the expansile character of this pulsation that actually erodes the bone. There may be a punched-out defect in the distal tuft. The margins of the erosive defect are generally smooth, while the cortical margin may be irregular. Osteoporosis may be an infrequent accompanying radiologic manifestation.

At times the underlying bone will show eburnation. When erosion is present, the remaining portion of the bone is generally calcified normally. It is felt that the erosive mechanism is similar to the mechanism of erosion by arterial aneurysms. If the tumor is interosseous, there may be honey-combed areas of decalcification.

Vogelsang utilized angiography to demonstrate the evasiveness of larger glomus tumors. He demonstrated that vessels become fuzzy in outline with serial x-rays and this is essential in making a diagnosis of glomus cell tumor.[282]

## Differential Diagnosis

The x-ray diagnosis of glomus tumors with bony involvement should not be confused with enchondromas which arise from within the bone itself, or from an epithelial cyst which arises at the finger tips or distal phalanx and may produce a defect closely resembling glomus tumors. Osteoid osteomas can generally be ruled out because they have pain occurring at night which can be relieved by aspirin.

The following diagnoses must also be considered when discussing the possibility of a glomus tumor: bone tumors, including enchondroma, bone cyst, and osteoid osteoma; bone lesions (non-neoplastic), including subungual exostosis and periostitis; benign vascular tumors, including hemangiomas, angiokeratoma, and lymphangiomas; malignant vascular tumors, including hemangiopericytoma, hemangiosarcoma, lymphangiosarcoma, Kaposi's sarcoma, and endothelioma; benign non-vascular soft tissue tumors, including eccrine spiradenoma, fibroma, neuroma, neurofibroma, leiomyoma, and blue nevus; malignant non-vascular soft tissue tumors, including fibrosarcoma; pigmented tumors, including blue nevus, malignant melanoma, subungual melanoma, metastasis melanoma; and miscellaneous lesions, including hematoma, Boeck's sarcoid, keloid, dermoid cysts, intradermal or sebaceous cysts, felon, and subungual wart.

## Pathology

The function of the glomus is not fully understood, but there are two types:

1. The first type does not involve a foot and is concerned with the carotid artery, the jugular vein, and similar structures. These are involved with diminution of oxygen tension, increase in carbon dioxide, alterations in pH, and other chemical changes in the blood.

2. The second type involves the extremities and has both local and general effects. These are involved with temperature and blood pressure regulation. They may affect just a single digit, an entire limb, or half the body.

These tumors are characterized by perivascular cupping of cuboidal epithelial-like cells. They vary in diameter from one to 30 millimeters, but are usually tiny.

Glomus tumors have three compositional elements that are almost always present: vascular spaces, nerve fibers (myelinated and non-myelinated), and smooth muscle fibers.

The tumor is an exaggerated structure of the normal glomus body with an overgrowth of all of its three elements;

vascular, epithelial, and nerve. The glomus cells are quite distinctive and have well defined cell outlines which are further accentuated by the delicate collagen fibers which separate every cell from its neighbor. It is a rare event to find a mitotic figure. At times the glomus cells have short muscle fibers within their cytoplasms.

The collagen fibers, which form a mesh work between the epithelial cells, pass out to join the stroma of the tumor which lies beneath the vascular complex. This stroma is generally loose textured and often shows mucinous degeneration. There are generally bundles of myelinated and non-myelinated nerves in or near the capsule of the tumor. These fibers pass among the epithelial cells and are in direct continuity with the cytoplasm of the cell.

In summary, the microscopic section of the epidermis is normal. The tumor is a circumscribed area between the corium and the subcutaneous tissue. At the periphery, there are numerous collagenous fibers that do not succeed in forming the capsule.

The lesions consist of irregular anastomoses of blood spaces lined by epithelial cells separated by collagenous tissue with a central cavity. Other cavities have layers of smooth muscles between endothelium and glomus cells. The vascular spaces are almost invariably similar to Sucquet-Hoyer canals. Neuro-fibrils are visible in most sections.

If the glomus tumor is encapsulated in bone, the histologic examination shows a loss of bone substance corresponding to the size and shape of the tumor, which was limited internally by the medullary canal and externally by the dense fibrous connective tissue. The tumor is almost entirely cellular, connective tissue almost non-existent, and nerve elements barely recognizable.

Histologically the glomus cell tumor can be categorized into four basic types: angiomatous form, a form with a few vessels and a large proportion of musculo-endothelial stroma; a form composed primarily of nerve fibers; and a degenerative form showing either edema, hyaline, or mucoid change.

Stout[263] found several of his patients with glomus cell

tumors, and noted that all the tumors had large Vater-Pacini corpuscles flattened out against the capsules. He believed these to be responsible for the pain. Believing that such a growth must represent hypertrophy of some sort of an organ because of its orderly arrangement and its rich connection, he examined serial sections of fingers and came upon peculiar arterial-venous anastomoses which exactly resembled the structure of the tumors. These were found everywhere in the deeper layers of the skin of the fingers and in greatest numbers associated with the corpuscles of Wagner-Meissner.

In the 1920's, Barre, the neurologist, described a patient with a glomus tumor of the distal phalanx with pain radiating to the elbow in association with Horner's syndrome. Masson (1920) noted the similarity between this and the glomus coccygeum and conceived of the arterio-venous anastomosis calling it the Sucquet-Hoyer canal. He noted the Paccinian corpuscle at the periphery of the capsule and believed this to be the source of the pain stimulus. He was the first to describe the tumor and recognize its origin from the neuro-myoarterial glomus. Clark later stated that one could see definitely that, when dilated, they permitted a large amount of blood to pass from artery to vein without passing through the capillaries.[49]

Stout contributed further to the microscopic interpretation of the tumor by means of tissue culture identification.[266] Lewis felt that the normal glomus regulated the arterio-venous circulation of the skin by shunting blood more superficially in deeper as it is needed for thermo-regulation.[86] Other authors later proposed that glomus bodies had a secretory function, controlled by pressure, and helped maintain the interstitial environment.

*Foot Involvement*

Popoff studied the number of glomic structures in a serial section of the great toe and found the following frequency: 18 glomic structures on the ventral surface, ten glomic structures on the lateral surface, 24 glomic structures on the nail bed, and 12 glomic structures in the nail matrix.[217]

Strahan reported 15 cases of glomus tumors. Twelve patients had solitary limb lesions, one patient had a glomus arising in a pilonidal sinus, and two members of the group had multiple lesions. Three were males and 12 were females, with ages ranging from 19–77 years. Pain was a presenting symptom for 14 of the 15 patients. Of the 15 cases, ten of the tumors were encapsulated; all of these were cured by simple enucleation of the tumor. The remaining five tumors were non-encapsulated; of these, only two were cured while three had to be re-excised. Four of the 15 cases were located on the foot; three on the plantar surface, and one subungual.[269] Galinski has also recently reported a case on the foot.[86]

*Treatment*

The glomus tumor is benign and its total removal results in a cure that is dramatically immediate, though in long standing cases the area of radiation of the former pain may remain sensitive for several months. Simple excision is the only recommended treatment. Amputation is an unwarranted mutilation. With complete excision, the lesions generally do not return.

If the lesion is interosseous, excision of the involved bone, generally the phalanx if the finger or toe is involved, will result in a complete cure. If the lesion is located subungually, the nail should be removed prior to excision of the tumor. If the nail is removed without excision of the tumor, pain will occur with greater intensity after regrowth of the nail than before the avulsion.

Various other authorities have suggested that x-ray therapy offers the best results although recurrence is likely sooner or later. Most of the symptoms, including pain and itching, will disappear promptly with x-ray treatment. Treatment with heat, cold, or sympathectomy has been shown to be of little or no value.

Ideally, with the excision of the glomus cell tumor, the pathology report should state that there is no evidence of any tumor on the resection margins.

*Prognosis*

With complete excision of the tumor, the prognosis for relief of pain and permanent non-recurrence of the mass is excellent. Treatment by any other means is generally not as satisfactory, and the prognosis not as favorable. For the rare malignant glomus tumor, prognosis is proportionate to the presence of metastases.

## Hemangioendothelioma

### Definition

Hemangioendothelioma is a rare vascular tumor that affects all age groups and is formed by malignant proliferation of the endothelium of capillaries. Vascular tumors occur in many locations, including muscle, tendon, nerve, bone, and fat, which gives rise to difficulty in diagnosis and treatment. The hemangioendothelioma can be and often is, locally invasive and destructive. The tumor, in many instances, has shown recurrences after surgical removal and it metastasizes to distant organs. The tumors can be single or multifocal in soft tissues or bone. In the latter case, the tumor can occur at any location in the bone, but mostly in the metaphyseal portion.[277]

### History

The term hemangioendothelioma was coined by Frank B. Mallory (1908) to designate malignant tumors in which the predominant cell was endothelial. Stout set the criteria for the histological classification of hemangioendotheliomas.[135] Garcia-Moral, in researching the literature, found the first probable case of endothelioma of bone, reported by Locke in 1866.[88] Golgi (1869) introduced the term endothelioma and Kolackzed (1895) used the term to denote tumors with blood between the acini. Marchwald (1895) reported a case of multiple intravascular endothelioma with symmetrical involvement of most of the bones, simulating multiple myeloma.[88]

Many authors stated that malignant vascular endothelial tumors are classified as one entity, hemangioendothelioma, due to their unpredictable course.[164,279] However, many dispute this and believe that other names should be utilized, i.e., angiosarcoma, angioendothelioma and hemangiosarcoma.[88,277] The histological picture is so varied that it is practically impossible to distinguish between these tumors.[277]

## Etiology

The true cause of hemangioendothelioma is unknown.

## Incidence

Dahlin (1967) reviewed 3,987 cases of primary neoplasms of bone from the Mayo Clinic and found seven cases of hemangioendothelioma, an incidence of 0.17 percent.[57] Bundens and Brighton, in reviewing 32 cases, found that males outnumbered females by two to one; and, in 60 percent of the cases studied, tumors occurred between the ages of 20 and 49 years of age.[37] Eleven of their patients were found to have multifocal origin, in contrast to Jaffe's statement that "multifocal lesions are more common than a solitary origin."[156] Otis and co-authors found the average age of their twelve patients to be 35 years.[206] Thomas and Garcia-Moral found the average age incidence to be in the fifth decade.[277,88]

There is a high incidence of hemangioendotheliomas affecting the long bones of the extremities, with the metaphyseal region being involved more than the diaphysis. The tumor was seen more often in the lower extremity than in the head and trunk, with the upper extremity being affected the least.

It is difficult to determine if the multicentric lesions are of multiple origins or whether they represent metastases from a primary site. Characteristically, multiple bone lesions involve several bones in one extremity, usually the wrist or ankle, in addition to one or more long bones.[206] In the majority of cases, blood-borne metastases occur where direct contact of the tumor cells with the circulating blood exists although lymph node metastases have been frequent.[96] Bundens and Brighton noticed that the femur was the most commonly involved long bone in their study of 32 cases.[37] Ramsey stated that the malignant hemangioendothelioma was nearly limited in occurrence to the cerebellum and spinal cord.[223] Thomas concurred by stating that there is a predilection for the vertebral column.[277] This would seem to mean that occurrence in these areas is common after metastases from the primary focus.

Kauffmann and Stout reviewed 129 reported cases of malignant hemangioendothelioma from the Columbia University College of Physicians and Surgeons, New York, during a 54 year period, and only nine cases involved children less than 16 years of age.[135] Therefore, (reported) malignant vascular tumors in children are exceedingly rare. Hemangioendotheliomas are more common in children than are hemangiopericytomas. The numbers of metastasizing tumors in each group are about the same. The incidence of benign hemangioendotheliomas found in the bones outnumber those that are malignant.[135]

There is no evidence that a benign hemangioendothelioma has ever undergone malignant transformation.[96] However, hemangioendotheliomas tend to recur after incomplete removal and usually show infiltrative, progressive growth and metastases. A reported case by Stout and Kauffmann stated that a seven year old child had nine recurrences of congenital malignant hemangioendothelioma of the eyelid, with no metastases.[135] Otis and co-authors noted in 12 patients with malignant hemangioendotheliomas of bone that the length of time from onset of symptoms until death ranged from 17 to 54 months, with the average time being 33 months.[206]

Dube and Fisher described a hemangioendothelioma that developed at the site of a metallic implant, that had been retained for 30 years at a tibial fracture, invading the soft tissues around the implant.[66]

In another case, the tumor caused rupture of the Achilles tendon in a 32 year old male, reported by Kullmann and Wouters.[146]

Benign hemangioendotheliosis has been considered by some to be an atypical pyogenic granuloma, rather than a reactive granuloma as stated by Petterson and Galtz.[210]

## Clinical Picture

Hemangioendotheliomas may occur as a solitary, firm, large nodule or as an infiltrating mass in the skin or subcutaneous tissue of the trunk or the extremities; or it can invade bone. However, it is rare in the soft tissues. These tumors are very vascular and friable, with a tendency for spontaneous hemorrhage if the lesion ulcerates through the overlying skin. The involved area on the skin may show dusky red plaques surrounded by erythema and small nodules. Ulceration of the plaque may occur. Physical examination is of little help in diagnosis, as is true with most bone tumors.

Thomas stated that the benign forms are slowly growing, regressive, and asymptomatic.[277] Therefore, they may either be unrecognized or may produce symptoms secondarily by pressure and growth. Pain exceeded swelling as the initial complaint in eight patients studied by Otis and co-authors.[206] In two other patients, swelling was noticed first, while limitation of movement was present in two additional cases. Numbness was the initial complaint in one case, with the tumor located in the parietal bone. Patients with tumors located in the vertebrae had evidence of spinal cord compression and complained of local tenderness and/or pain on movement.[277]

A history of previous injury was found in a few cases.[37,88] However, this may have been an incidental occurrence.

At the time of biopsy or surgery, profuse local bleeding has been recorded, but it is not a prominent finding.

## Diagnosis

Any lesion appearing to be osteolytic, multicentric, and located in the distal extremities in the metaphyseal regions, should alert the clinician to consider the possibility of hemangioendothelioma of bone.[37]

Radiographic findings can include a lytic lesion that erodes and expands the cortex and is associated with a mild periosteal reaction.[31]

There may be a possible correlation between vascularity and malignancy in the hemangioendothelioma. Excessive bleeding on biopsy and at surgery was noticed in two cases.[37]

Angiography is a diagnostic tool often used for vascular tumors, and has been employed since 1929. Three basic signs of malignancy are: 1) pathological—arteries newly formed, random, uneven diameter, and a less ordered pattern; 2) pooling—irregular, larger or smaller concentrations of contrast media, resembling pronounced vascular dilation or non-endothelia covered, interstitial pooling of blood in necrotic tumor tissue; 3) shunts—rapidly filling veins traversing the tumor.[76]

The diagnosis of hemangioendothelioma should be made only in lesions having well defined vascular spaces lined by atypical proliferating endothelioid cells.

Laboratory values may show an elevated level of alkaline phosphatase, as noticed by Otis and co-authors in their study of 12 patients. Their one case with a high level decreased to normal upon resection of the primary lesion. The cause of the elevation is best explained by the reactive bone formation.[206]

## Differential Diagnosis

It is difficult to diagnose a hemangioendothelioma if the cells are poorly differentiated by flattening or if they present in sheets or cords, or are spindle-shaped. Differential diagnosis includes fibrosarcoma, highly vascularized carcinomas, undifferentiated metastatic tumors, hemangiopericytomas, alveola rhabdomyosarcomas, and malignant synoviomas. This tumor appears to have variable degrees of malignancy depending upon its location. In a study of 14 cases involving children less than six years of age, all involving soft tissues or viscera, only four were known to be fatal, which is a death rate of 28 percent, about half the death rate in adults.[96]

## Pathology

Thomas described this tumor histologically as showing neoplastic blood vessel formation. He also stated that the vessels were lined by spindle to cuboidal cells with large nuclei. Anastomosing vessels were quite common, however, and there were areas of individual vessels with loose stroma with anastomosing channels. The stroma between the vessels invariably contained neoplastic cells. He noticed that the mitotic figures varied in number from frequent to uncommon. Thomas stated further that it was unusual to find zones with large blood-filled spaces lined by cells that were not necessarily strikingly atypical and easily identified as malignant. Generally, the low-grade tumor had a large amount of vasoformation with few mitotic figures. The high-grade tumors, however, had much less vasoformation with more mitotic figures and more atypia of the cells. The histogenesis of the vascular tumors tends to revert to the original primitive mesenchymal tissue. The histological picture varies greatly from that of the benign, well differentiated form to the obviously malignant.[277]

Thus, there are two groups, one characterized by a marked tendency toward vasoformation, which is probably of lower malignancy, and the other with little true vasoformation, but composed of atypical endothelial cells arranged in cords or sheets which show a high degree of anaplasia and malignancy.

Therefore, the essential feature of an angioblastic tendency, as evidenced by a vasoformation process of endothelial proliferation and the formation of new blood vessels, must be present in order to make the diagnosis, as stated by Thomas,[277] regardless of how bizarre the histological picture may be.

The gross appearance of the malignant hemangioendothelioma of bone is that of a dark red, highly vascular tumor, which has punched-out, well demarcated, discrete lesions, usually in the metaphysis and composed of hemorrhagic appearing spongy tissue and varying from soft to firm.[96,110,206] There are many variations cited in the literature, but this, apparently, is the most typical.

*Foot Involvement*

In the author's review of the literature, 17 cases of hemangioendothelioma were found to involve the foot. They most frequently involved the tarsals. The ratio was males three to one over females, with males being younger than females; the average age was 23.4 years. The most frequent presenting complaint was pain. Surgical treatment was performed in 16 cases, with only radiation treatment in one case.

Otis, Hutter, Foote, Marcove, and Stewart reported three cases involving the foot, out of 12 cases studied.[206] The first case involved a 54 year old female who presented with a mass, of five months duration, on the right foot and tibia. Soft tissue extension involving the popliteal artery was noticed. Normal laboratory data were found. The treatment included pre-operative radiotherapy in small doses. However, radiodermatitis (severe) resulted one year prior to amputation in the distal thigh. Postoperative radiotherapy of 2,800 roentgens was given. Metastases to the popliteal nodes were found. The patient is alive and well, with no evidence of disease, nine years from onset of symptoms.

A second case involved a 16 year old male who presented with pain, of two months duration, involving the right foot and fibula and the distal part of the right femur. Questionable soft tissue extension was noticed. The treatment was hip disarticulation, with no metastasis noted. The patient is alive and well, with no evidence of disease, five years from date of onset of symptoms.

In the third case, a 25 year old male presented with pain in the right foot of four months duration. No soft tissue extension was found. Midleg amputation was performed, with no evidence of metastases noted. The patient is alive and well, with no evidence of disease 17 years after surgery.

Kauffman and Stout cited a case which involved a 13 year old female. After excision of the original tumor, biopsy revealed a malignant hemangioendothelioma, and amputation of the toe was carried out. The diagnosis was made seven and a half months after the onset of symptoms. No metastases were noted. The patient is symptom-free one and a half years later.[135]

Thomas cited a case which involved a three year old male, with the location of the primary tumor in the tarsal bone.[297] Treatment involved amputation and radiation. No metastases were noted, and the patient is alive and well after six years.

Bundens and Brighton described two cases of malignant hemangioendothelioma that involved the foot.[37] The first case involved a three year old male with no history of trauma. The tumor was multifocal and involved the tarsal bones. The treatment consisted of amputation and radiation; there were no metastases noted, and the patient is alive and well after 13 years. Another case was that of a 25 year old male with multifocal involvement of the tarsal bones. The treatment was amputation with no metastases noted, and no recurrence after six years.

Hartmann and Steward described four cases in which the foot was involved.[110] In the first case a 25 year old male presented with a chief complaint of pain following injury lasting six to eight months, with bone involvement of the right foot in multiple sites. The therapy was biopsy and below-knee amputation. The patient is alive and well after eight years.

Case two was that of a 54 year old female with a chief complaint of pain lasting one year, following an injury and involved multiple foot bones and the tibial bone. Treatment included above-knee amputation and radiation therapy. The patient is alive and well after three years.

The third case involved a 41 year old male with a chief complaint of pain of unknown duration. There was multiple bone involvement of the left foot. The patient was treated with biopsy and radiation (3,000 roentgens), and is alive and well after a four year follow-up. The fourth case involving the tarsal bones of a young male was incomplete.

Thomas listed three cases of hemangioendothelioma of the foot, two benign and one malignant.[277] The first case was of a 35 year old male with involvement of the navicular bone. The x-ray appeared cystic, and treatment by curettement of the benign tumor left the patient symptom free after 11 years. The next case was a 15 year old male, with multiple sites involving the tibia, fibula, and tarsus. X-ray appearance showed fusiform expansions and cystic areas. Excision of the benign tumors left the patient symptom-free after 7 years. In the third case Thomas described a three year old male, with multiple involvement of the tarsus. The treatment consisted of curettement, radiation and amputation of the malignant hemangioendothelioma, with no recurrence after 13 years, and no known metastases.

Unni described a case involving a 15 year old female who had lesions on routine x-rays of approximately five years duration, with multiple bone involvement of the foot. The tumor was a "grade one" and treated with irradiation of two and one third years. Subsequently, the patient is well, with some healing noted on x-ray.

*Treatment*

It is generally agreed that surgery, whether it be by extirpation, amputation, curettage, or local resection is the best form of treatment. However, the therapy for each case must be individually determined by many factors—whether the lesion is solitary or multi-focal, benign or malignant, and its location. The mental and physical status of the patient must be also taken into consideration.

Most authors agree that radiation therapy is recommended when surgical removal is incomplete, when surgery is deferred, when the lesion is inoperable, or when only palliation is desired.

Chemotherapy with Actinomycin D and Nitrogen Mustrard has been used with little success.

Any combination of these treatment modalities can be utilized in patients with hemangioendotheliomas. However, they are not always successful.

*Prognosis*

Bundens and Brighton stated that the prognosis was poor in the 22 cases they studied with an eight year follow up.[37] Only eight were still alive and those that died did so from pulmonary metastases, with an average of two years from the time of onset. Morgenstern also found the average duration of life was two years for the malignant hemangioendothelioma.[199] This differs from Otis and co-authors whose study of 12 patients showed an average length of life of 33 months from the time of onset, with a range of 17 to 54 months.[206]

Tumors which showed a marked tendency toward vasoformation have a better prognosis than those without true vasoformation.[37,156,199,277]

There may be a possibility of a relatively benign course with long survival after surgical therapy; however, the tumors' unpredictable behavior cannot be overlooked.

## Hemangiopericytoma

### Definition

Hemangiopericytoma, by definition, is a tumor composed of spindle cells with a rich vascular network, which apparently arises from pericytes. It is related to the glomus tumor, but, unlike the latter, has no nerve elements.[64]

### History

The hemangiopericytoma is a rare tumor of vascular origin, characterized by a proliferation of capillaries, as first described by Stout and Murray (1942).[267] These masses of tumor cells take their origin from the pericytes, cells which are present around capillaries and small venules in almost every tissue of the body, but whose exact nature is not yet fully known. The anatomical considerations of the hemangiopericytoma are simple; they occur wherever capillaries are found. However, in reviewing the literature, there were only a few cases found in the foot. The tumors metastasize via the blood stream or the lymphatics, with pulmonary metastases by far the most prevalent.

There are both benign and malignant varieties of the hemangiopericytomas. The malignant kind is progressively malignant over a lifetime. The growth rate is variable and only in the most dramatic of the malignant tumors can rapid growth be correlated with malignant behavior.

The hemangiopericytomas have a rich vascular supply composed of numerous capillaries, with the neoplastic pericytes closely packed about the vessels. The pericytes, first described by the Swiss histologist, Zimmerman, resemble the vascular, smooth muscle cells.[267]

*Etiology*

No definite cause can be determined. Congenital hemangionomas have occurred, but they are not known to be malignant.

*Incidence*

Hemangiopericytomas can occur in the external soft tissues and internal tissues and bone. There is a slight preponderance of hemangiopericytomas occurring in the external soft tissues in the male. In the internal tissues, the female dominates. However, in children, the males have a higher incidence of the neoplasm.[266]

The hemangiopericytoma may occur at any age, but the incidence is greater in the first half of life. The malignant variety seems less common in the younger patients. In the literature, reports have involved patients from birth to 72 years old. There seems to be a higher incidence in the middle decades of life.

The anatomical distribution can occur anywhere capillaries are found, though the musculoskeletal system is most commonly involved. Local infiltration is a common occurrence. Metastases can occur by the hematogenous and lymphogenous routes; the former is more frequent in the lower extremity.[139]

*Clinical Picture*

Throughout the literature, the size of the neoplasm when first seen varied as greatly as did the rate of growth. Some hemangiopericytomas attain a weight of over 100 grams. In a study by Kennedy and Fisher, pain and limitation of function were entirely lacking as initial complaints. The presence of a lump, slowly increasing in size but without inflammatory changes, caused some of their patients to seek attention.[139]

Grossly, the tissue may be firm, traversed by a coarse trabeculae of fibrous tissue, or it may be interrupted by areas of necrosis or hemorrhage. Usually the tumor presents with a well defined capsule, which is firmly attached to muscle and fascia. Afferent and efferent blood vessels are present in abundance, yet subcutaneous tumors rarely show the external discoloration or redness to suggest their vascular nature.[139] The lack of discoloration sometimes is explained by the absence of blood-filled capillaries whose lumina are compressed by proliferating pericytes. On the other hand, the tumor can be a bright orange or gray to dark tan in appearance. Clinically, these tumors can be painless, growing masses, often nodular and circumscribed. There is pain only if the mass impinges on a nerve. In one case, studied by Kennedy and Fisher, the patient presented with an enlarged swelling of the right thumb, which had started as an innocent, mole-like warty growth.[139] Quite commonly, the patient notices the tumor due to its rapid growth, or because it may appear at a site of trauma although it is not usually related to the trauma. Hypoglycemia and hypertension have also been associated with the hemangiopericytoma.

The tumors have usually been firm, apparently circumscribed, and often nodular. Except in a few instances in which the tumor has been in the skin, there has been no external discoloration or redness to suggest its vascular nature. When excision is attempted, marked vascularity of the tumor is sometimes found. However, calcification in the tumor mass can occur on occasions, but actual necrosis of the tumor is apparently rare.

*Diagnosis*

The appearance of a painless or, sometimes, painful lump, increasing in size, on the trunk or extremities, which may feel encapsulated and which is devoid of any inflammatory reaction, may cause the clinician to consider a hemangiopericytoma in his differential diagnosis. The diagnosis must be confirmed by histological methods using the conventional hematoxylin and eosin stain, with differentiation facilitated by silver reticulin stain which demonstrates the extravascular nature of the pericytes.[12] If further confirmation is needed to obtain the diagnosis, electron microscopy is used to view the ultrastructure.

The extent and probable nature of the neoplasm can be further delineated with the help of arteriography. This technique will help to demonstrate the extent of the tumor, and its filling characteristics will suggest the diagnosis.

The radiologic changes are divided into three phases. The first or arterial phase shows numerous arterial twigs supplying the tumor mass. If no immediate filling of the veins occurs at this point, a direct arteriovenous shunt can be ruled out. The second or capillary phase shows a diffuse contrast "blush" outlining the tumor. The third or venous phase demonstrates the filling of enlarged, tortuous, draining veins, some running at right angles to the normal venous blood flow of the area, which Jaffe attributed to the malignancy of the lesion.[125] Stutton and Pratt suggested that the degree of malignancy may be correlated with the degree of vascularity.[271] Thus the hemangiopericytoma emerges as a neoplasm which does not have a sufficient amount of gross features to enable one to recognize it clinically.

Radiographically, hemangiopericytoma presents as a homogenous soft tissue mass. It may be well demarcated. Calcification within the mass may be present in the form of spicules or whorls; the latter suggests malignancy. Local erosion of bone may be present.[145]

*Differential Diagnosis*

The diagnosis of hemangiopericytoma depends upon its histologic differentiation among tumors of vascular origin and from highly vascular soft tissue tumors. Tumors exhibiting histologic similarity and, thus, cause confusion, include glomangioma, hemangioendothelial sarcoma, vascular leiomyoma, leiomyoblastoma, treated malignant melanoma, undifferentiated or metastatic carcinoma, and vascular portions of fibrosarcoma.[106]

Stout considered the pericytes to be the principal cell type in two closely related tumors, hemangiopericytoma and the glomus tumor.[267] Clinical and anatomical differences justify continuing to separate both tumors even though tumors of transitional structure occasionally occur.

## Pathology

Stout and Murray suggested that the tumor cells came from specialized cells normally present around the capillaries, the pericytes of Zimmerman.[267] They are rounded and spindle-shaped cells which have long branching processes applied to outer walls of capillaries. No myofibrils are present, yet they have contractile powers and have been assumed to have some kind of relationship to smooth-muscle cells.[74] The tumors varied grossly and histologically in most cases; however, some were uniform. Stout and Murray (1942) first proposed the pathologic entity hemangiopericytoma and emphasized the following two prerequisites for the diagnosis: (1) endothelial cells must retain their normal appearance and be separated from pericytes by a fibrous sheath; and (2) the proliferating tumor cell must be a pericyte.[106,267] The conventional hematoxylin and eosin stain was used convincingly to meet the first criteria, with differentiation facilitated by silver reticulin stain to give histologic confirmation. However, the second criteria is more difficult to establish. The function and nature of the pericyte was largely unknown then, and identification by morphology is difficult because the cell has few morphological features to distinguish it from endothelial cells, fibroblasts, or so-called primitive mesenchymal cells. Rhodin, in his paper, proposed a "primitive smooth muscle cell" which represents a transitional form between the pericytes and smooth muscle cells which takes its origin from the primitive mesenchymal cells.[228] He also speculated that the pericytes synthesize both their own basement membrane and nearby collagen fibers, that they provide mechanical support for capillaries, and that they serve as the precursor cell that may transform into smooth muscle cells. These pericytes are located along venous capillaries and precapillary venules and gradually give rise to those primitive smooth muscle cells which are likewise replaced by smooth muscle cells as the vessels increase in size.

Hahn, Dawson, Esterly, and Joseph stated that many tumor cells, which are morphologically identical to pericytes, and some cells, which show an increasing number of cytoplasmic fibrils, mimic the first step of differentiation from pericytes to smooth muscle cells.[106] This theory was used by Stout (1942) for his explanation of the confusing variations of the hemangiopericytoma.[267]

In a more recent paper, Battifora pointed out three basic patterns of growth that could be recognized, which he subdivided into three histologic types.[15] The divisions were based on the dominant patterns of growth of any given tumor. Type one is characterized histologically by many uniformly distributed, branching capillaries, with open, but sometimes slit-like, lumina and flattened endothelial cells. The cells of surrounding capillaries were rounded or oval. A fragile covering of reticulin could be demonstrated surounding the capillaries, but were fewer and inconsistant around individual pericytes. Collagen stains were weakly positive around the capillaries. This is the most characteristic histological type and coincides with the fleshy, light brown areas of the tumors. The ultrastructure of this type contains the best differentiated pericytes.[15]

Type two is characterized by wide open, round capillaries, surrounded by laminar layers of collagen of variable thickness which separated endothelial cells from pericytes. The pericytes were mostly spindle-shaped and frequently were separated from each other by abundant collagen and amorphous connective tissue.

Type three consisted of spindle-shaped pericytes alongside uniformly distributed capillaries with narrow and often inconspicuous lumina.

*Foot Involvement*

In the author's review of the literature reporting ten cases of hemangiopericytoma on the foot, bone was the most frequent site of involvement. The tumor appeared in six females and four males; the youngest patient was found at birth and the oldest was 65 years, with an average age of 28.9. Three of the lesions were malignant, and two had multifocal involvement. The treatment involved surgery in the majority of the cases, with six recurrences.

Kennedy and Fisher reported a case in which a 16 year-old girl presented with a painless nodule over the dorsal aspect of her left hallux. The nodule was excised locally. Recurrence led to the diagnosis of hemangiopericytoma, and the toe was amputated through the metatarsophalangeal joint. Two years later there was no evidence of recurrence. A second case reported involved a 43 year-old woman who had a below-knee amputation for a sarcoma of her right hallux. A careful review of the sections years later led to the diagnosis of hemangiopericytoma. This patient died 27 years later of carcinoma of the pancreas and no extension or recurrence of the hemangiopericytoma was found.[139]

Friedman and Egan reported a case as follows: a 50 year old white female suffered intermittent pains in the left foot for 20 years.[83] In 1957, a swelling appeared over the dorsum of her foot. X-rays demonstrated radiolucent areas in the navicular and first cuneiform bones, associated with a slight swelling of the adjacent soft tissues. A grayish granular tissue was found adjacent to the navicular and first cuneiform bones and was resected, but no defect was apparent in the cortex of either bone. In view of the x-ray findings, a small curette was inserted through an operative hole in the first cuneiform bone. The interior tissues were replaced by similar grayish granulation tissue, but no communication between the bone and soft tissue mass could be demonstrated. Only a portion of the tumor was removed. The histologic diagnosis was hemangiopericytoma. Following the operation, x-ray therapy was given. Pain on walking persisted, and additional irradiation was given. Gradual alleviation of pain ensued, and postoperative swelling was reduced. This patient has remained unchanged to date. The large x-ray dose was well tolerated, and resulted in only slight restriction of motion.

Kauffman and Stout reported three cases of benign hemangiopericytomas in children.[135] One case involved the toe of a 12 year old girl, the others were two males, with the lesions located on the foot.

Kuhn and Rosai reported hemangiopericytoma of the heel in a 41 year-old male, who had a history of previous nodules excised several times in 29 years.[145] Fisher studied 20 cases, three of which involved the hallux. All treatment involved amputation, and no metastasis was noted.[74] Stout (1956) reported five cases out of 98 cases of hemangiopericytomas, involving external tissues of the foot. One out of the five had metastases.[266]

*Treatment*

The unpredictable behavior of this tumor raises considerable problems for the clinician, because it infiltrates locally, has a high incidence of local recurrence, and has a varying rate of metastases. Any remnant of the neoplasm after local excision is capable of producing a recurrence of metastasis. Therefore, wide local or radical excision is the treatment of choice. Kennedy and Fisher recommend amputation if there is evidence of any recurrence after removal.[139] They also recommend immediate amputation as their treatment of choice for any large and/or deeply seated hemangiopericytoma. They also state that there is a 40 percent chance that the tumor in the lower extremities will metastasize. In five of their nine patients, after wide local excision, cobalt-60 therapy was given. In two of these cases there were early recurrences, almost before the course of cobalt-60 radiation was finished.[139]

In a study by O'Brien, x-ray therapy was preferred in conjunction with surgery.[203] In four patients studied, one was free of the disease four years and another 20 years postresection. The other two patients died, one eight and the other four years after diagnosis. No cases were treated with x-ray alone. No marked diminution in size of the metastases or successful palliation has been noted elsewhere with x-ray therapy alone. Two additional patients were treated with chemotherapy for an advanced stage of the disease. The drugs used were Actinomycin-D, Cyclophosphamide and Mitomycin-C, but no clinical response of the tumor was recorded.[203]

In a study by Backwinkel, treatment by surgical excision alone showed a cure rate of 53.1 percent, compared to a 13.3 percent cure rate for radiation and a 0 percent cure rate if cautery was used as the only method of treatment.[12] In addition, his study proved that radiotherapy does not improve the results of surgery, as shown in 27 cases treated by the combined method.

Ortega and co-authors reported a case of a child in whom the metastatic lesions of malignant hemangiopericytoma were successfully controlled with chemotherapy, after exploratory surgery and radiation therapy were tried for the lesions.[205] The child was treated with a combination of Actinomycin-D, Cyclophosphamide, and Vincristine, which at first appeared to be effective, since the abdominal mass regressed by 10 percent within two weeks. Metastasis occurred while the child was receiving this therapy but regressed in six months after Methotrexate was included in the drug regimen. The chemotherapy and radiation therapy caused sufficient regression of the tumor so that surgical excision could be performed.

Radiation therapy is an adjunct to surgical excision when surgical excision is incomplete, when operative treatment would involve an excessively mutilating procedure, or when the neoplasm is inoperable and palliation is desired. The lethal dose to the tumor is high, and delivery of a dose of this magnitude carries great danger and many complications. The recommended dose is in the range of 7,500 to 9,000 rads, but smaller doses may be administered for palliation.[145]

*Prognosis*

If the tumor is diagnosed early, treatment can be more effective through surgical, radiation and chemotherapy treatments or a combination of the three. However, recurrence is common. It was stated earlier that the malignant variety of the hemangiopericytoma is increasingly malignant over a lifetime, due to widespread metastasis. There appears to be an increase of metastases from the lower extremity. However, rapid death can occur despite radical treatment.

## Kaposi's Sarcoma

### Definition

Kaposi's Sarcoma is a form of vascular malignancy commonly referred to as multiple hemorrhagic sarcoma, usually starting on the hands and feet, with death most frequently occurring from hemorrhages from the lungs and gastrointestinal tracts.

### Synonyms

Angio-sarcoma multiplex; granuloma multiplex hemorrhagicum; Kaposi's disease; Kaposi's lymphoderma perniciosa; Kaposi's syndrome; lymphangiectoides. cutaneum; multiple hemorrhagic pigmented sarcoma; multiple hemorrhagic sarcomatosis; multiple idiopathic hemorrhagic sarcoma; sarcoma nodulosum cavernosum; parathelioma multiplex; sarcoma cutanium telangiectaticum multiplex.

### History

Kaposi's sarcoma (or idiopathic multiple hemorrhagic sarcoma) was first described by Kaposi (1872) as a clinical entity and is actually more common than the literature would indicate.

Kaposi's sarcoma is classified in the international statistical classification of diseases, injuries, and causes of death under Malignant Neoplasms of Connective Tissue.[297] Many studies, therefore, do not distinguish it separately. Haenzel was "obliged" to omit Kaposi's sarcoma from his study of cancer mortality in the foreign born in the United States.[105] Similarly, the statistical code for human tumors of the World Health Organization includes Kaposi's sarcoma along with multiple hemorrhagic hemangio-endotheliomas in the Rubric #50.5 (i.e. malignant neoplasms of blood vessels, infiltrating but rarely metastasizing). Kaposi's sarcoma is distinguished as a histo-pathologic type and assigned a separate Rubric, #52, in the tumor nomenclature and coding of the American Cancer Society.[178] This classification has been adapted by the AMA, the latter assigning it to the Rubric #852, among Tumors of Vascular Tissue.[131]

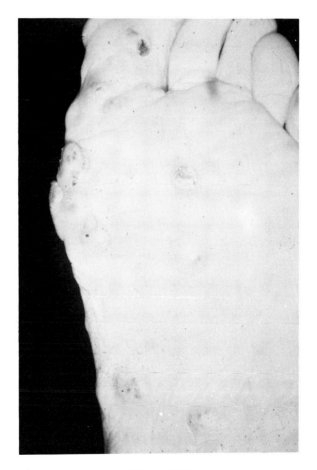

**Figure 5-10**
Kaposi's sarcoma. This illustration reveals multiple
Kaposi's lesions on the plantar surface. Also, the in-
dividual is affected on the medial dorsal aspect of the
foot. (Courtesy of Robert Rutherford, D.P.M., San
Francisco, Calif.)

## Etiology

Definite cause for this neoplasm has not been established.

## Incidence

This tumor normally has a marked preponderance in males, with figures varying from 75 percent to 94 percent in different series. The vast majority of cases are found in adults, with the peak incidence occurring in the 40 to 70 year age group in Europe and the United States, and in the 30 to 50 year age group in Africa. Only about four percent of the cases are found in children less than 16 years of age. Although nationals of all countries have been affected, there is an unusual preponderance of Negroes from certain parts of Africa, such as the Congo and Ruande-Urundi. However, Kaposi's sarcoma is rare in the American Negro.

In the South African Bantu, Kaposi's sarcoma is as common as melanoma and squamous cell carcinoma of the skin, and is the most frequent cancer of arms and legs. The disease was in existence in South Africa in 1912.[172] In Africa, Kaposi's sarcoma is most frequent in the north eastern Congo and least frequent in West Africa north of the Sahara. Unknown environmental influences are probably responsible for most cases.[240]

A few pedigrees are consistent with a dominant gene of poor penetrance. Kaposi's sarcoma sometimes occurs in assocation with chronic leukemia and lymphomas, nodular lymphoma, and Hodgkins disease, with the association being most striking in mycosis fungoides.[275]

The disease has very rarely been found in children of North America and Europe. This is in direct contrast to the children of Africa, where, according to Dörffel, the distribution of this disease is geographical and not racial.[29] Bluefarb, on the other hand, said that on the basis of recent data there was a denial of any racial predisposition.[29] However, McCarthy and Pack have found that 83 percent of their cases were Jews and Italians.[188] Rothman also believed that Kaposi's sarcoma was based on an inherent metabolic defect.[237]

Clinical observation showed that relative hypoxia of tissue is favorable for the initial development of the tumor since this development is in the acral areas. Malignant tissues showed a high anaerobic glycolysis and relatively high glycolysis also in the presence of oxygen. This was first discovered by Warburg and has since been confirmed. In candidates for Kaposi's sarcoma a congenital enzyme deficiency may well be present, promoting this tendency to anaerobic glycolysis, until some triggering factor brings about the disease.[237]

The total incidence of Kaposi's sarcoma in relation to other malignancies seems to be extremely variable in different geographic areas. The work of Quenum and Camain shows that the incidence of Kaposi's sarcoma in certain parts of Equatorial Africa is so high as to account for 10 percent or more of all malignancies.[220] This contrasts sharply with data from the University of Chicago, which show that in Chicago from 1946 to 1960, there were only eight Kaposi's sarcomas out of 13,700 malignancies. The data indicates that the incidence of Kaposi's sarcoma was 200 times more in the Congo than in Chicago.

Actual case histories of various sarcomas are extremely hard to find.

A study done in June, 1963, published in the British Journal of Cancer by MacClean, reviewed 45 cases discovered in Nigeria.[172] The distribution of these cases relative to age groups was as follows:

1. 0–14 years — 3 cases
2. 15–19 years — 2 cases
3. 20–24 years — 3 cases
4. 25–29 years — 5 cases
5. 30–34 years — 3 cases
6. 35–39 years — 6 cases
7. 46–44 years — 9 cases
8. 45–49 years — 5 cases
9. 50–54 years — 3 cases
10. 55–59 years — 3 cases
11. 60 years and above — 2 cases

Obviously, from these statistics, the reader can see that the age distribution of Kaposi's sarcoma on the African continent varies quite considerably from that of North America and Europe. Of 64 cases, also presented by MacClean, the following statistics relative to the site of the lesion are available: lower extremity, one or both, 47 cases; upper limb, 12 cases; head and neck, six cases; trunk, five cases; penis, five cases; lymph nodes, two cases; and viscera, one case.

Finally, one other statistical survey was done by MacKee and Cipolarro, (1936) in which they described nearly 350 patients, in whom the predominant incidence was in the sixth and seventh decades and in males. The breakdown according to sex was 325 males to only 21 females.[173] This type of statistical analysis confirms previous reports.

*Clinical Picture*

In cases beginning on the feet or hands, one usually can elicit a history of unilateral onset. Almost invariably, however, development of lesions is symmetrical, with the characteristic distribution on the hands and feet. Often, several lesions develop bilaterally, simultaneously; a dramatic illustration of multicentric origin. Aside from this approximate symmetrical arrangement, the distribution is haphazard. Occasionally, grouping of lesions does occur, common to the development of new nodules around the older lesions, producing a configuration reminiscent of tertiary syphilis and some deep mycoses.

In the majority of cases there are greater numbers of lesions on the extremities than on the head and trunk. The progression of cutaneous involvement is extremely variable. Many cases are on record in which single or just a few lesions have persisted for many years without any evident progression. As a rule, however, the lesion evolves slowly and progressively. When the first lesions appear on the feet and hands, lesions usually follow on forearms and legs, and later on the upper arms and thighs.[97] Since Kaposi first described it, this centripetal spread has often been noted. The total number of lesions may remain small for years, but periods of frighteningly rapid spread are also often seen. Cases with

306

more than one hundred lesions have been reported. However, the number and size of cutaneous lesions seem to be independent of internal involvement, again an indication of multicentricity.

It has been known, since Kaposi's first publication, that patients with lesions of the extremities, more usually the lower ones, have a strong tendency to develop edema. This complication often arises in connection with conspicuously few and insignificant lesions. It is not hard to imagine that in such situations the edema is caused mechanically by obstruction of major lymph vessels or veins due to pressure by the tumors. Hurlbut and Lincoln go so far as to say that in the presence of unexplained edema of the legs, one should consider Kaposi's sarcoma.[121]

In the white patient, there are two characteristic clinical features of the single cutaneous lesions of Kaposi's sarcoma—their color and their location. Early clinical diagnosis usually rests on these two features.

The dominant color is dark blue, violaceous or purplish, with or without the admixture of some brown tinge. This is hardly ever simulated by any other type of skin lesion. The histopathological concept of the lesion going through inflammatory and neoplastic stages is rarely expressed in the clinical appearance. The vivid red color of acute inflammation is never seen. The dusty red color of chronic inflammation, based on dilatation of the cutaneous arteriolar arcade, can sometimes be recognized but is usually masked by the dark color of the peculiar hemorrhage process which leads to hemosiderosis in the extra-vascular spaces. On clinical grounds, one would like to assume that the color change, due to extravasation of blood pigment, occurs very early or, at least, that it is this hemorrhage which makes the patient and the physician aware that something abnormal has developed.

The primary location on the feet, or less frequently, on the hands, is the second characteristic feature. It is known, of course, that Kaposi's sarcoma may start anywhere on the skin surface, on adjacent mucous membranes, or in any internal organ. Nevertheless, at least in patients of 19th century Europe and North America, the first cutaneous lesions have appeared on the feet in the great majority of caes. Of Kaposi's first five patients (1872), all five had lesions on the feet and some of them also on the hands.[132] In his text on skin diseases (1887), Kaposi wrote, "It starts on both feet and hands, soles and palms, dorsa of hands and feet and progresses with discrete lesions centripitally on arms and legs. After two to three years it appears also on the face and on the trunk."

Rothman says that the primary sites of the toes, fingers, and ears may be significant because these are areas of relatively poor blood supply and oxygenation.[237] These are the regions which are frostbitten first and freeze (with gangrene formation) as if they were being sacrificed for the sake of thermal economy of the whole body. This regulatory mechanism is made possible by the fact that these regions are richly supplied with arteriovenous anastomoses which keep the blood from reaching the surface and thus from cooling.

Concerning secondary changes in the development of single lesions, the most important fact is that they may involute. The dark bluish color gradually turns brown with the characteristic color of hemosiderin, which is familiar as the common sequelae of the venous stasis and eczema. The nodules flatten, the infiltrate disappears, and the lesions "heal" with the atrophic depressed scars retaining, however, their brown color for many years. The defense of the host tissue which leaves the fibrotic scarring is a purely local process. While some lesions involute, new lesions may appear on other sites; spread may be rapid.[286]

Ulceration of nodules is not infrequent and appears more often on the lower than the upper extremities. It is promoted by trauma and is more common in rapidly growing regions. The base of the ulcer is uneven and usually covered with necrotic, often purulent, yellowish masses. Ulcerations with stone-hard edges, particularly with rolled borders, should awaken suspicion that a true sarcoma has developed from Kaposi's sarcoma. Small lesions sometimes erode without true ulceration by losing their epidermal surface as a result of trauma or because of the invading infiltrate, and then highly vascularized granulation tissue appears on the surface.

In general, when viewing small protruding lesions, one often has difficulty in distinguishing Kaposi's from granuloma pyogenicum. The top of a lesion may be verrucous (meaning irregularly hyperkeratotic, with tips and valleys like those seen in common warts). One must assume that the disease process may stimulate the epidermis to excessive and irregular keratoses formation, which also occurs in other conditions on the lower extremities particularly in tuberculosis of the skin. Furthermore, it is clinically significant that verrucosities are sometimes seen in Kaposi's sarcoma, mainly on the sides of toes, before any typical feature of a Kaposi lesion has developed.[30]

Subjective symptoms are rare, but itching and burning have been reported. Pain on walking occurs when lesions are present on toes or heels, or pressure is exerted elsewhere on the foot. However, this is only observed after edema has developed, and then the pain is not confined to the single lesions. Circulatory disturbances in the lower extremities, which allegedly sometimes precedes the onset of the disease without obvious stasis, may cause sharp pain.[237]

## Diagnosis

X-rays can be helpful in the diagnosis of Kaposi's sarcoma, as there may be soft tissue changes. The soft tissue changes include tumors and scattered calcification. Peripheral arteriography shows the blood supply of the tumor and can demonstrate previously unsuspected nodules.[167] "Pooling" occurs and there is free connection between veins and lymphatics. Cortical erosion can be due to soft tumor pressure or can arise due to periosteal or cortical tumors. Thrombosis occurs in tumors which have healed spontaneously. Bone cysts are essentially from the marrow.

Bone changes are related to the severity and distribution of the disease and may be found anywhere. They are of three types—rarifaction, cysts, and cortical erosions.

The only way to establish the diagnosis is by excisional biopsy. Biopsies of angiosarcomas tend to be followed by fungation of the tumor toward the site of excision, but this has not been noted in Kaposi's sarcoma. Hemorrhage is likely to be brisk and arterial, for there are normally one or more bleeders at the base of the nodule which require ligation.

### Differential Diagnosis

Granuloma pyogenicum is a lesion which represents what appears to be highly vascularized tissue, but which is in fact a secondary, inflamed, capillary hemangioma. Its development often follows trauma and usually remains a single lesion. It bleeds easily, and its volume may shrink, but never subsides spontaneously. It is more common in children and is more often found on uncovered parts of the body. If an elderly person has a clinically typical granuloma phogenicum on the foot or hand, this should raise the suspicion of the possibility of an initial lesion of Kaposi's sarcoma.

The different kinds of benign angiomas are usually easily differentiated clinically, because they are soft rounded tumors, which hardly ever become hemorrhagic. Glomus tumors are usually tender, but pain may also occur with Kaposi's lesions.

In the differential diagnosis, the most important factor is the overall pattern of the disease, rather than the individual lesion. Leprosy, Madura foot, the reticuloses, neurofibromatosis, and hemangiomata are the most likely lesions to be confused with Kaposi's sarcoma.

### Foot Involvement

Some reported case histories are also very questionable as to the actual diagnosis. In a case of arteriovenous malformation with angiodermatitis, stasis dermatitis simulating Kaposi's sarcoma was discovered on the right leg of a 21 year old white male.[9] A case of acro-angiodermatitis of the foot was reported in a 45 year old white male, occurring on the dorsum of the right hallux and second toe.[176] Neither of the above cases can be definitely regarded as a true Kaposi's sarcoma.

There are familial cases of Kaposi's sarcoma such as that reported in father and son by Zeligman.[300] In this case a 73

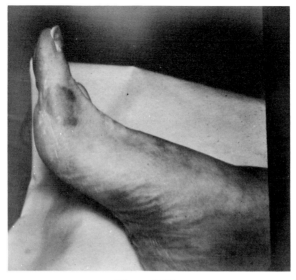

**Figure 5-11**

Kaposi's sarcoma. This photograph reveals a large lesion involving the base of the hallux and first metatarsal joint. (Courtesy of Israel Zeligman, M.D., Baltimore, Md.)

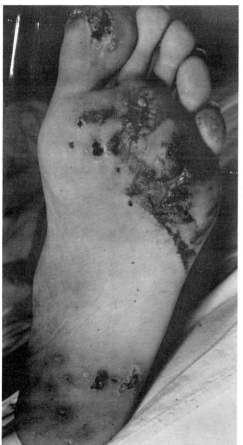

**Figure 5-12**

Angiosarcoma, revealing multiple hemorrhagic and necrotic areas on the entire plantar surface of the foot. (Courtesy of Armed Forces Institute of Pathology, Neg. No. 69-7643-1.)

year old white male had three red, smooth nodules on his right heel. His chief complaints were malaise, insomnia, and anorexia. At autopsy, there was found to be involvement of the right ankle, leg, and thigh, with spread to the pelvic lymph nodes and the adrenal cortex. The son developed similar symptoms on the left foot.

A case of Kaposi's sarcoma associated with chondrosarcoma of the tibia was reported in 1940 by Polliack and Even-Paz.[215] This 65 year old white male had lesions on the medial plantar aspect of his right foot, with swelling, pain, multiple sinuses, and purulent drainage. Biopsy of the right leg revealed lymphedema of the ankle, foot, and heel.

A case of Kaposi's sarcoma, associated with Hodgkin's disease and malignant melanoma was reported by Gilbert, Evjy, and Edelstein in a white male with lesions on the dorsum of his left foot.[97]

A study on vasoactive substances in Kaposi's sarcoma, described the most common symptoms as being prickling, discomfort, pain, itching, increased local sweating, and edema of the limbs.[25] Sometimes there was also abdominal pain. The clinical symptoms of nine patients were as follows: in one patient there was pain, sweating, plus edema of the left foot and leg; in two patients there was only edema of the left thigh; in five patients there was only edema of the left foot; and in eight patients, there was itching, pain, and sweating of both feet.

Another study of Kaposi's sarcoma, by O'Brien and Brasfield, followed 63 patients between the years 1935–1963.[203,204] Eighteen patients died of a second primary tumor. It has also been noted by Taylor (1971) that there are many clinical and pathologic similarities that exist between Kaposi's sarcoma and Hodgkin's sarcoma.[275] Southerland described Kaposi's sarcoma as presenting most commonly with lesions of the lower leg and foot,[257] which may also be associated with trauma of the leg and foot.

## Treatment

Wide excision of solitary lesions without any other treatment has been advocated by many and seems the rational approach. Such solitary lesions in our experience are, however, exceptional. One patient had an apparently single, ulcerated, conglomerate lesion treated by excision, but the wound healed poorly and satellite nodules soon appeared. This type of case is now treated with irradiation. Numerous excisions of isolated nodules have been performed for cosmetic and other reasons, and healing has been satisfactory. No recurrence has been noted at the site of excision. Some of the cases have been followed for more than ten years, and this tends to confirm the opinion expressed by others that wide excision of the solitary lesion may offer a reasonable chance for recovery.

Reparative surgery after radiotherapy can present difficulties. At one time, amputations had to be carried out for gangrene after irradiation therapy, but, with improvement in technique, this has become unnecessary within the last several years. However, there may be some difficulty with reparative surgery. After radiation therapy and chemotherapy careful evaluation is a necessity. After chemotherapy surgery is less of a problem for there appears to be less damage to surrounding normal tissues. Excision of groups of ulcerated nodules may be carried out so that split thickness skin grafts then give adequate cover to the area and insure a more likely recovery.

However, in the occasional case where radiation necrosis follows a large dose of x-rays, recovery may be less than adequate. To a vessel predominantly supplying the skin the problem is greatly exacerbated. The slough, which may extend to a considerable depth, must be excised and the rather poorly visualized recipient area grafted, preferably with full thickness grafts.[288]

Finally, surgery can be an adjunct to both chemotherapy and radiotherapy by reducing the tumor bulk. This type of surgery is extensively used in Africa, where tumors of all types may reach the surgeon in advanced stages.

Another form of Kaposi's sarcoma is fractional x-ray therapy directed to the involved site daily for ten days, for a total of 1400 roentgens. After six weeks flattening and subsidence of the edema was reported to have occurred in a 52 year old white male with bilateral involvement of the lower extremities.[112]

*Prognosis*

There is no certain clinical or histological criteria for establishing prognosis. Generally, the patient with a relatively stationary cutaneous picture has a better outlook. However, fatal internal involvement may also occur in the presence of only a few, nonprogressive skin lesions. We know that some patients have a fulminating course, while others may remain alive for 25 years or longer after the onset, some even in relatively good general health. McCarthy and Pack estimated the average survival to be eight years if the patients were treated.[188] Indeed, expert radiotherapy may considerably prolong life.[193]

## Reticular Cell Sarcoma

*Definition*

Kim defined the reticulum cell as being the following: a large cell with a pale, indented vesicular nucleus having a reticular chromatin pattern; a cell that produces reticulin; a cell of the stroma of the hematopoietic tissue; and, a cell of the reticuloendothelial system with phagocytic properties.[140]

*Synonyms*

Synonyms and related terms for reticulum cell sarcoma are: reticulosarcoma, reticulum cell lymphoma, stem cell lymphoma, clasmatocytic lymphoma, histiocytic lymphoma, monocytoma, reticulocytoma, and reticulothelial sarcoma.[70,262]

A look at these various synonyms illustrates the fact that there has been a considerable amount of debate over exactly what is meant by the term reticulum cell sarcoma. Subdivisions of this tumor have been based on the degree of immaturity and pleomorphism of the cells, along with their syncytial arrangement and the number of silver-staining fibers.

*History*

The credit for the first description of reticulum cell sarcoma is given to Roulet (1930).

*Etiology*

Etiology of this rare tumor is presently unknown.

*Incidence*

Reticulum cell sarcoma seems to predominate in males.[20,201] According to Mulligan, males outnumber females by a factor of two to one.[201] It occurs most commonly between the ages of 40 and 70.[70,201] However, Shrikhande and Sirsat found that males outnumber females only slightly, and the majority of their cases occurred between the ages of 30 and 55, the youngest being 17 years old.[246]

*Clinical Picture*

The most common clinical feature is lymphadenopathy.[52] Patients also present with swelling or a soft tissue mass in the affected area.[246,262] Some patients may show swollen, painful, ulcerated gums, and hemorrhage from mucous membranes.[201] Primary involvement of the reticuloendothelial system includes the lymph nodes, spleen, and thymus. Other organs which may be involved are nerve tissue, salivary gland, heart, alimentary tract, kidney, testis, lung, breast, skin, and bone. It has been associated with other diseases such as myelofibrosis, chronic myelogenous leukemia, multiple myelomatosis, and macroglobinemia.[52]

Cooper reported a case where reticulum cell sarcoma appeared to have occurred secondarily to Hodgkin's disease, follicular lymphoblastoma, lymphosarcoma, and chronic lymphocytic leukemia. He believes that a mutation could have caused this transition between cell types since there was a time lapse between the original diagnosis and the diagnosis of reticulum cell sarcoma.[52]

Cases have been reported in association with rheumatoid arthritis and pernicious anemia. Cooper reported a patient with Raynaud's phenomenon and severe hemolytic

315

anemia for seven years before reticulum cell sarcoma was diagnosed. He pointed out, however, that the association of auto-immune diseases may only be a chance occurrence.[52]

Reticulum cell sarcoma may produce skin lesions, which are, for the most part, discrete papulonodules and nodular plaques that may range from a translucent flesh-color to purplish but usually are reddish-brown.[140] Fungating growths occur but are not common.[140,246] Kim also reported two cases in which erythroderma was initially present.[140] Reticulum cell sarcoma has also been found in patients with mycosis fungoides.[140]

### Diagnosis

Diagnosis is usually made by aspiration of excisional lymph node or by tissue biopsy. The hematological picture is non-specific. Cooper found that 13 of 23 patients who presented with lymphadenopathy had a normochromic-normocytic anemia. Bone marrow examinations showed many different patterns. The sedimentation rate was elevated in many cases.[52]

### Differential Diagnosis

Because it is often difficult to distinguish between undifferentiated carcinomas, reticulum cell sarcoma may be confused with such carcinomas as amelanotic melanomas and juvenile alveolar rhabdomyosarcoma.[70] Also, all lymphomas would have to be included in the differential diagnosis, especially Hodgkin's disease and malignant histiocytoma. Shrikhande and Sirsat concluded that malignant histiocytoma and reticulum cell sarcoma should be classified together since they have the same incidence, location, appearance, and clinical features.[246] In Symmers' study of 226 cases diagnosed as reticulum cell sarcoma, 61 cases (27%) were found to be one of the following: Hodgkin's disease (most often), lymphosarcoma, and tumors such as squamous carcinoma, melanoma, lymphoepithelioma, seminoma, malignant glioma, dysgerminoma, hepatoma, granular cell myoblastoma, and non-chromaffin para-ganglioma. Non-neoplastic conditions have also been mistaken for reticulum cell sarcoma, including chronic (non-specific) lymphadenitis, infectious mononucleosis, dermatopathic lymphadenopathy, and drug-induced lymphadenopathy (due to phenytoin).[272]

*Pathology*

These tumors may become quite large and have a greyish-white, "fish-flesh" appearance. The microscopic descriptions of reticulum cell sarcomas generally indicate the presence of closely packed sheets of large, round cells with large, indented, and vesicular nuclei which may vary in size from ten to twelve microns to 20 microns or more.[183] The protoplasm stains weakly with acid or basic dyes.[183] Nucleoli are often prominent and mitotic figures may be seen.[183,240] Tissue stained with Gomori's silver stain shows abundant reticulin fibers which wrap around individual cells.[246]

Masson distinguishes three forms of reticulum cell sarcoma based on the degree of differentiation.[183] The first is the syncytial form, whose neoplastic base is the undifferentiated reticulum. This form, according to him, is found mostly in young patients around the twentieth year, with the cervical and pharyngeal lymphoid tissues being affected most often. Invasion may be diffuse or in cords. The second form that Masson described is the transitional form or syncytial form. This form contains not only the syncytial elements, but also the independent cells not encompassed by it but arising from it and released into the syncytial mass. Reticulin fibers are more abundant. Masson reports that the nature of this form is debatable. Some believe them to be abnormal lymphocytes and others consider them to be related to histiocytes (clasmatocytes of Gall and Mallory).[272] These cells are more basophilic. The third form is the dictyocytic form which is described as an "indefinite proliferation of independent cells."[183] The cells are large and irregular, and contain one or two prominent nucleoli. Again the reticulin fiber network is abundant and tends to divide the tissue into unequal areas of various shapes. In this form the tissue may have the appearance of Hodgkin's disease.[183]

As mentioned previously, Shrikhande and Sirsat believe

that reticulum cell sarcoma and histiocytoma should be classified together. The only difference they found was that reticulum cell sarcoma stroma contained reticulin fibers, and the histiocytoma tissue contained none.[246]

### Foot Involvement

The appearance of reticulum cell sarcoma on the foot is extremely rare. Spray reported a case which involved the soft tissue over the tibia and plantar aspect of the foot, and it appeared as a soft tissue mass.[259] Shrikhande and Sirsat, in their study of 18 cases, reported none on the foot but 55 percent on the thighs.[246] In Kim's study of 16 cases with primary skin lesions, one involved the shin, another the legs, and a third a thigh and again no foot involvement was reported.[140]

### Treatment

Treatment includes irradiation, chemotherapy, and surgery. The drugs often used are methotrexate and vincristine.[84,209] These drugs are often combined with x-ray therapy.[84] Kim found that skin lesions were radiosensitive and usually regressed quickly. However, more often than not, patients returned with recurrences and new lesions, which were often worse than before treatment and with decreased radiosensitivity.

### Prognosis

Kim indicated that cases with localized lesions have a better prognosis than with generalized involvement.[140] Prognosis is generally poor with late recognition and treatment.

## Arteriovenous Fistulae

### Definition

An arteriovenous fistula is an abnormal communication, single or multiple, between arteries and veins that causes arterial blood to enter directly into the vein without traversing a capillary network. The condition can be either congenital or traumatic.

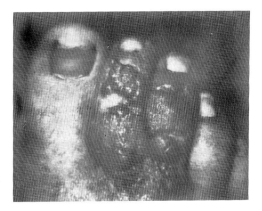

**Figure 5-13**

Multiple hemangiomas involving the second and third toes of the right foot with multiple arteriovenous fistula.

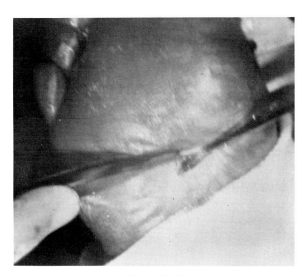

**Figure 5-14**

Varix. Surgical view revealing a thrombosed vessel, believed to be due to trauma.

## Synonyms

Pulsating angioma, cirsoid aneurysm, arteriovenous aneurysm, simple angioma, varicose aneurysm, cavernous angioma, aneurysm by anastomosis, arteriovenous varix, aneurysm serpentiva, plexiform angioma, and angioma arteriale.[5]

## History

An abnormal communication between an artery and a vein was first recognized by William Hunter (1757), who described the thrill and bruit.[120] Branman (1890) retarded a pulse upon closing a large fistula.[33] The first known case of foot involvement was reported by Gross (1867).[103]

## Etiology

Traumatic arteriovenous fistulae are almost always the result of a penetrating wound, such as gunshot, knife, glass, and many others.

Chronic arteriovenous fistulae are due to the failure of differentiation of the common embryonic analogues into arteries and veins. Most occur in the extremities.

## Clinical Picture

Symptoms of traumatic arteriovenous fistulae include bleeding, continuous thrill and bruit, symptoms of chronic venous insufficiency, ischemia and gangrene of distal parts, increased size of limb if arteriovenous fistula occurred before epiphyses closed, and increased skin warmth.

With congenital arteriovenous fistulae, thrill and bruit are not palpable. There may be the same effect as a post-phlebitic syndrome. Incidence is usually associated with port-wine type birth marks.

## Pathology

The intima of the vein becomes thickened with numerous, newly developed, elastic fibers arranged in a circular manner. The media is correspondingly thickened.

Besides a large amount of connective tissue, which on the side of the intima is developed more finely and contains numerous fine elastic fibers, a ring of circular, interlacing, muscular fibers develops within it. The transition into adventitia cannot be easily recognized, but a number of the elastic fibers, which must be considered as newly developed, are seen in this region as well as older, thick, stretched, elastic fibers. The changes are, in effect, those described after the transplantation of a segment of vein into an artery.

The opposite change occurs in the artery, whose wall becomes thinned, partly owing to the disappearance of elastic tissue and partly to the loss of the normal growth, muscular fibers.[5]

Different types of pathological changes include the direct communication between an artery and adjacent vein, an aneurysmal sac, interposed between an artery and vein, direct communication between an artery and vein plus an aneurysmal sac, aneurysm of an artery plus an aneurysm between an artery and vein, an artery and vein together enter into an aneurysm, and an artery and vein enter separately into an aneurysm.

### Foot Involvement

The first case of an arteriovenous fistula occurring on the foot, reported by S.W. Gross (1867), involved a 43 year old female with an arteriovenous fistula of the back of her foot.[103] She had been born with a nevus maternus of the left foot between the instep and toes. At the age of three, the foot began to enlarge, the superficial veins and arteries became tortuous and enlarged, and the skin temperature became elevated. Six years later an ulcer appeared, followed by ulcerations over her entire foot, especially near the medial malleolus. These bled freely on ambulation, but healed upon elevation of the foot. She also experienced occasional palpitations.

Examination showed an aneurysmal enlargement of the superficial veins of her left foot and leg, extending from the toes to the knee. A bruit and thrill were marked and observable. The internal saphenous vein appeared to be one inch in diameter. The great and second toes were doubled. There was a deep, excavated ulcer with a necrotic base on the dorsum of the foot. The foot had a "spongy" consistency due to the distended large veins. The circumference of the involved left foot was two inches greater at the instep than the right foot. The toes were distorted and painful. An amputation was performed by Gross, who noted that the internal saphenous vein looked like an artery. There was proximal dilatation of the posterior tibial artery. Following amputation, the patient unfortunately died of infection.

Vidal Puilachs (1952) demonstrated the relationship of arteriovenous fistulae of the foot and varices.[219] Mr. R.L. Lawton (1957) reviewed the history of arteriovenous fistulae and found that of 447 cases studied, only one (reported by Gross), was on the foot.[155]

Baer (1969) pointed out the need to consider an arteriovenous fistula of the foot when treating stasis dermatitis and varicose ulcerations. He reported a case of a 21 year old male who noted some discoloration of the skin of his left foot beginning nine years before. Varicose vein surgery had been unsuccessful for varicosities on his ankle. The evidence for an arteriovenous fistula consisted of a warmer left than right leg, and a stronger left dorsalis pedis pulse.[13]

E. Malan[174] differentiated three syndromes of blood diversion and summarized the surgical approaches and the indications for surgery which are recorded in the table on the following page.

## Treatment

Although arteriovenous fistulae occasionally close spontaneously, some form of surgical closure is usually necessary, to prevent chronic venous insufficiency, relieve cardiac strain and/or enlargement, and prevent overgrowth of an involved limb. However, surgery is somewhat difficult because of the large number of communications. Injections of sclerosing solution into superficial veins may be helpful.

The surgical approach to an acquired arteriovenous fistula used to be either multiple ligation or quadruple ligation and excision, but experience gained during the Korean War

| | Syndrome I | Syndrome II | Syndrome III |
|---|---|---|---|
| Site | AVA* of heel (anatomic dominance of P.T.† artery) | AVA of forefoot (dominance of A.T.†† artery) | AVA of sole (both A.T. and P.T. arteries involved) |
| Symptoms | Pain frequently localized in heel or entire foot, but may extend upward into leg during walking | Pain in forefoot in all cases, with parathesia of foot | Hypothermia due to capillary ischemia; calf pain while walking; burning sensation of entire foot and sole |
| Arteriography | P.T. artery is larger and sometimes elongated and tortuous with increased velocity of the blood flow, while that in the A.T. artery is markedly decreased | A.T. artery is larger and velocity of blood flow is increased | The A.T. and P.T. arteries are both visualized at the same time, and the maculae are visible on the entire sole |
| Plethysmography | Reduction of blood flow and pulse amplitude in great toe | Moderate increase in blood flow and amplitude | Marked increase in arterial flow in entire foot |
| Surgery | Sub-malleolar incision. Reduce short-circuiting of the blood by ligation of the P.T. artery | Detach fat pad of the sole from the aponeurosis of the forefoot through a plantar or lateral incision. The trans-metatarsal branches of the anterior tibial artery are ligated | Ligation of the afferent branches of the entire sole accomplished by a plantar detachment |

*AVA — arterio-venous anastomosis
†P.T. — Posterior Tibial
††A.T. — Anterior Tibial

323

showed that restoration of the arterial and venous continuity was much more desirable and precluded arterial and venous insufficiency following ligation and excision.

The surgical approach to each case is as varied as the lesion itself, and depends on the size, duration, character, associated aneurysms, collateral circulation available, and evaluation of the circulation during surgery. However, a grouping of the types of surgical procedures may be made, classified according to whether the fistula has been present for a short or long time. For arteriovenous fistulae of short duration, procedures include arteriorrhaphy, end-to-end anastomosis, graft, and/or sympathectomy. For aneurysms of long standing, procedures include mass ligation, quadruple ligation and excision, transverse arteriorrhaphy, resection of artery or vein, and ligation or transfixion of the fistula.[5]

### Prognosis

Small lesions usually end with a good surgical result; unfortunately, a high recurrence rate exists with larger lesions.

## Hamartomas

### Definition

A hamartoma may be defined as a non-neoplastic, tumor-like mass composed of the various tissues normally present in that area, but disarranged and disproportionate in growth.[36]

### History

In 1904, Albrecht coined the name "hamartoma" from the Greek, Hamartiona bodily defect, plus -oma, a swelling.[235] In his opinion, and many others since then, hamartomas are of congenital origin. Many such growths first manifest themselves at birth or within the first two years of life. A high percentage of these become apparent early in childhood, but some do not become clinically symptomatic or discovered until later in life.[36,235,292,295]

## Etiology

No etiological factors have been established as contributory at the present time.

## Incidence

Hamartomas are mostly found in the liver, lung and kidney, but seldom in the spleen or pancreas.[232,235] According to the literature, the incidence of hamartomas in the lower extremity, especially the foot, is extremely rare.[295]

We are not attempting to report the percentages or number of cases involved in different organs or tissues since there is no accurate report available. Many cases, which are now classified as hamartomas, most likely were either not reported or were classified under other names.

## Clinical Picture

Clinically, hamartomas range from soft to firm masses covered by normal skin which are freely moveable, but sometimes attached to the underlying tissue. There is usually a history of growth and increase in size without apparent pain. They may cause pain either by direct involvement of nerve tissue or by intruding upon and disturbing the function of nearby normal parts. Edema and heat may be part of the physical findings in some cases.[36,295]

## Diagnosis

Accurate clinical diagnosis of hamartoma is usually impossible, because it is a soft tissue mass without a specific gross appearance. It may be mistaken for a neoplasm.[6] X-rays may indicate involvement of bone.[295]

Laboratory findings are usually normal.[231,295] The only accurate diagnostic tool is the biopsy, and this is essential to prevent radical and/or unnecessary surgery.[2,36,127,231,295]

In vascular hamartoma (hemangioma), angiography provides valuable information for evaluating a patient and may provide the following information prior to surgery: 1) precise localization of best biopsy site, 2) boundaries and extent of the tumor, 3) involvement of adjacent bone, and 4) pattern of the major feeding vessels.

## Differential Diagnosis

The main differential, of course, is between hamartoma and malignant tumors.

## Pathology

These growths could vary from small nodules to huge, deforming masses with the appearance of malignant neoplasms. Depending on the tissue involved, microscopic examination reveals an increased number of cells for tissues normally found in the area, but disproportionately arranged. There may be interlacing with neighboring tissues. For example, in a case of lipofibromatous hamartoma of a nerve, the specimen may show mature adipose tissue covered by a thin fibrous membrane encircling the nerve, which shows numerous nerve fibers surrounded and separated by fatty connective tissue.[36,127,231,295]

## Foot Involvement

Involvement of the lower extremity is rare or, at least, is rarely reported.[231,295] The two cases reported in the recent literature are worth mentioning. Robbins, Hoffman, and Kahn (1970) reported an unusual case of fibrous hamartoma of the foot affecting a black child.[231] According to them, this case was important because, although most fibrous hamartomas appear clinically malignant, this was benign, because of its rarity in affecting a black female, and because of it occurrence in the foot. In a case reported by Wolf, a 50 year old white female complained of pain in her right great toe,[295] which was intermittent for several months—disappearing and recurring. It was painful and interfered with her walking. There was no history of significant trauma. Physical examination of her foot revealed a "hot," edematous, soft swelling on the dorsal surface of the right great toe. X-rays of the foot were unremarkable, except for some increased density of the soft tissues, consistent with edema. Laboratory findings were normal. The pathology was a lipo-neurofibromatous hamartoma.

Enzinger studied fibrous hamartomas and all but one of the 30 cases he reviewed occurred during the first two years of life. Seventy-three percent of the tumors were found in males, 27 percent in females. Only one of the 30 patients was a black, and none had involvement of the foot.[231]

## Treatment

Whether these lesions are treated depends on careful evaluation of several considerations, including the importance of a good cosmetic result, presence of pain, interference with function, and susceptibility to trauma.[2,127,231] After definitive therapy is indicated, surgical excision is the treatment of choice. However, cryotherapy, sclerosis, and radiation of x-ray therapy have been used in accessible tumors.[14,85,122]

## Prognosis

The prognosis is excellent when adequate treatment is rendered. However, recurrence is common if the mass is not destroyed or removed *in toto*.

## Bibliography

1. Ackerman, A.J. and Hart, M.S.: Multiple primary hemangioma of bones of extremity. *Amer. Jour. Roent.*, **48**: 47, 1942.
2. Aegerter, E. and Kirkpatrick, J.: *Orthopedic Diseases: Physiology, Pathology, Radiology*, 3rd Ed., W.B. Saunders Co., Phila., 1968.
3. Alberts, D.F.: Glomus tumor, a case report. *JAPA*, **61**: 23, 1971.
4. Alexander, A.M. and Koh, J.K.: Granuloma pyogenicum causing severe anemia. *Arch. Derm.*, **106**: 128, 1972.
5. Allen, E.V., Barker, N.W., and Hines, E.A.: *Peripheral Vascular Diseases*, 3rd Ed. W.B. Saunders Co., Phila., 1966, pp. 475–482.
6. Allen, A.C.: *The Skin, A Clinico-Pathological Treatise*, 2nd ed., Grune & Stratton, Inc., New York, 1967.
7. Angelopoulos, A.P.: Pyogenic granuloma of the oral cavity: statistical analysis of its clinical features. *Jour. Oral Surg.*, **29**: 840–847, 1971.
8. Angervall, L., Nilsson, L., Stener, B., and Wichbon, L.: Angiographic, microangiographic, and histologic study of vascular malformation in striated muscle. *Acta Radial*, **7**: 65, 1968.

9. Waterson, K.W., Shapiro, L., and Dannenbery, M.: Developmental A-V malformation with secondary angiodermatitis. Report of a case. *Arch. Derm. (Chicago)*, **110**: 297–302, 1969.

10. Ayella, R.J.: Hemangiopericytoma, a case report with arteriographic findings. *Radiology*, **97**: 611–612, 1970.

11. Ayers, S., Jr.: Granuloma pyogenicum giganteur. *Arch. Derm. Syph.*, **59**: 333, 1949.

12. Backwinkel, K.D. and Diddams, J.A.: Hemangiopericytoma, report of a case and comprehensive review of the literature. *Cancer*, **25**: 896–901, 1970.

13. Baer, A.C.: Multiple diffuse congenital A.V. aneurism appearing as stasis dermatitis. *Arch. Derm.*, **99**: 631–632, 1969.

14. Baque, O.C.: Un Caso De Nevus Vascular Verrugoso En Gorgonta Delphie. *Acta Derm. Syph.*, **35**: 117, 1943.

15. Battifora, H.: Hemangiopericytoma: ultrastructural study of five cases. *Cancer*, **34**: 1418–1432, 1973.

16. Beattie, W.M.: Glomangioma, three cases. *Lancet*, **2**: 137–138, 1945.

17. Becker, F.T.: Tumors of the neuromyoarterial glomus. *Minnesota Med.*, **23**: 78–82, 1940.

18. Beers, C.V. and Clark, L.A.: Tumors and short toe—a dihybrid pedigree: a family history showing the inheritance of hemangioma and metatarsus atavicus. *Jour. Hered.*, **33**: 366, 1942.

19. Berendez, V.: Genetics of skin tumors II. Multiple cutaneous leiomyoma, multiple glomus tumors and broom, rubber-bleb-nevus syndrome. *Arch. Derm. Forsch.*, **242**: 372–381, 1972.

20. Bergstrand, H.: Multiple glomic tumors. *Amer. Jour. Cancer*, **29**: 470–476, 1937.

21. Berlin, S.J.: Hemangioma of the foot, report of four cases and review of the literature. *JAPA*, **60**: 63–75, 1970.

22. Berlin, S.J., Block, L.D., and Donick, I.I.: Pyogenic granuloma of the foot. A review of the English literature and report of four cases. *JAPA*, **62**: 94–99, 1972.

23. Berlin, S.J. and Members of Maryland Podiatric Residency Research Committee: *Skin Tumors of the Foot: Diagnosis and Treatment.* Futura Publ. Co., Mt. Kisco, N.Y., 1974, pp. 135, 137, 148, 172, 203.

24. Berry, T.A.: Morton's metatarslagia due to cavernous angioma. *JBJS*, **39B**: 124, 1957.

25. Bhana, D., Hillier, K., Kerim, S.M., and Parm, B.: Vasoactive substances in Kaposi's sarcoma. *Cancer*, **27**: 233–237, 1971.

26. Bhashar, S.N. and Jacoway, J.R.: Pyogenic granuloma—clinical features, incidence and histology—report of 242 cases. *Jour. Oral Surg.*, **24**: 391, 1966.

27. Blanchart, A.J.: The pathology of glomus tumors. *Canad. Med. Assoc. Jour.*, **44**: 357–360, 1941.

28. Blinder, S.: Glomus tumor, report of a case. *Amer. Heart Jour.*, **17**: 238–242, 1939.

29. Bluefarb, S.M.: *Kaposi's Sarcoma.* C. Thomas Publishing Co., Springfield, Ill., 1957.
30. Blume, D.: Discussion to Andrews, G.C. Multiple ideopathic hemorrhagic sarcoma of Kaposi. *Arch. Derm. Syph.,* **38**: 452, 1938.
31. Bonvallet, J.M.: Angiomas Des Muscles Desquelette. *Presse Med.,* **58**: 535, 1950 (Fr.).
32. Boxer, L.A. et al: Angiomatous lymphoid hamartoma associated with chronic anemia, hypoferremia, and hypergammaglobulinenia. *Jour. Pediat.,* **81**: 66–70, 1972.
33. Branman, H.: Aneurismal varix of the femoral artery. *Inter. Jour. Surg.,* **3**: 250–251, 1890.
34. Bredt, A.B. and Serpick, A.A.: Metastatic hemangiopericytoma treated with vincristin and axtinomycin D. *Cancer,* **24**: 266–269, 1969.
35. Breschet, G.: Memoire Sur Les Aneurismes. *Mim Acod Rogale le Medicine. Paris,* **3**: 101–269, 1833.
36. Brunson, J.G. and Gall, E.A.: *Concepts of Disease, A Textbook of Human Pathology.* 1st Ed. Macmillan Co., N.Y., 1971, pp. 779–780.
37. Bundens, W.D., Jr. and Brighton, C.T.: Malignant hemangioendothelioma of bone, report of two cases and review of the literature. *JBJS,* **47**A: 762–772, 1965.
38. Burford, C.: Multiple glomus tumors. *Australia Jour. Derm.,* **1**: 35, 1974.
39. Bush, A.K.: Hemangiopericytoma, a report of two cases. *Amer. Surg.,* **35**: 351–357, 1969.
40. Buttner, A.: Die hemangiome peripheren Never. *Beitr. Klin. Chir.,* **173**: 129, 1942.
41. Callender, C.L.: Study of arterio venous fistula. *Amer. Surg.,* **71**: 428, 1920.
42. Caracostas, M.: Angioma of the soft parts of the sole of the foot. *Rev. Chir. Orthop.,* **47**: 674, 1961.
43. Carnevali, S.L.: Sugli Angiomi Dei Muscoli Striati. *Arch. Orthop.,* **54**: 476, 1938.
44. Carroll, R.E. et al: Glomus tumors of the hand: review of the literature and report on 28 cases. *JBJS,* **54**: 691–703, 1972.
45. Carter, J.M., Dickerson, R., and Needy, C.: Angiosarcoma of bone: a review of the literature and presentation of a case. *Ann. Surg.,* **144**: 107, 1956.
46. Cavshey, D.E. et al: Glomus tumors of the knee: report of a case. *JBJS Brit.,* **48**: 134–137, 1968.
47. Chandler, L.R.: Subcutaneous glomus tumor. *Cali. and West. Med.,* **47**: 156–158, 1937.
48. Chauvin and Roux (de Montpellier): Fibrochondrome de la gaine Tendineuse do l'extensus de quatriema orteil. *Bull. Mem. Soc. Anat. de Paris,* **90**: 75, 1920.
49. Clark, E.R.: Arteriovenous anastomoses. *Physiol. Rev.,* **18**: 229, 1938.

50. Cole, H.N.: In Discussion of Paper by Weidman and Wise, 1937.

51. Comline, J.C.: Painful subcutaneous tubercle. *Central African Jour. of Med.*, **3**: 308, 1957.

52. Cooper, I.A.: Clinical presentation of reticulum cell sarcoma, a disease with many faces. *Med. Jour. Aust.*. **1**: 697–704, 1970.

53. Coskey, R.J. and Mehregan, A.H.: Granuloma phygenicum with multiple satellite recurrences. *Arch. Derm.*, **96**: 71, 1967.

54. Couch, J.H.: Glomus tumors, clinical picture and physiology. *Canad. Med. Assoc. Jour.*, **44**: 356–357, 1941.

55. Crow, H.E.: In Discussion of Paper by Chandler. 1937.

56. Curr, J.F.: Arteriovenous aneurysm due to glomangioma. *Journal of the Royal College of Surgeons*, **19 (6)**: 374–376, 1964.

57. Dahlin, D.C.: *Bone Tumors: General Aspects and Data on 3,987 Cases*, 2nd Ed. C.C. Thomas Publishing Co., Springfield, Ill., 1967.

58. Davies, J.H.T., Hellier, F.F., and Klaber, R.: The glomus tumor; doubts and difficulties in diagnosis. *Brit. Jour. Derm.*, **51**: 312–318, 1939.

59. Davis, J.S.: Primary hemangiomata of muscle. *Bull. Johns Hopkins Hosp.*, **19**: 74, 1908.

60. Davis, J.S. and Kitlowski, E.A.: Primary intramuscular hemangiomas of striated muscle. *Arch. Surg.*, **20**: 39, 1930.

61. Desforges, J.A.: Nonsurgical reduction of granuloma and keloids. *JAPA*, **48**: 384, 1958.

62. Doane, C.P.: Glomus tumor (glomangioma). *JAMA*, **112**: 1049–1050, 1939.

63. Dockerty, M.B.: Certain small painful tumors of the extremities. *Lancet*, **73**: 57–62, 1953.

64. *Dorlands Illustrated Dictionary, 24th Ed.* Saunders Co., Phila., 1965.

65. Drake, H., Sudler, M.T. and Canuteeson, R.I.: Pyogenicum: case of staph actinophytosis (botryomycosis) in man: tenth reported human case. *JAMA*, **123**: 339, 1943.

66. Dube, V.E., and Fisher, D.E.: Hemangioendothelioma of leg following metallic fixation of the tibia. *Cancer*, **30**: 1260–1266, 1972.

67. Duhlop, J.: Primary hemangiopericytoma of bone, a report of two cases. *JBJS*, **55**: 854–857, 1973.

68. Eisen, D.: Pyogenic granuloma, four cases treated by roentgen rays. *Canadian Med. Assoc. Jour.*, **42**: 528, 1940.

69. Evans, C.D. and Warin, R.P.: Pyogenic granuloma with local recurrences. *Brit. Jour. Derm.*, **69**: 106, 1957.

70. Evans, R.V.: *Histological Appearance of Tumors*, 2nd Ed. William and Wilkins Co., Baltimore, 1966, pp. 256, 245–248.

71. Eyster, W.H. and Montgomery, H.: Multiple glomus tumors. *Arch. Derm. Syph.*, **62**: 893–906, 1950.

72. Ferguson, L.K.: Neuromyoangioma of the leg with sumptoms similar to glomus tumor. *Amer. Jour. Surg.*, **91**: 1021, 1956.

73. Finnerud, C.W.: Pyogenicum in children. *Med. Clin. N.A.*, **13**: 1285, 1930.

74. Fisher, J.H.: Hemangiopericytoma, a review of twenty cases. *Canad. Med. Assoc. Jour.*, **83**: 1136, 1960.

75. Fitzpatrick, T.B. and Walker, S.A.: *Dermatologic Differential Diagnosis.* Year Book Medical Publishers, Inc., Chicago, 1962, pp. 272–273.

76. Flester, A., Rosenklint, T., Rersing, N., Stephergen, E., and St. St. Chistersen: Angiography in tumors of the extremities. *Acta Orthop.*, **42**: 152–161, 1971.

77. Folickman, S.R. and Sokolowski, K.E.: Pyogenic granuloma—a case report. *JAPA*, **63**: 99–100, 19??.

78. Forrest, J. and Straple, W.T.: Synovial hemangioma of the knee. Demonstration by arthrography and arteriography. *Amer. Jour. Roent.*, **112**: 512, 1971.

79. Forty, F.: Vascular tumor seated in extenson hallucis brevis muscle. *Lancet*, **2**: 676, 1936.

80. Fragiadakis, E.D. et al: Gomus tumor in the fingers. *Hand*, **3**: 172–174, 1971.

81. Freedman, H.: Multiple glomus tumors. *Brooklyn Hosp. Jour.*, **8**: 4–13, 1950.

82. Freudenthal, W., Anderson, R.G., and Weber, F.P.: Glomus and the glomus tumor (Masson); with the clinical account of a case. *Brit. Jour. Derm.*, **49**: 151–163, 1937.

83. Friedman, M. and Egan, J.W.: Irradiation of hemangiopericytoma of stout. *Radiology*, **74**: 721–730, 1960.

84. Fromer, J.: Reticulum cell lymphoma. *Arch. Derm.*, **102**: 124, 1970.

85. Fulton, M.N. and Sosman, M.C.: Venous angiomas of skeletal muscle in four cases. *JAMA*, **119**: 319, 1942.

86. Galinski, A.W. and Vlahos, M.: Glomus tumors or glomangioma in podiatric medicine. *JAPA*, **65**: 167–170, 1975.

87. Gandy, D.T.: In Discussion of Paper by Fowlkes, R.W. and Pepple, A.W.: Tumors of glomus. *Southern Med. J.*, **33**: 269–274, March, 1940.

88. Garcia-Moral, C.A.: Malignant hemangioendothelioma of bone, review of world literature and report of two cases. *Clin. Orth.*, **82**: 70–79, 1972.

89. German, W.: Glomus tumors of the triceps muscle. *Amer. Jour. Clin. Path.*, **15**: 199–201, 1945.

90. Germansky, G.: Glomus tumor. *Bull. Hosp. Joint Dis.*, **6**: 160–164, 1945.

91. Gerstmann, K.E. and Nimberg, G.A.: Angiographic studies of hemangiopericytoma, a case report. *Clin. Orth.*, **68**: 108–111, 1970.

92. Gerwing, W.H.: Glomus tumor. *M. Ann. Dist. of Columbia*, **16**: 135–137, 1947.

93. Geschickter, C.F. and Keasbey, L.E.: Tumors of blood vessels. *Amer. Jour. Cancer*, **23**: 568, 1935.

94. Geschickter, C.F. and Maseritz, L.H.: Primary hemangioma involving bones of the extremities. *JBJS*, **20**: 887, 1938.

95. Ghei, P.N. et al: Glomus tumor. *JAPA*, **55**: 198–200, 1965.

96. Gibler, E.F., Jones, B., and Majzoub, H.S.: Malignant hemangioendothelioma of bone in childhood, report of a case and review of the literature. *Amer. Jour. Dis. Child.*, **121**: 410–414, 1971.

97. Gilbert, T., Evjy, J.T., and Edelstein, L.: Case report of multiple primary malignancies. *Cancer*, **28**: 293, 1971.

98. Giugiaro, A. and Bertola, L.: Emangioma Del Muscoli Del Piede Ed Emangioma Primitivo Del Nerve Plantare Mediale. *Arch. Sci. Med.* (Torino), **106**: 113, 1958.

99. Glasscok, M.E., III et al: Glomus tumors: diagnosis and treatment. *Laryngoscope*, **84 (11)**: 2006–2032, 1974.

100. Goidonich, F.I. and Campanicci, M.: Vascular hamartoma and infantile angioblastic osteohyperplasia of the extremities. A study of 94 cases. *JBJS*, **44A**: 815, 1962.

101. Gordon, H.B. et al: Multiple non-tender glomus tumors. *Arch. Derm.*, **83**: 640–643, 1961.

102. Grassi, A.: Su di un Angioma Cavernoso Diffuso Del Piede. *Riforma Med.*, **54**: 1154, 1938.

103. Gross, S.W.: A remarkable case of congenital aneurismal varix of the leg and foot. *Prac. Path. Soc. Phil.*, 86, 1867.

104. Gupta, R.K. et al: Multiple painful glomus tumors of the skin. Views on histogenesis. *Arch. Derm.*, **92**: 670–673, 1965.

105. Haenzel, W.: Cancer mortality among the foreign born in the U.S. *Jour. Nat. Can. Inst.*, **26**: 37–132, 1961.

106. Hahn, J.J., Dawson, R., Esterly, J.A., and Joseph, D.J.: Hemangiopericytoma, an ultrastructural study. *Cancer*, **34**: 255–261, 1973.

107. Hare, P.J.: Granuloma pyogenicum. *Brit. Jour. Derm.*, **83**: 513–515, 1970.

108. Harkins, H.N.: Hemangioma of a tendon or tendon sheath. Report of a case with a study of 24 cases from the literature.

109. Harris, W.R.: Erosion of bone produced by glomus tumor. *Canad. Med. Assoc. Jour.*, **70**: 684–685, 1954.

110. Hartmann, W.H. and Steward, F.W.: Hemangioendothelioma of bone: unusual tumor characterized by indolent course. *Cancer*, **15**: 846–853, 1962.

111. Hartzell, M.B.: Granuloma pyogenicum. *Jour. Cut. Dis.*, **22**: 520, 1904.

112. Haylock, A.: Angiography in Kaposi's sarcoma. *Clin. Radio.*, **14**: 304, 1963.

113. Herzberg, D.L. and Schreiber, M.H.: Angiography in mass lesions of the extremities. *Amer. Jour. Roent.*, **3**: 541, 1971.

114. Hill, J.H.: Radical onychectomy, partial with onychoplasty and sterilization. *Jour. Foot Surg.*, **8**: 34, 1969.

115. Hodges, F.M.: The treatment of pyogenic granulomas and hemangiomas. *N.C. Med. Jour.*, **14**: 11, 828, 1953.
116. Hoeffel, J.C., Chardot, C., Parache, R., Brauer, B., Delagoutte, J., Henry, M., and France, N.: Radiologic patterns of hemangiopericytoma of the leg. *Amer. Jour. Surg.*, **123**: 591–593, 1972.
117. Hollingsworth, J.F. et al: A multi-focal diffuse glomus tumor. A case report and review of the literature. *Amer. Sur.*, **38**: 161–167, 1972.
118. Hopkins, G.S. and Olsen, A.K.: Subungual glomus tumor, case. *Guthrie Clin. Bull.*, **18**: 83–86, 1948.
119. Horton, C. et al: Glomus tumors. *A.M.A. Arch. Surg.*, **71**: 712–716, 1955.
120. Hunter, W.: Observations upon a particular species of aneurisms. *Med. Obs. Soc. Phy. London*, **2**: 350–414, 1762.
121. Hurlbut, W.B. and Lincoln, C.S., Jr.: Multiple hemorrhagic sarcoma and diabetes mellitus. *Arch. Int. Med.*, **84**: 738–750, 1949.
122. Imperial, R. and Helwig, E.B.: Verrucous hemangioma: a clinico-pathologic study of 21 cases. *Arch. Derm.*, **96**: 247, 1967.
123. Jeker, L.: Symmetricial hemangioma of both feet with rheumatic changes—case report. *Schweiz. Med. Wschr.*, **67**: 633, 1937.
124. Jenkins, H.P. and Delaney, P.A.: Benign angiomatous tumors of skeletal muscles. *Surg. Gyn. Obst.*, **55**: 464, 1932.
125. Joffe, J.: Hemangiopericytoma: angiographic findings. *Radiol.*, **33**: 614, 1960.
126. Johnson, E.W., Jr., Ghormley, R.K., and Dogherty, M.B.: Hemangiomas of the extremities. *Surg. Gyn. Obst.*, **102**: 531, 1956.
127. Johnson, R.J. and Bonfigio, M.: Lipofibromatous hamartoma of the median nerve. *JBJS*, **51**: 984–990, 1969.
128. Jones, K.G.: Cavernous hemangioma of striated muscle. Review of the literature and report of four cases. *JBJS*, **35A**: 717, 1953.
129. Kandil, E. and Bassile, F.: Granuloma pyogenicum—report of a case of intra-lesional tuamrinolave acetonide. *Derm.*, **138**: 477, 1969.
130. Kaplan, I.W. and Karlin, S.: Glomus tumor—a report of two cases. *Amer. Jour. of Surg.*, **86**: 192–195, 1953.
131. Kaposi, M.: Acta. Univ. Int. Contre Cancre 14.
132. Kaposi, M.: Idiopathisches Multiplex Pigment Sarcoma der Haut Ardin. *F. Dermatologie, (Berlin)*, **4**: 265–273, 1872.
133. Katz, H. and Goetz, R.H.: Glomus tumor: diagnosis and pathology. *South African Med. Jour.*, **23**: 290–298, 1949.
134. Kauffman, S. and Stout, A.P.: Hemangiopericytoma in children. *Cancer*, **13**: 695–710, 1960.
135. Kauffman, S. and Stout, A.P.: Malignant hemangioendothelioma in infants and children. *Cancer*, **14**: 1186–1196, 1961.
136. Kay, S.: Sarcoma of the soft parts: experience with 85 cases. *Virginia Med. Monthly*, **78**: 619–626, 1960.
137. Kendall, A.W. and Thomson, S.: Glomus tumors. *Lancet*, **1**: 1102–1104, 1938.

138. Kendrick, J.L., Bergfield, J.A., Alfidi, R.J., and Beven, E.G.: Angiography in the surgical management of vascular hamartoma with respective cases. *Clin. Orth.*, **77**: 193, 1971.

139. Kennedy, J.C. and Fisher, J.H.: Hemangiopericytoma: its orthopedic manifestations. *JBJS (British)*, **42B**: 80–85, 1960.

140. Kim, R.A., Winkelman, R.K., and Dockerty, M.: Reticulum cell sarcoma of the skin. *Cancer*, **16**: 646, 1963.

141. King. B.: Personal Communications. Dept. of Path. Md. General Hosp., Balt., Md., 1975.

142. Kleinberg, S.: Angioma of the foot. *JBJS*, **24**: 367, 1942.

143. Kline, P.R., Brody, M., and Brody, E.R.: The glomus tumor, report of two cases. *Ohio State Med. Jour.*, **35**: 1317–1319, 1939.

144. Kondo, S.: Hemangioendotheliama, soft part of the knee joint, case report. *Osaka Med. School*, **16**: 160–168, 1970.

145. Kuhn, C., III and Rosai, J.: Tumors arising from pericytes. Ultrastructure and organ culture of a case. *Arch. Path. (Chicago)*, **88**: 653–663, 1969.

146. Kullmann, L. and Wouters, H.W.: Muscle hemangioendothelioma causing rupture of the Achilles tendon. *Clin. Orth.*, **4**: 154–158, 1972.

147. Kummel, B. et al: Overgrowth of an extremity caused by a glomus tumor. *Clin. Ortho.*, **82**: 80–81, 1972.

148. Lampe, L. and Latourette, H.B.: The management of cavernous hemangiomas in infants. *Post. Grad. Med.*, **19**: 262–270, 1956.

149. Lampe, L. and Latourette, H.B.: The management of cavernous hemangiomas in infants. *Pediat. Clin. North Amer.*, **6**: 511, 1959.

150. Larsen, I.L. et al: Hemangioma of synovial membrane. *JBJS*, **51**: 1210–1215, 1969.

151. LaSorte, A.F.: Cavernous hemangioma of striated muscle—review of the literature and report of one case. *Amer. Jour. Surg.*, **100**: 593, 1960.

152. Lasser, E.C. and Stapel, W.T.: Synovial hemangioma of the knee.: demonstration by arthrography and arteriography. *Amer. Jour. Roent.*, **112**: 512, 1971.

153. Lattes, R. and Bull, D.C.: Angioneuromyoma, a case of glomus tumor with primary involvement of bone. *Ann. Surg.*, **127**: 187–191, 1948.

154. Law, W.B.: An example of painful subcutaneous tubercle. *Brit. Med. Jour.*, **4983**: 30, 1956.

155. Lawton, R.L. et al: A clinical pathological study of multiple congenital A.V. fistula of the lower extremities. *Angiology*, **8**: 161, 1957.

156. Lea and Febiger: *Tumors and Tumorous Conditions of the Bones and Joints.* Publishers. Phila., 1958, pp. 224–239, 341–349.

157. Lee, F.D.: Comparative study of Kaposi sarcoma and granuloma pyogenicum in Uganda. *Jour. Clin. Path.*, **21**: 119, 1967.

158. Lehman, W.J. and Kraisal, C.J.: Glomus tumor within bone. *Surg.*, **25**: 118–121, 1949.

159. Lemmer, K.E.: Glomus tumors, summary of 15 cases. *Arch. Surg.*, **57**: 531–538, 1948.

160. Lendrum, A.C. and Mackey, W.A.: Glomangioma, a form of painful subcutaneous tubercle. *Brit. Med. Jour.*, **2**: 676–681, 1939.

161. Lenet, G. et al: Our experience with the diagnosis and therapy of tumors and tumor formations of the feet. *Magy, Traumatol. Orth.*, **17**: 19–25, 1974 (English Abstract).

162. Levin, D.C., Watson, R.C., and Baltake, H.A.: Arteriography in diagnosis and management of acquired peripheral soft tissue masses. *Radio.*, **104**: 52, 1972.

163. Leyden, J.J. and Master, G.H.: Oral cavity pyogenic granuloma. *Arch. Derm.*, **108**: 226–228, 1973.

164. Lichenstein, L.: *Bone Tumors, 3rd Ed.* C.V. Mosby Co., St. Louis, 1965, pp. 160–174.

165. Lidholm, S.O., Lindbon, A., and Spjut, H.J.: Multiple capillary hemangioma of the bones of the foot. *Acta. Path. Micro. Scand.*, **51**: 9, 1961.

166. Losli, E.J.: Intrinsic hemangiomas of the peripheral nerves; a report of two cases and a review of the literature. *Arch. Path.*, **55**: 226, 1952.

167. Losser, J., Rasin, A., Rusing, T., Stephenson, N., and Strove-Christonsen: Angiography in tumors of the extremities. *Acta Orthop. Scand.*, **42**: 152–161, 1971.

168. Love, J.G.: Glomus tumors: diagnosis and treatment. *Proc. Staff Meet., Mayo Clinic*, **19**: 113–116, 1944.

169. Love, J.G.: Glomus tumors. *Minn. Med.*, **32**: 275–277, 1949.

170. Love, J.G.: Glomus tumors. *Heart Bull. (Houston)*, **8**: 13–15, 1959.

171. Lumley, J.S. et al: Infiltrating glomus tumor of the lower limb. *Brit. Med. Jour.*, **1**: 484–485, 1972.

172. MacClean, C.M.: Kaposi's sarcoma in Nigeria. *Brit. Jour. Cancer*, **17**: 195, 1963.

173. MacKee, G.M. and Cipollarro, A.C.: Idiopathic multiple hemorrhagic sarcoma. *Amer. Jour. Cancer*, **26**: 1227, 1936.

174. Malan, E.: History and different clinical aspects for A.V. communication. *Jour. of Cardio-Vasc. Surg.*, **13**: 491–494, 1972.

175. Maley, E.D. et al: Bilateral subungual glomus tumors. *Plast. Recon. Surg.*, **55** (4): 488–489, 1975.

176. Mali, J.W., Kuiper, J.D., and Hamers, A.: Aeroangiodermatitis of the foot resembling Kaposi's sarcoma in chronic venous insufficiency. *Nederl. Tijdschr Geneesk.*, **110**: 791–796, 1966.

177. Manning, E.L.: Pyogenic granulomas. *Arch. Otol.*, **70**: 502, 1959.

178. *Manual of Tumor Nomenclature and Coding.* American Cancer Soc., 119, 1951.

179. Marcia-Roja, R.A.: Primary hemangiopericytoma of bone, review of the literature and report of the first case with metastases. *Cancer*, **13**: 308–311, 1960.

180. Margileth, A.M. and Museles, M.: Current concept in diagnosis and management of congenital cutaneous hemangiomas. *Pediat.*, **36**: 410, 1965.

181. Margileth, A.M. and Museles, M.: Cutaneous Hemangioma in children. *JAMA*, **194**: 523, 1965.

182. Martens, V.E. and MacPherson, D.J.: Fibroangioma: a proposed descriptive term for granuloma pyogenicum, granuloma gravidarum, juvenile angiofibroma and urethral carbuncle. *Arch. Path.*, **61**: 120, 1956.

183. Masson, P.: *Human Tumors,* translated by Sidney D. Kobernick. Wayne State Univ. Press. 1970.

184. Mathis, W.H., Jr. and Schulz, M.D.: Roentgen diagnosis of glomus tumors. *Radiol.*, **51**: 71–75, 1948.

185. Matorelli, F.: Glomus tumor. *Angiology*, **1**: 451–456, 1950.

186. Mau, C.: Development of clubfoot following epiphyseal growth damage due to radium therapy of hemangioma. *Z. Orth.*, **81**: 34, 1951.

187. McCain, L. and Galinski, A.W.: Dermal hemangioma of the foot (case report). *JAPA*, **57**: 561, 1967.

188. McCarthy, W.D. and Pack, G.T.: Malignant blood vessel tumors, 56 cases. *Surg. Gyn. and Obst.*, **91**: 465–482, 1950.

189. McGregor, A.: Pyogenicum treated with penicillin. *Med. Jour. Aust.*, **2**: 43, 1947.

190. McNeil, T.W. and Chan, G.E.; Cope, K.V. and Ray, R.D.: The value of angiography in the surgical management of deep hemangiomas. *Clin. Orth. and Related Research*, **101**: 176–181, 1974.

191. McNeil, T.W. and Ray, R.D.: Hemangioma of the extremities, review of 35 cases. *Clin. Orth. and Related Research*, **101**: 154–165, 1974.

192. Meyerding, M.W. and Varney, J.H.: Glomus tumors, two cases. *Minn. Med.*, **30**: 159–160, 1947.

193. Meyers, D.S. and Jacobson, LD.C.: Multiple hemorrhagic sarcoma of Kaposi. *Amer. Jour. Path.*, **3**: 321–328, 1927.

194. Michelson, H.E.: Granuloma pyogenicum, a clinical and histological review of 29 cases. *Arch. Derm.*, **12**: 492, 1925.

195. Mieschen, G.: Eruptive glomus tumors. *Derm.*, **91**: 233–234, 1945.

196. Montgomery, D.W. and Culver, D.: Pyogenicum and high blood pressure. *Jour. Cutaneous Dis.*, **35**: 338, 1917.

197. Montgomery, D.W. and Culver, D.: Pyogenic granuloma. *Arch. Derm. Syph.*, **26**: 131, 1932.

198. Mordovtsev, V.N. et al: Case of multiple familial glomus tumors. *Vestin. Derm. Venerol.*, **38** (7): 82–85, 1974 (English Abstract).

199. Morgenstern, P. and Westing, S.W.: Malignant hemangioendothelioma of bone, 14 year follow up in a case treated with radiation alone. *Cancer*, **23**: 221–224, 1969.

200. Mueller, S.C.: Subungual glomus tumor. *Minn. Med.*, **22**: 708–723, 1939.

201. Mulligan, R.M.: *Syllabus of human neoplasms.* Lea and Febiger, Phila., 1951, pp. 72–73.

202. Nabarro, J.D.N.: A case of glomus tumor with observation on variations of pain with temperature. *Brit. Med. Jour.,* **2**: 416, 1940.

203. O'Brien, P. and Brasfield, R.D.: Hemangiopericytoma. *Jour. Indian Med. Assoc.,* **43**: 447–449, 1964.

204. O'Brien, P. and Brasfield, R.D.: Hemangiopericytoma. *Cancer,* **18**: 249–252, 1965.

205. Ortega, J.A., Finkelstein, J.Z., Isaacs, H., Jr., Hittle, R., and Hastings, N.: Chemotherapy of malignant hemangiopericytoma of childhood, report of a case and review of the literature. *Cancer,* **27**: 730–735, 1971.

206. Otis, J., Hutter, R.V.P., Foote, F.W., Jr., Marcove, R.C., and Stewart, F.W.: Hemangioendothelioma of bone. *Surg. Gyn. Obst.,* **127**: 295–305, 1968.

207. Oughterson, A.W. and Tennant, R.: Angiomatous tumors of the hands and feet. *Surg.,* **5**: 73–100, 1939.

208. Pack, T.T. and Miller, T.R.: Hemangiomas classification, diagnosis and treatment. *Angiology,* **1**: 405, 1950.

209. Peekhaus, M.F. and Cooper, E.H.: The pattern of cell growth in reticulum cell sarcoma and lymphosarcoma. *European Jour. Cancer,* **6**: 453–463, 1970.

210. Petterson, W.C., Jr. and Galty, R.: Atypical granuloma, a case of benign hemangioendothelioma. *Arch. Derm.,* **90**: 197, 1964.

211. Peyri, J.M.: Glomal tumors; relation to solitary cutaneous myomas. *Acta. Derm.,* **35**: 56–66, 1943.

212. Pillsbury, D.M., Shelley, W.B. and Kligman, A.M.: *Dermatology.* W.B. Saunders Co., Phila., 1968, pp. 1112–1113.

213. Pinkus, H. and Rudner, E.: How we treat granuloma pyogenicum. *Post Grad. Med.,* **45**: 270–271, 1969.

214. Plewes, B.: Multiple glomus tumors, four in one finger tip. *Canadian Med. Assoc. Jour.,* **44**: 364–365, 1941.

215. Polliack, Z. and Even-Paz: Kaposi's sarcoma with chondrosarcoma of the tibia. *Derm.,* 23–29, 1940.

216. Pomerantz, M.M. and Tunich, L.S.: Visualization and obliteration of angiomata by radiopaque solutions. *Ann. Surg.,* **114**: 1050, 1941.

217. Popoff, N.W.: The digital vascular system, with reference to the state of glomus in inflammation, arteriosclerotic gangrene, diabetic gangrene, thromboangitis obliterans and supernumerary digits in man. *Arch. Path.,* **18**: 295–330, 1934.

218. Pringigalli, S.: Contributo Alla Conoscenza Dei Tumori Delle Guaine Tendinee. *Chir. Organi.,* **Mov. 17**: 128, 1932.

219. Puilachs, V.: Wrodzona Przetoka Tetmizo—Zylna Stapy. Tygodnik Leparski, 1966.

220. Quenum, A. and Camain, R.: Les Aspects Africians Des La Maladie

337

De Kaposi, Reticulopathie Malignie Systematisee. *Ann. Anat. Path.*, 3: 337–368, 1958.

221. Radash, H.E.: Glomus tumors. *Arch. Path.*, 23: 615–633, 1937.

222. Raisman, V.: Glomus tumors (angioneuromyoma). *Bull. Hosp. Joint Dis.*, 1: 107–115, 1940.

223. Ramsey, H.: Fine structure of hemangiopericytoma, and hemangioendothelioma. *Cancer*, 19: 2005–2018, 1966.

224. Reeves, D.L.: Glomus tumor; clinical and pathologic report of a case. *Bull. Los Angelos Neurologic Soc.*, 14: 40–45, 1949.

225. Reid, M.R.: Studies of abnormal arteriovenous communications, acquired and congenital. *Arch. Surg.*, 10: 601–638, 1925.

226. Reis, I.J.: A case of granuloma of the nail bed of the great toe. *Jour. Nat. Assoc. Chir.*, 13: 10, 1923.

227. Reis, I.J.: Granuloma pyogenicum. *Jour. Nat. Assoc. Chir.*, 26: 16, 1936.

228. Rhodin, J.A.G.: Ultra structure of malnmaliam venous capillaries, venules and small collecting veins. *Jour. Ultrastruct. Res.*, 25: 452–500, 1968.

229. Riley, K.: Dermatological don'ts, case of six granuloma pyogenicum. *J.S.C. Med. Assoc.*, 58: 485, 1962.

230. Riveros, M. and Pack, G.T.: Glomus tumor, 20 cases. *Ann. Surg.*, 133: 394–400, 1951.

231. Robbins, L B., Hoffman, S., and Kahn, S.: Fibrous hamartoma of infancy, a case report. *Plast. Recon. Surg.*, 46: 197–200, 1970.

232. Robbins, S.L.: *Pathology.* W.B. Saunders Co., Phila., 1967.

233. Ronchese, F.: Granuloma pyogenicum. *Amer. Jour. Surg.*, 109: 430, 1965.

234. Rosenberg, R.E.: Cavernous hemangioma of the foot. *JAPA*, 57: 382, 1967.

235. Ross, C.F. and Schiller, K.F.R.: Hamartoma of spleen associated with thrombocytopenia. *Aour. Path.*, 105: 62–64, 1971.

236. Ross, S.B.: Subungual granuloma pyogenicum. *Jour. Nat. Assoc. Chir.*, 45: 17, 1955.

237. Rothman, S.: (Symposium of Kaposi( *Acta Univ Int. Contre Cancer*, 18: 400, 1962.

238. Rowe, L.: Granuloma pyogenicum differential diagnosis. *Arch. Derm.*, 78: 341, 1958.

239. Rowntree, T.: Multiple painful glomus tumors. *Brit. Jour. Surg.*, 40: 142–144, 1952.

240. Ryalwazi, S.R., Bhana, D., Sr., and Master, S.P.: Actinomycin D in malignant Kaposi's sarcoma. *East African Jour. Med.*, 48: 16–26, 1971.

241. Salter, R.B.: *Testbook of Disorders and Injuries of the Musculoskeletal System.* Williams and Wilkins, Co., Balt., 1971.

242. Saunders, T.S. and Fitzpatrick, T.B.: Multiple hemangiopericytomas. *Arch. Derm.*, 76: 731–734, 1957.

243. Shallow, T.A., Eger, S.A., and Wagner, F.B., Jr.: Primary hemangiomatous tumors of skeletal muscle. *Ann. Surg.*, **119**: 700, 1944.

244. Sheils, W.C. et al: Subungual glomus tumors. A cause of pain beneath the fingernail. *Jour. Med. Assoc. Ga.*, **61**: 268–270, 1972.

245. Shim, W.K.T.: Hemangiomas of infancy complicated by thrombocytopenia. *Ameri. Jour. Surg.*, **116**: 896–904, 1968.

246. Shrikhande, S.S. and Sirsat, M.V.: Reticulum cell sarcoma and malignant histiocytoma of the soft tissues. *The Indian Jour. Cancer*, **9**: No. 4, 1972.

247. Shtern, R.D. et al: Malignant glomus tumor of the stomach. *Arkh. Patol.*, **36 (1)**: 60–63, 1974.

248. Sibulkin, D. et al: Invisible glomus tumor. *Arch. Surg.*, **109**: 111–112, 1974.

249. Siege, M.W.: Interosseous glomus tumor. *Amer. Jour. Orth.*, **9**: 68–69, 1967.

250. Silva, J.F. et al: Solitary glomus tumors of the fingers. *Hand*, **6**: 204–207, 1974.

251. Simko, M.V.: Chemo-surgery for subungual granuloma: a case report. *JAPA*, **52**: 512, 1962.

252. Simpson, A.R.: Proceedings: giant glomangioma. *Brit. Jour. Derm.*, **90**: 229–231, 1974.

253. Slepyan, A.H.: The glomus tumor; report of two cases with histologic observations. *Arch. Derm. Syph.*, **36**: 77–84, 1937.

254. Slepyan, A.H.: Multiple painful and painless glomus tumors. *Arch. Derm. Syph.*, **50**: 179–182, 1944.

255. Solland, A.: Sarcoma of the skin, malignant glomic tumors. *U.S. Nav. Med. Bull.*, **35**: 85–86, 1937.

256. Sommer, R.: Uber cavernose angioma am peripheren nervensystem. *Deutsch. Z. Chir.*, **173**: 65, 1922.

257. Southerland, N.: Description of Kaposi's sarcoma. *Acta. Univ. Int. Contre Cancer*, **18**: 508, 1962.

258. Spector, G.J. et al: Glomus tumors of the hand and neck. Analysis of clinical manifestations. *Ann. Otol. Rhinol. Laryngol.*, **84**: 73–79, 1975.

259. Spray, J.B.: Tumors of the lower extremities. *JAPA*, **62**: No. 6, 1972.

260. Stabins, S.J., Thornton, J.J., and Scott, W.J.M.: Changes in the vasomotor reaction associated with glomus tumors. *Jour. Clin. Invest.*, **16**: 685–693, 1937.

261. Steiner, G.C. and Dorfman, H.D.: Ultrastructure of hemangioendothelioma of bone. *Cancer*, **29**: 122–135, 1972.

262. Stout, A.P.: *Atlas of Tumor Pathology*, Tumors of the Soft Tissues. Armed Forces Institute of Pathology. Sect. 11, Fascele 5.

263. Stout, A.P.: Tumours of the neuromyoarterial glomus. *Amer. Jour. Cancer*, **24**: 255–272, 1935.

264. Stout, A.P.: The painful subcutaneous tubercle (tuberculum dolorosum). *Amer. Jour. Cancer*, **36**: 25–33, 1939.

265. Stout, A.P.: Hemangiopericytoma, a study of 25 new cases. *Cancer*, **2**: 1027–1054, 1949.

266. Stout, A.P.: Tumors featuring pericytes. *Lab. Investigations*, **5**: 217–223, 1956.

267. Stout, A.P. and Murray, M.R.: Hemangiopericytoma, a vascular tumor featuring Zimmermann's pericytes. *Ann. Surg.*, **116**: 26–33, 1942.

268. Stout, A.P., Murray, M.R., Bianchi, O., et al: *Cutaneous Hemangiopericytoma. Tijdschrift voor Gastro-Enterologie*, **12**: 159–167, 1969.

269. Strahan, J. et al: Glomus tumors: a review of 15 clinical cases. *Brit. Jour. Surg.*, **59** (**2**): 91–93, 1972.

270. Sull, W.J. and Brown, H.W.: Malignant hemangioenthelioma. *Int. Surg.*, **57**: 417–421, 1972.

271. Sutton, D. and Pratt, A.E.: Angiography of hemangiopericytoma. *Clin. Radiol.*, **18**: 324, 1967.

272. Symmers, W. St. C.: Survey of the eventual diagnosis in 226 cases referred for a second histological opinion after an initial biopsy diagnosis of reticulum cell sarcoma. *Jour. Clin. Path.*, **21**: 654–655, 1968.

273. Symmers, W. St. C.: Glomus tumors. *Brit. Med. Jour.*, **2**: 50–51, 1973.

274. Taylor, J.F. and Templeton, A.C.: Clinical and pathological similarities between Kaposi's sarcoma and Hodgkins sarcoma. *Brit. Jour. Cancer*, **58**: 577, 1971.

275. Taylor, J.F., Templeton, A.C., Rylwazi, S. et al: Kaposi's sarcoma in pregnancy. *Brit. Jour. Surg.*, **58**: 577–579, 1971.

276. Theis, F.V.: Subungual neuromyoarterial glomus tumor of toe; effect of increased peripheral temperature. *Arch. Surg.*, **34**: 1, 1937.

277. Thomas, A.: Vascular tumors of bone, pathological and clinical study of 27 cases. *Surg. Gyn. Obst.*, **74**: 777, 1942.

278. Toker, C. et al: Glomangioma, an ultra-structural study. *Cancer*, **28**: 487–492, 1969.

279. Unni, K.K.: Hemangiopericytoma and hemangioendothelioma. *Cancer*, **27**: 1403–1414, 1971

280. Vidrine, A., Jr.: Hemangiopericytoma, a report of five cases. *Surg.*, **56**: 912–918, 1964.

281. Vlasov, W.I.: Glomus tumors. *Khirurgia*, (**2**): 102–105, 1975.

282. Vogelsang, H.: Angiography in glomus tumors (Authors translation). *Z. Larygnol. Rhinol. Otol.*, **52**: 807–812, 1973.

283. Waddell, G.F.: A hemangioma involving tendons. *JBJS*, **49B**: 138, 1967.

284. Waisman, M.: Common hemangioma: to treat or not to treat. *Post Grad. Med.*, **43**: 183–188, 1968.

285. Warner, J. and Jones, E.W.: Pyogenic granuloma, recurring with multiple satellites: a report of 11 cases. *Brit. Jour. Derm.*, **80**: 218, 1968.

286. Warren, S. and Gates, O.: Multiple primary malignant Tumors. *Amer. Jour. Cancer*, **16**: 1358–1414, 1942.

287. Webster, C.V. and Geschickter, C.F.: Benign, capillary hemangioma of digital flexortendon sheath, case. *Ann. Surg.*, **122**: 444, 1945.

288. Wechsler, H.: Kaposi's sarcoma angiographic finding before and after orthovoltage treatment. *Arch. Derm. (Chicago)*, **96**: 67–70, 1967.

289. Wile, J.J.: Granuloma pyogenicum. *Jour. Cutan. Dis.*, **28**: 663, 1910.

290. Wiley, A.M.: Ganglion and hemangioma as a cause of plantar neuritis. *Post Grad. Med. Jour.*, **34**: 489, 1958.

291. Williams, D.L.: Pachyonychia and multiple epidermal hamartomata (Boxley, J.D. for Williams, D.L., Royal Society of Medicine, Section of Derm.) *Brit. Jour. Derm.*, **85**: 289–298, 1971.

292. Willis, R.A.: *The Borderland of Embryology and Pathology.* Butterworth and Co., LTD, London, 1958.

293. Winkler, M.A.: Black cancerous and non-cancerous lesions of the skin. *R.I. Med. Jour.*, **41**: 490, 1958.

294. Wohl, M.G.: Granuloma pyogenicum. *N.Y. Med. Jour.*, **105**: 106, 1917.

295. Wolf, W.B.: Lipo-neurofibromatous hamartoma of the foot, a case report. *JAPA*, **62**: 313–314, 1972.

296. World Health Organization. Expert Committee on Health Statistics. Sub-committee on the registration of cases of Cancer as well as their statistical presentation. Statistical Code for human tumors. WHO/HS/CANC. **24** (1): 46, 1956.

297. World Health Organization. *Manual of the International Statistical Classification of Diseases, Injuries and Causes of Death.* Geneva **1**: 393, 1957.

298. Yelin, F.S. et al: Glomus tumor assimulating nerve root compression and Raynaud's phenomenon. A case report. *Jour. Neurosurg.*, **29**: 645–647, 1968.

299. Zayid, I. and Farras, S.: Granuloma pyogenicum—a hitherto unrecognized complication of smallpox vaccination. *Brit. Jour. Derm.*, **90**: 293–299, 1974.

300. Zeligman, I.: Kaposi's sarcoma in father and son. *Johns Hopkins Hosp. Bull.*, **107**: 208–212, 1960.

# Index

345